Circumcision, Public Health, Genital Autonomy and Cultural Rights

Circumcision is one of the oldest and most common surgical processes being practised for a range of medical, social and religious reasons, on up to 30 per cent of males worldwide. It is currently being promoted by a range of health bodies as a means of tackling HIV in developing countries. Yet, there is significant concern about sexual, physiological and psychological effects and complications, and its prophylactic effectiveness. In examining a case in which a failed circumcision was performed for religious reasons, the Regional Court in Cologne decided that the practice contravened the bodily autonomy of minors and was subject to the same legislation used to classify female genital cutting as assault. This, understandably, aroused serious concerns among various religious communities who practise circumcision. At the same time as religious groups seek to protect circumcision from comparisons with female genital cutting, there is a trend, particularly in post-colonial thought in the US, to revise negative understandings of female genital cutting by making cautious, positive comparisons with circumcision.

This collection considers the apparent contradictions and complications of the contemporary status and deployment of the many forms of genital cutting, raising a serious, wide-reaching question: what scope should society have to impose physically invasive rites on people?

This book was originally published as a special issue of *Global Discourse*.

Matthew Johnson is a Lecturer and British Academy Postdoctoral Fellow in Politics, Philosophy and Religion at the University of Lancaster, UK. He is interested in the evaluation of culture and the effect of forms of intervention on wellbeing. He has authored *Evaluating Culture* and edited *The Legacy of Marxism*.

Megan O'Branski is a PhD student in Politics at Newcastle University, UK.

Circumcision, Public Health, Genital Autonomy and Cultural Rights

Edited by
Matthew Johnson and Megan O'Branski

Routledge
Taylor & Francis Group
LONDON AND NEW YORK

First published 2014
by Routledge
2 Park Square, Milton Park, Abingdon, Oxon, OX14 4RN, UK

and by Routledge
711 Third Avenue, New York, NY 10017, USA

Routledge is an imprint of the Taylor & Francis Group, an informa business

British Library Cataloguing in Publication Data
A catalogue record for this book is available from the British Library

ISBN 13: 978-0-415-73544-5

Typeset in Times New Roman
by Taylor & Francis Books

Publisher's Note
The publisher accepts responsibility for any inconsistencies that may have arisen during the conversion of this book from journal articles to book chapters, namely the possible inclusion of journal terminology.

Disclaimer
Every effort has been made to contact copyright holders for their permission to reprint material in this book. The publishers would be grateful to hear from any copyright holder who is not here acknowledged and will undertake to rectify any errors or omissions in future editions of this book.

Contents

Citation Information vii
Notes on Contributors xi

Introduction: Circumcision, public health, genital autonomy and cultural rights
Matthew Johnson and Megan O'Branski 1

1. Infant male circumcision in the public square: applying the public reason of John Rawls
Robert Van Howe 4

2. Infant male circumcision in the public square: applying the public reason of John Rawls (a reply to Robert Van Howe)
Susan Mendus 20

3. How reasonable is intactivism?: a reply to Van Howe
Martyn Griffin 24

4. Promoting genital autonomy by exploring commonalities between male, female, intersex, and cosmetic female genital cutting
J. Steven Svoboda 27

5. Discourses on sexual pleasure after genital modifications: the fallacy of genital determinism (a response to J. Steven Svoboda)
Sara Johnsdotter 46

6. Critiquing circumcision: in search of a new paradigm for conceptualizing genital modification
Zachary T. Androus 56

7. A reply to "Critiquing circumcision: in search of a new paradigm for conceptualizing genital modification"
Jennifer Coffman 71

8. New lives for old: modernity, biomedicine, traditional culture and HIV prevention in Lesotho
Nicola L. Bulled 74

9. New lives for old: modernity, biomedicine, traditional culture and HIV prevention in Lesotho (a response to Nicola L. Bulled)
Louise Vincent 90

10. The production of sexual mutilation among Muslim women in Cairo
Maria Frederika Malmström 96

11. A reply to 'The production of sexual mutilation among Muslim women in Cairo', by Maria Frederika Malmström
Debra L. DeLaet 112

Symposium on German Court ruling on Circumcision **117**

12. Thinking about infant male circumcision after the Cologne court decision
Geoffrey Brahm Levey 119

13. Circumcision: what should parents and states do? An essay
Ayelet Banai 125

14. Legislation on male infant circumcision in Europe: a call to avoid paternalism and to promote evidence-based, patient-centred care
Maria Kristiansen and Aziz Sheikh 135

15. The goose and the gander: the genital wars
Richard A. Shweder 141

Review symposium on *The New Politics of Male Circumcision: HIV/AIDS, Health Law and Social Justice* by Marie Fox and Michael Thomson **161**

16. Review symposium: "The New Politics of Male Circumcision: HIV/AIDS, Health Law and Social Justice" By Marie Fox and Michael Thomson
Sydney Calkin, Richard Mullender, Sander L. Gilman, Marie Fox and Michael Thomson 163

Index 179

Citation Information

The chapters in this book were originally published in *Global Discourse*, volume 3, issue 2 (June 2013). When citing this material, please use the original page numbering for each article, as follows:

Introduction
Circumcision, public health, genital autonomy and cultural rights
Matthew Johnson and Megan O'Branski
Global Discourse, volume 3, issue 2 (June 2013) pp. 211–213

Chapter 1
Infant male circumcision in the public square: applying the public reason of John Rawls
Robert Van Howe
Global Discourse, volume 3, issue 2 (June 2013) pp. 214–229

Chapter 2
Infant male circumcision in the public square: applying the public reason of John Rawls (a reply to Robert Van Howe)
Susan Mendus
Global Discourse, volume 3, issue 2 (June 2013) pp. 230–233

Chapter 3
How reasonable is intactivism?: a reply to Van Howe
Martyn Griffin
Global Discourse, volume 3, issue 2 (June 2013) pp. 234–236

Chapter 4
Promoting genital autonomy by exploring commonalities between male, female, intersex, and cosmetic female genital cutting
J. Steven Svoboda
Global Discourse, volume 3, issue 2 (June 2013) pp. 237–255

Chapter 5
Discourses on sexual pleasure after genital modifications: the fallacy of genital determinism (a response to J. Steven Svoboda)
Sara Johnsdotter
Global Discourse, volume 3, issue 2 (June 2013) pp. 256–265

Chapter 6
Critiquing circumcision: in search of a new paradigm for conceptualizing genital modification
Zachary T. Androus
Global Discourse, volume 3, issue 2 (June 2013) pp. 266–280

Chapter 7
A reply to "Critiquing circumcision: in search of a new paradigm for conceptualizing genital modification"
Jennifer Coffman
Global Discourse, volume 3, issue 2 (June 2013) pp. 281–283

Chapter 8
New lives for old: modernity, biomedicine, traditional culture and HIV prevention in Lesotho
Nicola L. Bulled
Global Discourse, volume 3, issue 2 (June 2013) pp. 284–299

Chapter 9
New lives for old: modernity, biomedicine, traditional culture and HIV prevention in Lesotho (a response to Nicola L. Bulled)
Louise Vincent
Global Discourse, volume 3, issue 2 (June 2013) pp. 300–305

Chapter 10
The production of sexual mutilation among Muslim women in Cairo
Maria Frederika Malmström
Global Discourse, volume 3, issue 2 (June 2013) pp. 306–321

Chapter 11
A reply to 'The production of sexual mutilation among Muslim women in Cairo', by Maria Frederika Malmström
Debra L. DeLaet
Global Discourse, volume 3, issue 2 (June 2013) pp. 322–325

Chapter 12
Thinking about infant male circumcision after the Cologne court decision
Geoffrey Brahm Levey
Global Discourse, volume 3, issue 2 (June 2013) pp. 326–331

Chapter 13
Circumcision: what should parents and states do? An essay
Ayelet Banai
Global Discourse, volume 3, issue 2 (June 2013) pp. 332–341

Chapter 14
Legislation on male infant circumcision in Europe: a call to avoid paternalism and to promote evidence-based, patient-centred care
Maria Kristiansen and Aziz Sheikh
Global Discourse, volume 3, issue 2 (June 2013) pp. 342–347

Chapter 15
The goose and the gander: the genital wars
Richard A. Shweder
Global Discourse, volume 3, issue 2 (June 2013) pp. 348–366

Chapter 16
Review Symposium: "The New Politics of Male Circumcision: HIV/AIDS, Health Law and Social Justice" By Marie Fox and Michael Thomson
Sydney Calkin, Richard Mullender, Sander L. Gilman, Marie Fox and Michael Thomson
Global Discourse, volume 3, issue 2 (June 2013) pp. 367–382

Please direct any queries you may have about the citations to clsuk.permissions@cengage.com

Notes on Contributors

Zachary T. Androus is a US anthropologist based in Florence, Italy, where he conducts independent research and teaches for international higher education programs.

Ayelet Banai is a Research Fellow at the Centre for Advanced Studies 'Justitia Amplificata', Goethe University, Frankfurt am Main, Germany. Her research and publications are in international political theory, including the right of self-determination, democracy and diversity, and minority rights. Her publications include 'Europe of the regions and the problem of boundaries in liberal democratic theory' (*Journal of Political Ideologies*, 2012) and 'Political self-determination and global egalitarianism' (*Social Theory and Practice*, 2013). She is co-editor of the volume *Social Justice, Global Dynamics: Theoretical and Empirical Perspectives* (Routledge, 2011).

Geoffrey Brahm Levey is an Australian Research Council Future Fellow and Associate Professor in Political Science at the University of New South Wales, Sydney, Australia. He was the foundation director of the UNSW Program in Jewish Studies. His publications include *Secularism, Religion and Multicultural Citizenship* (2008), co-edited with Tariq Modood.

Nicola L. Bulled holds a PhD in Applied Critical Medical Anthropology at the University of Connecticut, USA. Her research focused on how the dissemination of biomedical HIV knowledge amidst prevention efforts impacts the practices, understandings and identities of youth in Lesotho.

Sydney Calkin is a PhD candidate in Politics at the University of York, UK.

Jennifer Coffman is Associate Executive Director of International Programs and Associate Professor of Integrated Science and Technology at James Madison University, USA. She is the founder and Director of JMU's Kenya Field School. Coffman's research in Kenya examines the politics of land access and ownership, concepts of sustainability, and resource distribution.

Debra L. DeLaet is Professor of Politics and International Relations at Drake University in Des Moines, Iowa, USA. She has published several books as well as numerous articles and book chapters on topics related to human rights, global health and gender in world politics.

Marie Fox is Professor of Socio-legal Studies at the University of Birmingham, UK. In addition to this current project on genital cutting, her research focuses more generally on how law regulates human and animal bodies and embodiment. She is also interested in the ethico-legal regulation of veterinary practice.

Sander L. Gilman is a distinguished Professor of the Liberal Arts and Sciences and Professor of Psychiatry at Emory University, USA.

Martyn Griffin is a Research Officer at Durham University Business School, UK. He holds a PhD in politics from the University of Newcastle-upon-Tyne where he also received his Masters and undergraduate degree. He previously worked at the University of Central Lancashire as a Research Assistant in Applied Education and has a multi-disciplinary background.

Matthew Johnson is a Lecturer and British Academy Postdoctoral Fellow in Politics, Philosophy and Religion at the University of Lancaster, UK. He is interested in the evaluation of culture and the effect of forms of intervention on wellbeing. He has authored *Evaluating Culture* and edited *The Legacy of Marxism*.

Sara Johnsdotter PhD (Social Anthropology, Lund University, 2002) is Professor in Medical Anthropology at the Faculty of Health and Society, Malmö University, Sweden. Her research is concerned with genital modifications, particularly female circumcision. Since 1997 she has worked closely with gynaecologist Dr. Birgitta Essén on issues of sexuality and reproductive health in a migration context.

Maria Kristiansen is Assistant Professor at the Department of Public Health, University of Copenhagen, Denmark, and Honorary Fellow at the University of Edinburgh, UK. She is involved in studies exploring the relationship between ethnic, religious and social inequality in health and access to health care.

Maria Frederika Malmström is a Researcher at the Nordic Africa Institute, Uppsala, Sweden. She is also a Senior Lecturer at the Department of School of Global Studies at University of Gothenburg, Sweden. Additionally, she is a Visiting Scholar at New York University, New York City, USA (2010–2012) at the Center for the Study of Gender and Sexuality, and from 2012 at the Performance Studies, Tisch School of Arts.

Susan Mendus is Morrell Professor Emerita in Political Philosophy at the University of York, UK. She has been a member of the Morrell Centre for Toleration at York since 1985 and has published extensively on modern political philosophy, and especially on problems of toleration.

Richard Mullender is Professor of Law and Legal Theory at Newcastle Law School, UK.

Megan O'Branski is a PhD student in Politics at Newcastle University, UK.

Aziz Sheikh is Professor of Primary Care Research & Development and Co-Director of the Centre of Population Health Sciences at the University of Edinburgh, UK. He has a long-standing interest in the interfaces between religion, health and health care delivery and has published widely on these issues.

Richard A. Shweder is a cultural anthropologist and the Harold Higgins Swift Distinguished Service Professor in the Department of Comparative Human Development at the University of Chicago, USA. His recent research examines the scope and limit of cultural pluralism in Western liberal democracies.

J. Steven Svoboda founded Attorneys for the Rights of the Child (ARC) in 1997. He has written on issues relating to genital autonomy in the *Journal of Medical Ethics*, *Journal of the Royal Society of Medicine*, *Medical Anthropology Quarterly*, all eight Springer/Kluwer circumcision symposium proceedings volumes and has presented the only known document ever accepted by the United Nations focusing on male circumcision.

Michael Thomson is Professor of Law at the University of Leeds, UK. His research focuses on health care decision-making with children, legal embodiment, and the ethico-legal regulation of public health interventions.

Robert Van Howe, Paediatrician, is a Clinical Professor in the Department of Pediatrics and Human Development at Michigan State University College of Human Medicine, USA. He also holds a Master's Degree in Biostatistics. Dr. Van Howe is an expert on circumcision, has spoken internationally on that topic, and has published numerous articles and studies, including 'How the Circumcision Solution in Africa Will Increase HIV Infections' (*Journal of Public Health in Africa* (*JPH*), 2012).

Louise Vincent is a Qualitative Researcher with a particular passion for narrative research. Her research is principally in the field of the corporeal politics – an interest in ways in which social and political power relations can be understood to be written on the bodies of citizens. This interest has expressed itself in a variety of projects in which she attempts to read South Africa's democratic transition through a corporeal lens. She is Professor of Political Studies in the Department of Political and International Studies at Rhodes University in South Africa.

INTRODUCTION

Circumcision, public health, genital autonomy and cultural rights

Circumcision is one of the oldest and most common surgical practices, being practised, for a range of medical, social and religious reasons, on up to 30% of males worldwide. At present, it is being promoted by a range of international health bodies, such as the World Health Organization, as a means of tackling HIV in developing countries. Yet, there is significant concern, both, about sexual, physiological and psychological effects and complications and the prophylactic effectiveness of the practice. In Western countries, in particular, a range of 'intactivist' organizations and campaign groups have emerged, drawing qualitative parallels with female genital cutting. For these groups, a right to bodily, or more specifically, genital integrity, is invoked to protect minors from invasive surgery. This movement has emerged at a time in which circumcision rates in states such as the US have declined and many medical bodies have sought either to exercise caution on claims of medical benefits, while deferring to parental choice in non-therapeutic instances, such as the British Medical Association (BMA), or to reject the practice in all but the most essential medical cases, such as the Royal Dutch Medical Association (KNMG).

This position was advanced most significantly and controversially in Germany in 2012. In examining a case in which a botched circumcision performed for religious reasons, the Regional Court in Cologne decided that the practice contravened the bodily autonomy of minors and was subject to the same legislation used to classify female genital cutting as assault. This, understandably, aroused serious concerns among various religious communities who either practise circumcision or regard the decision as an infringement on liberty of faith. Amidst claims of anti-Semitism and Islamophobia, the German government responded by seeking to introduce legislation to exempt circumcision from judicial inquisition.

At the same time as religious groups seek to protect circumcision from comparisons with female genital cutting, certain bodies, particularly in the US, are attempting to revise negative understandings of female genital cutting by making cautious comparisons with circumcision in order to challenge the 'passion' of anti-mutilation activists. The Public Policy Advisory Network on Female Genital Surgeries in Africa (2012), for example, highlight the diversity of female genital cutting practices, arguing that some are not particular invasive, do not irreversibly eradicate sexual functioning, are viewed as enhancements rather than mutilations by practising communities, are often seen as parallel to male genital rites, are not always associated with, or inevitable consequences of, patriarchy, are often controlled and managed by women, and are not clearly associated statistically with perinatal and maternal mortality.

This attempt to caution sensationalist criticism of female genital cutting is often associated with postcolonial or culturally sensitive approaches which seek to interrogate unreflective colonial mindsets. Interestingly, while the core concerns of genital autonomy appear to be of persisting relevance to the efforts of international health bodies to tackle HIV transmission through circumcision, there is also scope for concern regarding potential implications of imposing a practice on non-circumcising peoples. Whereas attempts to challenge female genital cutting in areas of Africa have been met with criticism by multiculturalist thinkers, such as Yael Tamir, for their imperialist implications, there has been little by way of opposition to the introduction of circumcision to non-circumcising peoples by Western bodies.

The apparent contradictions and complications of the contemporary status and deployment of the many forms of genital cutting raise serious, wide-reaching questions: Should gender be of significance in considering claims for genital autonomy? To what extent can law assist in challenging apparently invasive cultural practices? Which values or goods should be of importance when considering the status of invasive practices? Are there any particular interests or ethnocentric tendencies that motivate the promotion or proscription of the practice? What costs are involved in reforming or eradicating practices?

The papers in this issue attempt to address these sorts of questions. Robert Van Howe (2013) examines the reasonableness of circumcision with regard to political liberalism. Susan Mendus (2013) and Martyn Griffin (2013) respond. Steven Svoboda (2013), with a reply by Sara Johnsdotter (2013), and Zachary Androus (2013), with a reply by Jennifer Coffman (2013), seek to find means of categorizing practices across gender. Nicola Bulled (2013) presents an account of the shifting place of circumcision in Lesotho, which Louise Vincent (2013) explores further with regard to the effect of medicalization on the cultural value of the practice. Maria Malmström (2013) examines the ambivalence and conflicting feelings of modern Egyptian women towards female genital cutting. Debra DeLaet (2013) replies, exploring feminist arguments on the topic. Next, is a symposium on the German court ruling, featuring essays by Geoffrey Brahm Levey (2013), Ayelet Banai (2013), Aziz Sheikh and Maria Kristiansen (2013) and Richard Shweder (2013). Finally, there is a review symposium on the recent work by Marie Fox and Michael Thomson on genital autonomy, public health and social justice. This features reviews by Sydney Calkin (2013), Richard Mullender (2013) and Sander L. Gilman (2013) with a reply by Fox and Thomson (2013).

References

Androus, Z. T. 2013. "Critiquing Circumcision: In Search of a New Paradigm for Conceptualizing Genital Modification." *Global Discourse* 3 (2): 266–280.

Banai, A. 2013. "Circumcision: What Should Parents and States Do? An Essay." *Global Discourse* 3 (2): 332–341.

Brahm Levey, G. 2013. "Thinking About Infant Male Circumcision After the Cologne Court Decision." *Global Discourse* 3 (2): 326–331.

Bulled, N. L. 2013. "New Lives for Old: Modernity, Biomedicine, Traditional Culture and HIV Prevention in Lesotho." *Global Discourse* 3 (2): 284–299.

Calkin, S. 2013. "'The New Politics of Male Circumcision: HIV/AIDS, Health Law and Social Justice'. Review." *Global Discourse* 3 (2): 367–370.

Coffman, J. 2013. "Reply to Critiquing Circumcision: In Search of a New Paradigm for Conceptualizing Genital Modification." *Global Discourse* 3 (2): 281–283.

De Laet, D. L. 2013. "A Reply to the Production of Sexual Mutilation Among Muslim Women in Cairo, by Maria Frederika Malmström." *Global Discourse* 3 (2): 322–325.

Fox, M., and M. Thomson. 2013. "Response to Calkin, Gilman and Mullender." *Global Discourse* 3 (2): 378–382.

Gilman, S. L. 2013. "'The New Politics of Male Circumcision: HIV/AIDS, Health Law and Social Justice'. Review." *Global Discourse* 3 (2): 376–378.

Griffin, M. 2013. "How Reasonable is Intactivism? A Reply to Van Howe." *Global Discourse* 3 (2): 234–236.

Johnsdotter, S. 2013. "Discourses on Sexual Pleasure after Genital Modifications: The Fallacy of Genital Determinism (a Response to J. Steven Svoboda)." *Global Discourse* 3 (2): 256–265.
Kristiansen, M., and A. Sheikh. 2013. "Legislation on Male Infant Circumcision in Europe: A Call to Avoid Paternalism and to Promote Evidence-Based, Patient-Centred Care." *Global Discourse* 3 (2): 342–347.
Malmström, M. F. 2013. "The Production of Sexual Mutilation Among Muslim Women in Cairo." *Global Discourse* 3 (2): 306–321.
Mendus, S. 2013. "Infant Male Circumcision in the Public Square: Applying the Public Reason of John Rawls (a Reply to Robert Van Howe)." *Global Discourse* 3 (2): 230–233.
Mullender, R. 2013. "Exploring Normative Space with Fox and Thomson." *Global Discourse* 3 (2): 371–376.
The Public Policy Advisory Network on Female Genital Surgeries in Africa. 2012. "Seven Things to Know About Female Genital Surgeries in Africa." *Hastings Center Report* 42 (6): 19–27.
Shweder, R. 2013. "The Goose and the Gander: The Genital Wars." *Global Discourse* 3 (2): 348–366.
Svoboda, J. S. 2013. "Promoting Genital Autonomy by Exploring Commonalities Between Male, Female, Intersex, and Cosmetic Female Genital Cutting." *Global Discourse* 3 (2): 237–255.
Van Howe, R. 2013. "Infant Male Circumcision in the Public Square: Applying the Public Reason of John Rawls." *Global Discourse* 3 (2): 214–229.
Vincent, L. 2013. "A Reply to New Lives for Old: Modernity, Biomedicine, Traditional Culture and HIV Prevention in Lesotho by Nicola Bulled." *Global Discourse* 3 (2): 300–305.

Matthew Johnson
University of Lancaster

Megan O'Branski
Newcastle University

Infant male circumcision in the public square: applying the public reason of John Rawls

Robert Van Howe

Department of Pediatrics and Human Development, College of Human Medicine, Michigan State University, Marquette, MI, USA

John Rawls is perhaps the most influential political philosopher of the twentieth century. His philosophy is based on the idea of justice as fairness and emphasizes the importance of basic liberties, including the right to bodily integrity and the use of rationality in making ethical determinations. His political philosophy addressed the challenges a secular society faces when its citizens adhere to a variety of comprehensive doctrines and religious beliefs yet requires social cooperation for the benefit of all. Public policy is determined through 'public reason' in which reasonable proposals are considered and compromises made. Using the decisional approaches that Rawls developed, this article explores how the process of public reason would consider the reasonableness of surgically altering the genitals of male minors for non-therapeutic ends. It will incorporate the issues of the basic liberties of minors and the weaknesses of a utilitarian defense of this practice.

Why circumcision?

Circumcision of male infants and minors is a divisive cultural practice that is ubiquitous in the United States and common among Jewish, Muslim, and other communities throughout the world. It involves the amputation of the foreskin from the penis, leaving the child with a permanent scar. This practice was introduced into Anglophone societies by the medical profession at a time when foundational doctrines in bioethics such as the needfulness of informed consent had not been developed. The practice has persisted long after its initial quasi-medical indication – that is, the prevention of masturbation – evaporated as either a medical or a moral concern and despite the fact that subsequent medical indications have either been dismissed or recognized as insufficient to warrant recommending the procedure (Hodges 1997; Darby 2005; AAP 2012). Since the medicalization of circumcision in the late nineteenth century, women have been enfranchised, infants and children have been recognized as having full moral standing (Convention on the Rights of the Child 1989), and the autonomy of the patient has been recognized as the driving force of bioethics (O'Neill 2002). By contrast, the notion that monarchs, religious leaders, slave owners, or parents have the sovereignal freedom to exercise power over another individual is fading as the Enlightenment principle of individual freedom takes wider hold (Patterson 1991). This shift has not taken place without conflict. Parents have traditionally enjoyed broad authority to do as they pleased with their children; but in modern, secular, pluralistic societies, a parental right to beat, coerce, or mark children as members of a cultural or religious group[1] is no longer recognized because the child is considered to have full moral standing. The ethical issue posed by circumcision[2] is whether it is morally permissible, considering that it ignores the welfare interests and autonomy of the child and that there are less harmful means of achieving the objective of raising responsible citizens.

In 2012, the Cologne regional court ruled that circumcision violated a child's right to bodily integrity and freedom of religion (Landgericht Köln 2012). This judgment exposed the tension between human rights interests and that of the adherents of religions that mandate circumcision of children. A heated debate ensued in which Germany's official pediatric association denounced circumcision (Hartman 2012), while defenders of the practice declared the ruling 'fatal to the future of religion' (Raftery 2012). Eventually, this debate resulted in legislation (Jordans 2012) that sought to clarify the legality of circumcision, but which may yet be found unconstitutional (Walter 2012).

With the Cologne ruling, the circumcision debate has entered the public square. In this article, I explore the issue by applying the philosophy of John Rawls, which is the most comprehensive approach to handling the conflicts over values that are inevitable in modern, pluralistic societies.[3] I begin with a critique of A. M. Viens's (2004) defense of circumcision and use this to show how Rawls intended 'public reason' to be used.

Justice as fairness

Rawls believed that a conception of rights should be a set of principles that is 'general in form and universal in application' and publicly recognized as a method of ordering conflicting claims (Rawls 1971, 135). Rawls developed the principles of justice as fairness to repudiate the limitations of utilitarianism (Rawls 1971, 27).[4] Although he redirects attention to the individual (missing from utilitarianism), individuals must coexist with others. To address this, he formulated a structure called political liberalism. Because no society can embrace all ways of life, a secular community must allow citizens with different cultural backgrounds and belief structures to live together (Rawls 2001, 154). Rawls notes that although factions of the public have reasonable disagreements (Rawls 2001, 35), an aim of moral philosophy is to seek areas of agreement where none seem to exist (Rawls 1971, 582). Questions and policy should be disputed in the public square with 'public reason', in the hopes of creating a reasonable pluralism:

> citizens are to conduct their fundamental discussions within the framework of what each regards as a political conception of justice based on values that the others can reasonably be expected to endorse and each is, in good faith, prepared to defend that conception so understood. (Rawls 2005, 226)

Using public reason, the merits of public policy are determined by reasonableness:

> The values of public reason not only include the appropriate use of the fundamental concepts of judgment, inference, and evidence, but also the virtues of reasonableness and fair-mindedness as shown in abiding by the criteria and procedures of commonsense knowledge and accepting the methods and conclusions of science when not controversial. (Rawls 2005, 139)

In the process, each comprehensive doctrine or system of moral beliefs (philosophical or theological) explains how its idea of the reasonable connects with its concept of truth, and a reasonable attempt is made to formulate a consensus that accommodates the diversity.

Circumcision is 'reasonable'

Viens appeals to Rawls's public reason approach to demonstrate that circumcision is indeed reasonable. The question posed is whether a parental right to determine their children's best interests and to raise them in their chosen religion gives them the power to have their son circumcised. He answers in the affirmative, not because parents are necessarily the best arbiters of their child's best interest, but because parents should be allowed this freedom.[5] This question should not be approached using any one person's concept of the good, but by means of a different justificatory class: whether the practice is reasonable using public reason. The aim is to advance a policy that no one could reasonably reject.

Viens notes that the traditional justifications for circumcision are religious, that the law allows it, and that it is based on parental concepts of the good. It is not clear whether he is abandoning these justifications or believes they contribute to his overall argument, but he argues that what matters most is whether circumcision is reasonable. The onus is thus placed on those who oppose circumcision to demonstrate that it is unreasonable, 'unequivocally harmful', that the 'majority' of circumcised males are harmed, or that there is a compelling interest in protecting boys that outweighs parental wishes. He concludes that anticircumcision proponents fail on all accounts.[6]

In making his case for the reasonableness of circumcision, Viens cites the importance of preserving parental rights; he notes that national medical organization consider the procedure to be justified; he lists positive non-medical factors; and he argues that the procedure is performed with 'optimal' pain measures, that the complication rate is low, that the harm (which he admits is a highly subjective measure) has not been demonstrated, that international human rights documents either do not apply to circumcision or do not apply to children, that parental interests in having their sons circumcised and the child's interest in bodily integrity are either not in conflict or parental interests outweigh the child's, and that prohibition of circumcision would be opposed by religious organizations and result in more procedures generating serious complications.

Applying the philosophy of John Rawls

Viens's arguments allow us to show how Rawls's philosophy integrates with the process of public reason and how he would approach the issue of circumcision. The thrust of Viens' argument is unclear. Does he believe circumcision is reasonable because circumcision opponents are unable to demonstrate that the practice is unreasonable[7] or because of the reasons he provides? By addressing the latter, I will also address the former.

Analysis of Viens's arguments

(1) Preserve parental rights.

Viens repeatedly states that circumcision is reasonable because of the importance of preserving parents' right to define their child's best interest and 'the freedom to raise their children under the tenets of a particular religious doctrine or community' (Viens 2004, 242). These unsupported assertions have several problems, most notably the circular nature of the argument. Viens assumes that parents have this right to demonstrate the importance of this right to parents, families, and society. But the concept of parental rights has been questioned, with some describing it as a dead or a zombie dogma (Dwyer 2006; Van Howe 2013). Dwyer argues that parents do not need a 'right' to be responsible for the protection of the rights and interests of their children (Dwyer 1994, 2006). Viens must justify his claim that parents have these rights without an appeal to religious dogma, an appeal to laws,[8] or an appeal to tradition, but he makes no attempt to do so.[9]

Rawls advocates a different approach to how parents should treat their children. Society places an enormous burden on the shoulders of parents, who are given moral and social authority to nurture a child (Rawls 2001, 163) and provide an 'orderly production and reproduction of society and of its culture from one generation to the next' (Rawls 2001, 162). Their reproductive labor is socially necessary as it provides for the raising of and caring for children and ensures their moral development, education, and assimilation into the wider culture (Rawls 2001, 162–163).

Children are initially subjected to the authority of their parents, with the understanding that the parents' love will translate into proper care (Rawls 1971, 463). Within the family, children recognize the parents' love as being based on the parents' assurances of the children's worth as persons. Consequently, they are aware that they are appreciated for their own sake by, what to them are, the most powerful persons in the world (Rawls 1971, 464). While it is hoped that parents will have the motivation and the skills to properly care for their children, there is no empirical evidence that they are uniquely qualified to do so. The child has little opportunity to negotiate. He is subject to the authority of his parents and is not in the position to assess the validity of their decisions. Because he lacks the knowledge, understanding, and opportunity to challenge them, he cannot doubt the proprietary nature of parental injunctions (Rawls 1971, 463). Any calculus of the power structure between parents and children must acknowledge the intrinsic imbalance when those in a position of strength can advance their interests unjustly without being shown to be out of bounds (Rawls 1971, 320). This runs counter to one of our societal ideals – that no one takes unfair advantage of human weakness (Rawls 1971, 515). While political principles do not apply directly to the internal life of the family, Rawls argues that they impose constraints on the family not to violate the basic rights, liberties, and fair opportunities of all its members (Rawls 1997, 468–470, 2001, 164, 166). If one accepts the reality of parental rights, it is apparent that these are fettered by the duties parents owe their children. As trustees for their children, parents have a duty to respect their basic rights (Dwyer 1994; Rawls 2001, 11, 102).

There is also a wide gap between Viens's view that parents have the right to make decisions on behalf of their children based on 'the parent's concept of the good' and Rawls's approach to proxy decision-making. Rawls advocates the substitute judgment approach:[10]

> Those who care for others must choose for them in the light of what they will want whatever else they want once they reach maturity. Therefore following the account of primary goods, the parties presume that their descendants will want their liberty protected. (Rawls 1971, 208–209)

The best proxy would replicate what a child would presumptively choose on the basis of his individual characteristics and generic interests if fully competent and able to determine and advance his interests (Dwyer 2006, 130–131). In making these decisions, the decision maker should be able to argue that with the development of our rational powers, he would accept the decision made on our behalf and agree that it was the best (Rawls 1971, 249). This approach brings a proxy decision as close as possible to an autonomous individual choosing for himself.

To avoid the major shortcoming of substitute judgment (that decisions on a child's behalf are more likely to reflect what the decision-maker would choose for himself), Rawls argues that such decisions should be made from the standpoint of the 'original position' (Rawls 1971, 249).[11] In the case of a child, decision makers should put themselves in his place and ignore all other interests. Most would presume that children would want their basic liberties preserved (Rawls 1971, 209).[12]

(2) The positions of national medical organizations justify circumcision.
Despite Viens's nonchalant approach to the topic, not a single national medical organization recommends circumcision (Canadian Paediatric Society 1996; American Medical Association 1999; British Medical Association 2004; Royal Australasian College of Physicians 2010; American Academy of Pediatrics 2012), and several national medical organizations have come out strongly against it (Royal Dutch Medical Association 2010; Behrtel 2011 (*Circumcision of Babies for Proposed HIV Prevention*. Letter to Dean Ferris from The Human Rights, Law & Ethics Committee of the South African Medical Association, June 23.); Smith 2011; Suomen Lääkäriliitto 2011; Hartman 2012; Slovenia Human Rights Ombudsman 2012; Swedish Pediatric Society 2012). But these pronouncements did not deter Viens from asserting that the lack of a recommendation is the same as saying the procedure is 'justified'. None of these organizations provide a 'justification' for circumcision. Even the blatantly pro-circumcision[13] 2012 American Academy of Pediatrics statement did not assert that infant circumcision was justified (American Academy of Pediatrics 2012). It merely appeals to parental discretion:

> In cases such as the decision to perform a circumcision in the newborn period (where there is reasonable disagreement about the balance between medical benefits and harms, where there are nonmedical benefits and harms that can result from a decision on whether to perform the procedure, and where the procedure is not essential to the child's immediate well-being), the parents should determine what is in the best interest of the child. (American Academy of Pediatrics 2012, e759)

Viens has confused the concepts of 'permissible' and 'justified'. This appeal to authority does not make infant circumcision reasonable.

(3) Circumcision has non-medical benefits.
This claim that circumcision has non-medical benefits, primarily the moral significance of belonging to a community, needs empirical support. Even if this claim could be substantiated, the presence of benefits does not make something reasonable. For example, a benefit of slavery is that the slaves were not unemployed.[14]

(4) 'Optimal' pain control measures are available for infant circumcision.
Viens, without knowing the facts, assumes that infant circumcision can be performed using 'optimal' pain relief measures. All studies of topical and local anesthetics demonstrate that the procedure still remains stressful and painful (Van Howe 1997; Paix and Peterson 2012). Newborns are at greater risk for complications from general anesthesia, which could provide 'optimal' pain relief, so elective surgical cases are typically delayed until the infant is 6 months old, when the risks are reduced. Benatar and Benatar, who make the same erroneous assumption as Viens, argue that infant circumcision must be pain-free to be morally permissible (Benatar and Benatar 2003b). The medical evidence is that circumcision performed on infants is not pain-free.

(5) Circumcision has a low complication rate.

Like many of his arguments, this argument fails to gain traction because the numbers Viens cites reflect his bias rather than the medical literature. Meatal stenosis (narrowing of the urethral opening from which urine is expelled) has been reported in 5% to 20% of circumcised males (Van Howe 2006; Joudi, Fathi, and Hiradfar 2011). But haggling over the rate of complications is an unnecessary diversion. What Viens appears to be driving around (instead of directly at) is a utilitarian defense of infant circumcision.

In many ways, Rawls's entire philosophy was a reaction against utilitarianism. A utilitarian argument in favor of infant circumcision would posit that the benefits would outweigh the harms.[15] One of the weakness of the utilitarian approach is that the difficulty in placing a value on religious or cultural conviction and whose conviction (the parents' or the child's) should be considered (Gray 2004). This also creates a dilemma for adjudication in a secular society.

Another problem with utilitarianism is that it treats persons as both ends and means (Rawls 1971, 182). In other words, a utilitarian calculation showing that the denial of a basic legal right would maximize utility should not interfere with someone exercising a basic moral right (Dworkin 1977). Rawls does not endorse treating people instrumentally to bolster overall utility, but rather adopts an ethic of mutual respect (Rawls 1971, 256).

Finally, while Rawls's third principle of justice as fairness is most commonly applied to economic decisions, the proposition that an improvement in overall utility should not come at the expense of those who are the worst off may apply here.[16] Application of this principle of justice in the case of circumcision would mandate that the weakest and most vulnerable not be further weakened. In other words, no complications for any individual infant would be acceptable.

(6) Circumcision does not result in harm.

Here, Viens presents another argument based on unsupported assertions that ignore empirical evidence. For added measure, he posits that the determination of harm is based on cultural popularity.[17] The harm is easy to demonstrate. Circumcision involves removing 30–50% of the penile skin system, nearly all of the fine-touch neuroreceptors in the penis (Taylor, Lockwood, and Taylor 1996; Cold and Taylor 1999) and the most sensitive portion of the penis (Sorrells et al. 2007).[18] The infant's skin is broken and a body part is removed. Even if it could be documented that functionality was not affected, there is harm merely in amputating a body part that has intrinsic worth.[19] There is, however, growing evidence that circumcision adversely affects both form and function (Frisch, Lindholm, and Grøbæk 2012; Bronselaer et al. 2013).

By stating that circumcision does not result in harm, Viens ignores the rationality at the core of Rawls's philosophy. It is not the height of passion nor the determination of the conviction that give weight to claims, but its rationality (Rawls 2005, 34). The process of deliberation begins in what Rawls called the 'original position' (Rawls 1971, 518). In the original position, a question is considered in its most basic form, free of any prejudicing embellishments, and, using what Rawls calls 'considered judgment', the universal implications are considered and a decision is made. The process is to be rational. There can be no appeals to tradition or self-evidence of general conceptions or particular convictions (Rawls 1971, 21). At this level, any principles or laws that facilitated instrumental treatment of any human being, regardless of age, would be rejected. Any law that placed children in situations for the purpose of gratifying certain adults or advancing diffuse societal aims rather than what best serves the child's interests would be rejected (Dwyer 2006, 153). The fatal flaw in Viens's case is that he begins by asserting the reasonableness of circumcision but skips the preliminary steps prescribed by Rawls.[20] The first involves the distinction between rational and reasonable. Rawls states:

> In everyday life we employ schemes of deliberation acquired from our culture and modified during the course of our personal history. But there is no assurance that these forms of reflection are rational. (Rawls 1971, 553)

So in a situation with conflicting values, how do we ascertain that another's conscience and not our own is mistaken (Rawls 1971, 518)? Rawls recommends using our intellect and imagination, the capacity to be impartial and to take a wider and more inclusive view, as well as sensitivity to the concerns and circumstances of others (Rawls 2001, 170). Rationality is important for Rawls because a departure from generally recognized methods of reasoning would result in a privileged place for the views of some over others, creating an exceptionalism for those whose decisions and behaviors are not rational (Rawls 1971, 213).

The first step is to exclude the unreasonable or irrational (Rawls 2005, 93, 144). This means going to the original position where cultural considerations and parental wishes to project their belief systems onto the child are put aside. The fundamental question becomes whether a child, given the choice, would forgo his right to bodily integrity and to an open future,[21] have the most sensitive portion of his penis amputated, and accept all of the inherent risks. By using Rawls's original position, we should be solicitous of the interests of children and place substantial restrictions on the ability of others to control them (Dwyer 2006, 149–150). The problem is that Viens adds parental power to the mix. When that happens, the decision is based entirely on the parents' values, not what the child would be likely to choose for himself if competent. In reality, the child is being circumcised to fulfill a parental religious obligation, because the community demands it, or to obtain a cosmetic outcome desired by the parents.[22] Consequently, the child is being used as a means to obtain an end determined by the parents. Rawls would summarily reject such instrumental use of children.

Viens argues that critics must demonstrate that circumcision is unreasonable[23] and that any attempt to limit parental liberties would require a justification that is 'exceedingly robust and fair'. The rational rejection of circumcision in the original position should sufficiently address Viens's challenge.

(7) Circumcision is not a human rights violation.

Although this is the most important topic in the ethics of circumcision, Viens simply states that some people do not believe that children have rights, while others think that circumcision does not violate the right to bodily integrity.[24] Using this logic, these people are in essence arguing that infants do not have the right not to be punched, kicked, or shaken. Yet as a matter of both law and logic, when the foreskin is crushed or cut without medical need or the direct consent of the person, bodily integrity is, by definition, violated.

For Rawls, equal liberties form his first principle of justice as fairness: all citizens have basic liberties or rights, and these basic liberties take priority over social and economic concerns (Rawls 2001, 57, 85; Rawls 2005, 77). Basic rights and liberties are the logical result of possessing the status of a moral person (being human) and are generated from the original position. Moral rights identify and protect interests that are important in themselves and are given overriding force. The principles of justice 'require that equal basic rights be assigned to all persons' (Rawls 1971, 505) – presumably regardless of age: we do not deprive the weak of the full protection of justice (Rawls 1971, 509). Rawls maintains that being a moral agent or having the capacity to become a moral agent entitles persons to the full protection of the principles of justice. He notes specifically that infants and children, because they have the capacity to become moral agents, do possess basic rights (Rawls 1971, 505, 509). If the basic liberties and rights of some are restricted, social cooperation on the basis of mutual respect becomes difficult (Rawls 2001, 115; Rawls 2005, 337). Consequently, basic rights and liberties should never be jeopardized or sacrificed for 'the greater public good' (Rawls 2001, 111, 295).

Rawls sees the basic liberties as a family of liberties that has overall priority and does not acknowledge the priority of a single right or liberty by itself (Rawls 2005, 356). A basic liberty can be limited only to enhance one or more of the other liberties (Rawls 2005, 356). Among the basic rights identified are freedom of thought and liberty of conscience; the liberty and integrity of the person (both physical and psychological – violated, for example, by slavery and serfdom and by the denial of freedom of movement and occupation) (Rawls 2001, 44, 113; Rawls 2005, 291, 335); and freedom from physical pain (Rawls 2005, 182). These rights have been consistently codified in a number of international declarations that attempt to secure rights for all humans, including children (Convention on the Rights of the Child 1989).[25]

The argument that infants do not have rights is based on the Will/Power Theory that they lack the power to make claims that obligate others to recognize these claims (O'Neill 1992). The logical consequence of denying basic liberties to children is that they then lack the moral worth of a human and are thus not fully human. This demotes the child to the status of chattel, which can be used instrumentally as the owner sees fit (Olsen 1992; Rawls 1995, 431, 1997, 447, 468, 2001, 165, 166; Dwyer 2006, 179). If a child does enjoy a right to bodily integrity, cutting or crushing the foreskin violates this right.

(8) Parental rights and the child's interests either do not conflict or parental rights trump the child's interests.

Viens's argument based on unsupported assertions has little substance. Using the structure Rawls supplies, one should argue that basic liberties are the same for all citizens and the question of how to compensate for a lesser liberty does not arise (Rawls 2001, 149). In other words, to compensate for the violation of a child's human right to bodily integrity, some other basic human right of the child (not the parents) would need to be enhanced. Since this does not happen, the intervention is not morally permissible. In discussing the differences between rational and reasonable, Rawls states:

> there is no reason for any of them to accept principles that assign to them lesser basic rights than the rest. Those who insist on imposing such principles on others, moved say by their greater power or stronger bargaining position, are being unreasonable, yet given their interests, they may be perfectly rational. (Rawls 2001, 191)

In this context, it would not be reasonable for an infant to waive his basic right to bodily integrity to allow a significant portion of his penis to be excised merely because his parents have the power to make him submit. This is unlikely to be the plan he would pursue if he had full knowledge of his situation and the alternatives (Rawls 1971, 409).[26] As Rawls states,

> Clearly the morality of authority must be subordinate to the principles of right and justice which alone can determine when these extreme requirements, or analogous constraints, are justified. (Rawls 1971, 467)

Similarly, the only right of the parents at play is the freedom of thought and liberty of conscience. Not circumcising a child does not violate that liberty. First Amendment rights are about 'self-determination' not 'other-determination'. The right to freedom of religious belief and practice does not include a carte blanche to actions that affect others (UDHR 1948, Articles 29(2), 30).

(9) Religions that mandate circumcision would object.

The heart of Viens's case is that the religious requirement of circumcision would be considered reasonable using public reason as outlined by Rawls. But for Rawls, political liberalism is based on the primacy of basic rights and liberties and a rational approach. The irrationality of circumcision in the original position and its violation of basic human rights would prevent it from being considered reasonable in the public square. For the purposes of this discussion, these nuisances will be set aside.

The goal is to formulate a general consensus on what is reasonable. This process is dependent on the parties' willingness to propose and abide by the fair terms of social cooperation and their willingness to accept 'the consequences of the burdens of judgment' (Rawls 2005, 93).

This process may be difficult. Disagreement can result from a lack of reasonableness or rationality, prejudice, self-interest, or the group-interest of the parties involved (Rawls 2005, 58, 121). It is also possible that the convictions and passions of the majority interfere with liberty (Rawls 1971, 451). Attempts to achieve a consensus of reasonable doctrines may be overwhelmed by doctrines and religious beliefs that resist rational discussion (Rawls 2005, 126). Often, 'the deeper the conflict, the higher the level of abstraction to which we must ascend to get a clear and uncluttered view of its roots' (Rawls 2005, 46). Consequently, it is not surprising that Rawls excluded comprehensive religious and philosophical doctrines in isolation from being specified as public reason (Rawls 2001, 90). Comprehensive doctrines and religion can also run afoul of public reason if they are unable to support a reasonable balance of political values (Rawls 1997, 483, 2005, 243):

> given the fact of reasonable pluralism, citizens cannot agree on any moral authority, whether a sacred text, or institution. Nor do they agree about the order of moral values, or the dictates of what some regard as natural law. (Rawls 2005, 97)

Rawls recognizes that comprehensive doctrines have an impact on our society and lead to conflict:

> Deeply religious and moral conflicts characterize the subjective circumstances of justice. Those engaged in these conflicts are surely not in general self-interested, but rather, see themselves as defending their basic rights and liberties which secure their legitimate and fundamental interests. Moreover, these conflicts can be the most intractable and deeply divisive, often more so than social and economic ones. (Rawls 2001, 85)

Consequently, Rawls argues that comprehensive religious and philosophical doctrines should not be specified as public reason (Rawls 2001, 90):

> fundamentalist religious doctrines and autocratic and dictatorial rulers will reject the ideas of public reason and deliberative democracy. They will say that democracy leads to a culture contrary to their religion, or denies the values that only autocratic or dictatorial rule can secure. They assert that the religiously true, or the philosophically true, overrides the politically reasonable. (Rawls 1997, 488)

The difficulty in using public reason to justify a religious ritual that adherents believe to be non-negotiable is that there is no room for discussion (Rawls 1971, 206).

Rawls is quite careful about where religion fits into public reason. Since religion is a private matter, people have the freedom to abandon or change their religious adherence; only in totalitarian and theocratic monocultures is apostasy a crime (Rawls 2001, 93, 156). The aim of developing a system of political justice necessitates that we are not directed by tradition or the opinions of others, but rather that we strive to hold a conception of right based on reasonable grounds that can be set out individually for ourselves (Rawls 1971, 516).

Viens has trouble differentiating between the private influence of a particular comprehensive doctrine in reaching a decision and making a public appeal. He assumes that the comprehensive doctrine that influences individuals privately will have public appeal, without establishing that it does. The problem is that one should oppose non-publicly backable coercion even in one's private decisions (Greenawalt 1995).

(10) Risks from non-medical circumcision.
Brusa and Barilan make a similar utilitarian argument that cultural and religious circumcision should be at public expense because the risk of having the procedure performed outside the medical system would exceed the costs of paying for it (Brusa and Barilan 2008). This assertion requires empirical data to support it. Neither they nor Viens provide any. Their claim might be part of an argument that circumcision should not be illegal; it has no relevance to an argument over whether it should be funded by the taxpayer through the health budget.

How not to argue about circumcision[27]

For Viens to prove his case, several elements are needed. It has to be documented that statements he makes have a factual basis, that children do not have basic human rights, that the foreskin has no intrinsic value, that circumcision has value, that parents have the authority to make this decision, that informed deliberation takes place and this discussion makes a difference, that the child's future exercise of autonomy is being respected, that the infant's security of person is not violated, that he would choose circumcision if competent, that circumcision of a non-consenting child is rational, and that violating his right to bodily integrity is reasonable. This only leaves the possibility of a demonstration of reasonableness based on a history of tolerance and indifference: a defense similar to that used by slave owners in the antebellum South. Religious practices are not rational. Some are reasonable, but some, like circumcision, are not.

Where are we now?

Governments are faced with the dilemma that a popular, religiously mandated ritual is also a human rights violation. Courts have the duty to apply the protections guaranteed by human rights doctrines, while legislatures have to muster the courage to challenge influential interest groups, whether they be religious organizations or medical organizations who profit financially from the procedure.

One of the reasons I have characterized circumcision as a divisive as opposed to a controversial issue is that both the defenders and critics of circumcision want a rule that applies to everyone. Critics of circumcision believe that the protection of human rights applies to everyone, including cultural and religious groups that are most committed to the practice, the most loath to give it up, and who are willing to fight fiercely to perpetuate the practice. The defenders of circumcision formulate their arguments in favor of circumcision in terms that apply to all boys, not just boys in their own subculture. To appease circumcising subcultures, without actually admitting that this is what they are doing, medical organizations, such as the American Academy of Pediatrics, have produced a policy that allows any parent to have any boy circumcised for any reason (AAP 2012). Consequently, all boys have been placed at risk for an unnecessary procedure to preserve circumcision for a minority subculture that traditionally circumcises. Rawls recognized the danger of an influential element in society with an intransigent posture based on their comprehensive doctrine or religious beliefs. In this case, the tail is wagging the dog and telling the dog this is reasonable. Unfortunately, demonstrating that circumcision is unreasonable does not resolve the divisiveness.

Acknowledgements

I thank Brian Earp, MSc, and James G. Dwyer, JD, PhD, for their input and insightful comments while preparing this manuscript.

Notes

1. This would include, but not be limited to, scarification of the face as practiced in some parts of Africa (R v Adesanya), female genital cutting (Boulware-Miller 1985), or tattooing (Lopez 2010).
2. Unless otherwise specified, circumcision means non-therapeutic circumcision of male infants or other minors.
3. This article will deal predominantly with the later writings of Rawls with some references to his earlier material.
4. Rawls argued that utilitarianism did not assign adequate value to the rights and autonomy of moral persons, and an increase in the average utility of a population may have devastating impact on those at the bottom end of the distribution curve.
5. Viens offers no argument to support this statement.
6. Viens conveniently ignores the relevant analogy of how we would view incursions on the bodily integrity of an incompetent adult as a *per se* harm absent, compelling justification tied to that person's urgent welfare needs. Imagine if a guardian for an incompetent adult wanted very much to have that adult circumcised for cultural reasons or because of belief in the various medical claims that have been made about its benefits. What should the legal rule be for permissibility of the guardian doing so? (Dwyer 2006)
7. This is an example of the 'burden of proof' fallacy.
8. Ironically, Viens cites the law as justification for parental rights, yet he believes that relying on legal remedies to prohibit circumcision uses the law to enforce 'a particular value judgment in a way that appears to remove the moralism inherent in its source' (Viens 2004, 245).
9. Viens is begging the question here. His argument can be restated thus: not allowing parents' 'other-regulating' conduct to violate their infant's bodily integrity limits the parents' liberty to violate their infant's bodily integrity. Viens also appears to have trouble thinking of infants and children as persons distinct from their parents. Consequently, he repeatedly engages in *ad hoc* assertions of position that he would not apply to anyone other than children.
10. This approach is explored extensively by Dwyer (2006) and Lebit (1992).
11. Rawls's 'original position' is discussed later in the manuscript.
12. Nearly all rational people would not choose to have their basic liberty to bodily integrity violated or to have sensitive parts of their genital amputated without their input. The empirical evidence is that in developed countries, competent male rarely choose to be circumcised unless there is a medical indication (Wallerstein 1980). Some circumcision apologists have summarily rejected substitute judgment as nonsensical without discussion (Friedman Ross 1999; Diekema 2004). They argue the impossibility of determining what an infant or a child would want, yet it does not take much insight to determine that a child would choose to live, to be fed, to have shelter, and to maintain their bodily integrity. Others have argued that parents do

not have the authority to provide proxy consent for infant circumcision (Svoboda, Van Howe and Dwyer 2000). In the case of circumcision, it must also be considered that when males become adults, they generally place high value on protection of their genitals and the quality of sexual experience.

13. Thirty-eight prominent European clinicians called the report of the 2012 AAP Task Force 'culturally biased' (Frisch et al. 2013).
14. A similar ineffectual argument favoring infant circumcision based on a 'double effect' has also been floated (Clark, Eisenman, and Szapor 2007) and refuted (Van Howe and Svoboda 2008).
15. Although this has been repeated been asserted by pro-circumcision activists (Schoen, Wiswell, and Moses 2000), including the members of the 2012 AAP Task Force (American Academy of Pediatrics 2012), this conclusion has not generally been accepted (Frisch et al. 2013; Svoboda and Van Howe 2013). As noted earlier, national medical organization uniformly have not found sufficient evidence to recommend it. Likewise, cost-utility analyses that follow established standards for identifying articles, making calculations, and reporting results (Gold 1996) that looked at the full array of potential benefits and known risks have not found circumcision to be cost-effective or to have sufficient benefits (Ganiats et al. 1991; Lawler, Bisonni, and Holtgrove 1991; Chessare 1992; Van Howe 2004; Schoen, Colby, and To 2006). One exception is a study by Sansom et al. (2010) that found that circumcision would be cost-effective in preventing HIV infections in the United States. This study only looked at one issue, did not adequately consider the risks of the procedure, overestimated the incidence of HIV infection, and assumed that circumcision was 40–80% effective in preventing HIV infection when studies in the United States have consistently failed to demonstrate an association between circumcision status and HIV infection (Chiasson et al. 1991; Laumann, Masi, and Zuckerman 1997; Thomas et al. 2004; Mor et al. 2007; Warner et al. 2009; Rodriguez-Diez et al. 2012). A further critique of the analysis by Sansom et al. can be found at http://www.plosone.org/annotation/listThread.action?root = 9371 and http://www.plosone.org/annotation/listThread.action?root = 301.
16. While many see Rawls as a political philosopher, it is fairly evident that Rawls, with the publication of the first edition of *A Theory of Justice*, was looking to establish a universal, rational, ethical system. He stated, 'Justice as fairness is a theory of our moral sentiments as manifested by our considered judgments in reflective equilibrium' (Rawls 1971, 120).
17. If one only looks at the benefits and ignores the harms, one could justify penectomy as a more effective intervention than circumcision (Van Howe and Svoboda 2008).
18. Even if the foreskin was not most sensitive portion of the penis, removing it would still be an unacceptable violation of basic human liberties.
19. Healthy tissue has intrinsic worth from a biological perspective, in that it has blood vessels, nerve endings, lymphatics, *et cetera*.
20. Another problem with jumping immediately to a justification based on the 'reasonable' is that 'reasonable' also changes with time. Slavery used to be considered reasonable. Sometimes this determination is made by those in power rather than those affected by the decision; consequently, the views of those in power (the parents) will usually prevail. The first principle of justice is there to protect the basic liberties of all and the interests of the least powerful from the tyranny of those in power.
21. The right to an open future involves leaving decisions with permanent, irreversible consequences that can safely wait until the child is old enough to decide for himself (Feinberg 1980; Davis 2000; Darby 2013).
22. In cultures in which circumcision is popular, many men say that they prefer to be circumcised and that they are glad that it was done when they were an infant, so that they did not have to consciously experience the surgery. This attitude is likely the result of cultural conditioning and indoctrination. Given the opportunity, very few adult men choose to be circumcised, even though general anesthetic is available (Wallerstein 1980). No one is suggesting that adult men would not have that choice available to them.
23. This represents the logical fallacy of putting the burden of proof on the circumcision opponents rather than providing the necessary proof to support his own position.
24. At the risk of providing an argument based on popularity, the 'choice-protecting' view of rights expressed by the Will/Power Theorists enjoys little acceptance among rights theorists and the 'interest-protecting' views are now dominant (Dwyer 2006).
25. Note that religious practices are not included.

26. The counter argument is given the religious and cultural pressures to be circumcised; many men within circumcising cultures would choose to have been circumcised as infants. This argument was typically given by men who were circumcised as infants. This projection of one's value system on an infant infringes on what Singer calls the principle of equal consideration of interests (Singer 2011). Likewise, the religious or cultural affiliation of the parent would not be a factor when addressing this issue in the original position. The empirical evidence indicates a very low rate of elective circumcisions among adult males in the United States (Wallerstein 1980) and substantial rate of adults who do not adhere to the religion of their upbringing (PEW 2008).
27. Apologies to Benatar and Benatar (2003a).

References

American Academy of Pediatrics Task Force on Circumcision. 2012. "Male Circumcision." *Pediatrics* 130: e759–e785.

American Medical Association Council on Scientific Affairs. 1999. *Report 10: Neonatal Circumcision*. Chicago, IL: American Medical Association.

Benatar, D., and M. Benatar. 2003a. "How Not to Argue About Circumcision." *American Journal of Bioethics* 3 (2): W1.

Benatar, M., and D. Benatar. 2003b. "Between Prophylaxis and Child Abuse: The Ethics of Neonatal Male Circumcision." *American Journal of Bioethics* 3 (2): 35–48.

Boulware-Miller, K. 1985. "Female Circumcision: Challenges to the Practice as a Human Rights Violation." *Harvard Women's Law Journal* 8: 155–177.

British Medical Association. 2004. "The Law and Ethics of Male Circumcision: Guidance for Doctors." *Journal of Medical Ethics* 30: 259–263.

Bronselaer, G. A., J. M. Schober, H. F. L. Meyer-Bahlburg, G. T'Sjoen, R. Vlietinck, and P. B. Hoebeke. 2013. "Male Circumcision Decreases Penile Sensitivity as Measured in a Large Cohort." *BJU International* 111: 820–827.

Brusa, M., and Y. M. Barilan. 2008. "Cultural Circumcision in EU Public Hospitals – An Ethical Discussion." *Bioethics* 23: 470–482.

Chessare, J. B. 1992. "Circumcision: Is the Risk of Urinary Tract Infection Really the Pivotal Issue?" *Clinical Pediatrics (Philadelphia)* 31: 100–104.

Chiasson, M. A., R. L. Stoneburner, D. S. Hildebrandt, W. E. Ewing, E. E. Telzak, and H. W. Jaffe. 1991. "Heterosexual Transmission of HIV-1 Associated with the Use of Smokable Freebase Cocaine (Crack)." *AIDS* 5: 1121–1126.

Clark, P. A., J. Eisenman, and S. Szapor. 2007. "Mandatory Neonatal Circumcision in Sub-Saharan Africa: Medical and Ethical Analysis." *Medical Science Monitor* 13 (12): RA205–RA213.

Cold, C. J., and J. Taylor. 1999. "The Prepuce." *BJU International* 83 (suppl. 1): 34–44.

Convention on the Rights of the Child. UN GA Resolution 44/25, November 20, 1989.

Darby, R. 2005. *A Surgical Temptation: The Demonization of the Foreskin and Rise of Circumcision in Britain*. Chicago, IL: University of Chicago Press.

Darby, R. 2013. "The Child's Right to an Open Future: Is The Principle Applicable to Non-Therapeutic Circumcision?" *Journal of Medical Ethics*. Published Online First: January 30, 2013. doi:10.1136/medethics-2012-101182.

Davis, D. S. 2000. *Genetic Dilemmas: Reproductive Technology, Parental Choices, and Children's Futures*. 2nd ed. Oxford: Routledge.

Diekema, D. S. 2004. "Parental Refusals of Medical Treatment: The Harm Principle as Threshold For State Intervention." *Theoretical Medicine* 25: 243–264.

Dworkin, R. 1977. *Taking Rights Seriously*. London: Duckworth.

Dwyer, J. G. 1994."'Parents' Religion and Children's Welfare: Debunking the Doctrine of Parents' Right." *California Law Review* 82: 1371–1447.

Dwyer, J. G. 2006. *The Relationship Rights of Children*. Cambridge: Cambridge University Press.

Feinberg, J. 1980. "The Child's Right to an Open Future." In *Whose Child? Children's Rights, Parental Authority, and State Power*, edited by W. Aiken and H. LaFollette. Totawa, NJ: Littlefield, Adams.

Fetus and Newborn Committee, Canadian Paediatric Society. 1996. "Neonatal Circumcision Revisited." *Canadian Medical Association Journal* 154: 769–780.

Friedman Ross, L. 1999. *Children, Families, and Health Care Decision Making*. Oxford: Oxford University Press.

Frisch, M., Y. Aigrain, Y. Barauskas, R. Bjarnason, S.-A. Boddy, P. Czauderna, R. P. E. de Gier, et al. 2013. "Cultural Bias in the AAP's Technical Report and Policy Statement on Male Circumcision." *Pediatrics* 131: 796–800.

Frisch, M., M. Lindholm, and M. Grønbæk. 2011 "Male Circumcision and Sexual Function in Men and Women: A Survey-Based, Cross-Sectional Study In Denmark." *International Journal of Epidemiology* 40: 1367–1381.

Ganiats, T. G., J. B. Humphrey, H. L. Taras, and R. M. Kaplan. 1991. "Routine Neonatal Circumcision: A Cost-Utility Analysis." *Medical Decision Making* 11: 282–293.

Gold, M. R., J. E. Siegel, L. B. Russell, and M. C. Weinstein. 1996. *Cost-Effectiveness in Health and Medicine*. Oxford: Oxford University Press.

Gray, D. T. 2004. "Neonatal Circumcision: Cost-Effective Preventive Measure or 'The Unkindest Cut of All'?" *Medical Decision Making* 24: 688–692.

Greenawalt, K. 1995. *Private Consciences and Public Reasons*. Oxford: Oxford University Press.

Hartman, W. 2012. "Stellungnahme Dr.med:Wolfram Hartmann, Präsident des Berufsverbands der Kinder- und Jugendärzte, zur Anhörung am 26. November 2012 zum Gesetzentwurf der Bundesregierung: 'Entwurf eines Gesetzes über den Umfang der Personensorge bei einer Beschneidung des männlichen Kindes' und zum Gesetzentwurf der Abgeordneten Marlene Rupprecht, Katja Dörner, Diana Golze, Caren Marks, Rolf Schwanitz, weiterer Abgeordneter: 'Entwurf eines Gesetzes über den Umfang der Personensorge und die Rechte des männlichen Kindes bei einer Beschneidung'." Accessed April 7, 2013. http://www.kinderaerzte-im-netz.de/bvkj/kinpopup/psfile/pdf/70/121126_Ste50aa5e211e6a6.pdf

Hodges, F. M. 1997. "A Short History of the Institutionalization of Involuntary Sexual Mutilation in the United States." In *Sexual Mutilations A Human Tragedy*, edited by G. C. Denniston and M. F. Milos, 17–40. New York: Plenum Press.

Jordans, F. 2012. "Germany Approves Bill to Protect Male Circumcision." Accessed December 19, 2012. http://start.localnet.com/article.php?category=topstories&article=a028ec0da5f4458fa200891071 b65d0d

Joudi, M., M. Fathi, and M. Hiradfar. 2011. "Incidence of Asymptomatic Meatal Stenosis in Children Following Neonatal Circumcision." *Journal of Pediatric Urology* 7: 526–528.

Laumann, E. O., C. M. Masi, and E. W. Zuckerman. 1997. "Circumcision in the United States: Prevalence, Prophylactic Effects, and Sexual Practice." *Journal of the American Medical Association* 277: 1052–1057.

Lawler, F. H., R. S. Bisonni, and D. R. Holtgrave. 1991. "Circumcision: A Decision Analysis of its Medical Value." *Family Medicine* 23: 587–593.

Landgericht Köln. May 7, 2012. Urteil Ns 169/11.

Lebit, L. E. 1992. "Compelled Medical Procedures Involving Minors and Incompetents and Misapplications of the Substituted Judgment Doctrine." *Journal of Law & Health* 7: 107–130.

Lopez, P. 2010. "Fresno Father Who Tattooed Son Given Prison Time." *Fresno Bee*. Accessed January 23, 2013. http://www.mcclatchydc.com/2010/07/20/97834/fresno-father-who-tattooed-son.html

Mor, Z., C. K. Kent, R. P. Kohn, and J. D. Klausner. 2007. "Declining Rates in Male Circumcision Amidst Increasing Evidence of its Public Health Benefit." *PLoS ONE* 2: e861.

O'Neill, O. 1992. "Children's Rights and Children's Lives." In *Children, Rights and the Law*, edited by P. Alston, S. Parker and J. Seymour, 24–42. Oxford: Clarendon Press.

O'Neill, O. 2002. *Autonomy and Trust in Bioethics*. Cambridge: Cambridge University Press.

Olsen, F. 1992. "Children's Rights: Some Feminist Approaches to the United Nations Convention of the Rights of the Child." In *Children, Rights and the Law*, edited by P. Alston, S. Parker and J. Seymour, 192–220. Oxford: Clarendon Press.

Patterson, O. 1991. Freedom in the Making of Western Culture, as summarized in Patterson, O. 2008. "Freedom, Slavery and the Modern Construction of Rights." In *The Cultural Values of Europe*, edited by H. Joas and K. Wiegandt, 115–151. Liverpool: Liverpool University Press.

R v Adesanya. 1975. 24 ICLG 136.

Raftery, I. 2012. "German Court Bans Male Circumcision, Sparks Outrage Among Jews, Muslims." *World News on NBC News.com*. Accessed April 7, 2013. http://worldnews.nbcnews.com/_news/2012/06/27/12446284-german-court-bans-male-circumcision-sparks-outrage-among-jews-muslims?lite

Rawls, J. 1971. *A Theory of Justice (Original Edition)*. Cambridge, MA: Harvard University Press.

Rawls, J. 1995. "Reply to Habermas." from *Journal of Philosophy* 92 (3), In *Political Liberalism: Expanded Edition*, edited by J. Rawls, 372–434. New York: Columbia University Press.

Rawls, J. 1997. "The Idea of Public Reason Revisited." *University of Chicago Law Review*, 64: 765–807, in *Political Liberalism: Expanded Edition*, edited by J. Rawls, 435–490. New York: Columbia University Press.

Rawls, J. 2001. *Justice as Fairness: A Restatement*. Cambridge, MA: Harvard University Press.

Rawls, J. 2005. *Political Liberalism: Expanded Edition*. New York: Columbia University Press.

Rodriguez-Diaz, C. E., M. C. Clatts, G. G. Jovet-Toledo, R. L. Vargas-Molina, L. A. Goldsamt, and H. García. 2012. "More than Foreskin: Circumcision Status, History of HIV/STI, and Sexual Risk in a Clinic-Based Sample of Men in Puerto Rico." *Journal of Sexual Medicine* 9: 2933–2937.

Royal Australasian College of Physicians. 2010. *Circumcision of Infant Males*. Sydney: Royal Australasian College of Physicians.

Royal Dutch Medical Association. 2010. *Non-Therapeutic Circumcision of Male Minors*. Utrecht: KNMG.

Sansom, S. L., V. S. Prabhu, A. B. Hutchinson, Q. An, I. Hall, R. K. Shrestha, A. Lasry, and A. W. Taylor. 2010. "Cost-Effectiveness of Newborn Circumcision in Reducing Lifetime HIV Risk Among U.S. Males." *PLoS One* 5 (1): e8723.

Schoen, E. J., C. J. Colby, and T. T. To. 2006. "Cost Analysis of Neonatal Circumcision a Large Health Maintenance Organization." *Journal of Urology* 175: 1111–1115.

Schoen, E. J., T. E. Wiswell, and S. Moses. 2000. "New Policy on Circumcision – Cause for Concern." *Pediatrics* 105: 620–623.

Singer, P. 2011. *Practical Ethics*. 3rd ed. Cambridge: Cambridge University Press.

Slovenian Human Rights Ombudsman. 2012. "Obrezovanje fantkov iz nemedicinskih razlogov je kršitev otrokovih pravic" [Circumcision of boys for non-medical reasons is a oiolation of children's rights]. *Varuh Clovekovh Pravich*, February 3. Accessed February 27, 2012. http://www.varuh-rs.si/medijsko-sredisce/aktualni-primeri/novice/detajl/obrezovanje-fantkov-iz-nemedicinskih-razlogov-je-krsitev-otrokovih-pravic/?cHash=7364092ccb

Smith, J., S. Velaphi, A. Horn, Y. Joolay, and A. Madide. 2011. "Neonatal Circumcision." *South African Journal of Bioethics and Law* 4: 50–51.

Sorrells, M. L., J. L. Snyder, M. D. Reiss, C. Eden, M. F. Milos, N. Wilcox, and R. S. Van Howe. 2007. "Fine-Touch Pressure Thresholds in the Adult Penis." *BJU International* 99: 864–869.

Suomen Lääkäriliitto. (2011). "Poikien ympärileikkaus." http://www.laakariliitto.fi/uutiset/kannanotot/ymparileikkaus.html, cited in Askol, H. 2011. "Cut-off point? Regulating male circumcision in Finland." *International Journal of Law Policy and Family* 25: 100–119.

Svoboda, J. S. and R. S. Van Howe. 2013. "Out of Step: Fatal Flaws in the Latest AAP Policy Report on Neonatal Circumcision." *Journal of Medical Ethics*.

Svoboda, J. S., R. S. Van Howe, and J. G. Dwyer. 2000. "Informed Consent for Neonatal Circumcision: An Ethical and Legal Conundrum." *Journal of Contemporary Health Law and Policy* 17: 61–133.

Swedish Paediatric Society. 2012. "Swedish Docs in Circumcision Protest: Circumcision of Young Boys for Religious and Non-Medical Reasons Ought to be Banned in Sweden, Urged the Swedish Paediatric Society (Svenska barnläkarföreningen, BLF)." *The Local Sweden's News in English*, February 19. Accessed February 27, 2012. http://m.thelocal.se/39200/20120219/

Taylor, J. R., A. P. Lockwood, and A. J. Taylor. 1996. "The Prepuce: Specialized Mucosa of the Penis and its Loss to Circumcision." *British Journal of Urology* 77: 291–295.

The Pew Forum on Religion & Public Life. 2008. *U.S. Religious Landscape Survey Religious Affiliation: Diverse and Dynamic*. Washington, DC: The Pew Forum on Religion & Public Life.

Thomas, A. G., L. N. Bakhireva, S. K. Brodline, and R. A. Shaffer. 2004. "Prevalence of Circumcision and its Association with HIV and Sexually Transmitted Infections in a Male US Navy population." Naval Health Research Center Report No. 04-10.

Van Howe, R. S. 1997. "Anesthesia for Neonatal Circumcision: Who Benefits?" *Journal of Prenatal and Perinatal Psychology and Health* 12 (1): 3–18.

Van Howe, R. S. 2004. "A Cost-Utility Analysis of Neonatal Circumcision." *Medical Decision Making* 24: 584–601.

Van Howe, R. S. 2006. "Incidence of Meatal Stenosis Following Neonatal Circumcision in a Primary Care Setting." *Clinical Pediatrics (Philadelphia)* 45: 49–54.

Van Howe, R. S. 2013. "Infant Circumcision: The Last Stand for the Dead Dogma of Parental (Sovereignal) Rights." *Journal of Medical Ethics*. epub ahead of print.

Van Howe, R. S. and J. S. Svoboda. 2008. "Neonatal Circumcision is Neither Necessary Nor Ethically Permissible: A Response To Clark et al. Comment to: Mandatory Neonatal Circumcision in Sub-Saharan Africa: Medical and Ethical Analysis Peter Clark, Justin Eisenman, Stephen Szapor *Med Sci Monit* 2007; 13 (12): RA205-13." *Medical Science Monitor* 14 (8): LE7–LE13.

Viens, A. M. 2004. "Value Judgment, Harm, and Religious Liberty." *Journal of Medical Ethics* 30: 241–247.

Wallerstein, E. 1980. *Circumcision An American Health Fallacy*. New York: Springer.

Walter, T. 2012. "Der gesetzentwurf zur beschneidung – kritik und strafrechtliche alternative." *Juristenzeitung* 22: 1110–1017.

Warner, L., K. G. Ghanem, D. R. Newman, M. Macaluso, P. S. Sullivan, and E. J. Erbelding. 2009. "Male Circumcision and Risk of HIV Infection Among Heterosexual African American Men Attending Baltimore Sexually Transmitted Disease Clinics." *Journal of Infectious Diseases* 199: 59–65.

Infant male circumcision in the public square: applying the public reason of John Rawls (a reply to Robert Van Howe)

Susan Mendus

Department of Politics, University of York, York, UK

This is a reply to:

Van Howe, Robert. 2013. "Infant male circumcision in the public square: applying the public reason of John Rawls." *Global Discourse.* 3 (2): 214–229. http://dx.doi.org/10.1080/23269995.2013.805515.

In his spirited and wide-ranging article, Robert van Howe (2013) mounts a sustained attack on defenders of infant male circumcision. His primary target is Viens who, in his 2004 paper, 'Value Judgement, Harm and Religious Liberty', argues that 'as there are reasonable doctrines held by individuals that contain deeply held social, cultural and religious views concerning the value of having their son undergo circumcision, current attempts to advance a policy which prohibits the provision of this procedure that fail to take these value judgements seriously would be unjustified' (Viens 2004). In short, Viens is in favour of a permissive attitude towards infant male circumcision, and his support for it springs primarily from his endorsement of parental rights and parental authority, together with his acknowledgement of the significance of circumcision in some religions – notably, but not exclusively, in the Jewish and Muslim faiths.

Van Howe, by contrast, is vigorously opposed to infant male circumcision, and his case against it is made along three distinct yet inter-related lines: first, he argues that a male circumcision is mutilating and constitutes a serious harm; second, he argues that an appeal to parental rights cannot justify the mutilation even if it is a requirement of religious faith; and finally he argues that since religious belief is a private matter, it should not be used to justify a public policy. So where Viens emphasises the importance of parental rights and religious liberty, van Howe emphasises the rights of the child and the violations of those rights, which, he says, are inherent in male circumcision.

One very intriguing feature of the debate between Viens and van Howe is that, in making their respective arguments, each prays in aid the political liberalism of John Rawls. In particular, each notes the challenge (Rawls's challenge) involved in trying to secure agreement amongst people with very different and conflicting conceptions of the good, and each invokes Rawls's account of public reason as a way of securing consensus against a background of diverse conceptions of the good. In other words, both Viens and van Howe use the apparatus of modern political liberalism in order to address their central questions, yet they arrive at very different, indeed conflicting, answers to those questions. It might be thought that this merely shows us that one is right and the other wrong, and that our task now is to decide which is which. However, there is another, and more interesting, possibility, which is that the case of infant male circumcision is peculiarly problematic for liberals because it brings together issues on which liberalism is itself conflicted and uncertain. In my reply to van Howe, I will explore this possibility and my focus will be on the three themes he himself identifies: parental rights, the concept of harm, and the status and significance of religious belief. Through a discussion of these themes, and of the way in which van Howe engages with them, I hope to illuminate the nature of the challenges which modern liberalism faces and which the case of male infant circumcision throws into stark relief.

I begin with parental rights.

Parental rights

In his 2004 article, Viens notes that 'the law generally provides parents with the freedom and discretionary authority, in the course of raising their children, to decide what is in the interest of their children (within reason, of course) … justifiable reasons to circumcise or not to circumcise their son will be based on the parents' conception of the good' (Viens 2004, 242–243). Ignoring, for the moment, the vexed question of what counts as 'within reason', we should note that the argument in favour of circumcision is the one which invokes parents' right to exercise authority over their children, and also to instil their own conception of the good into their children. It is this claim to parental authority, which van Howe disputes in his article. Referring to the doctrine of parental rights as 'dead dogma' he emphasises instead the importance of parental duty, and, following Rawls, he proposes that parents choose for their children 'in the light of what they [the children] will want whatever else they want once they reach maturity' (Rawls 1971, 208–209). So where Viens appeals to parental rights in order to justify infant male circumcision, van Howe appeals to parental duty and to the concept of the autonomous individual in order to deny its justifiability.

Although the two strategies deliver conflicting conclusions, both exemplify a problem that is internal to liberalism itself. This is that, as an individualist political theory, it struggles to say how decisions should be made in the case of those whom the theory does not classify as individuals. Should decisions be taken on the basis of what they (the non-individuals or not-yet individuals) would choose were they now asked, or should they be taken on the basis of what they would choose if they were fully informed and rational? If the former, then why not allow them the status of individuals now; if the latter, then on what grounds do we, the decision-takers, declare something rational or irrational? This problem within liberal individualism has long been recognised by feminists, and it is the problem which both Viens and van Howe encounter in judging the permissibility of infant male circumcision. Van Howe is clear that an appeal to rationality is the correct approach and that it will deliver a judgement against circumcision, but Viens is equally clear that what is rational is partly determined by culture and context and this, he says, speaks in favour of the permissibility of circumcision in cases where the practice is part of a wider religious or cultural commitment.

Either way, the case of infant male circumcision is a specific case of a very general problem within a liberal political theory, and that problem concerns the ways in which we might decide on behalf of those who, for whatever reason, are not themselves accorded the status of individual or of citizen by the theory itself.

Beneath that problem, however, there is a further one, which revolves around the ambiguities inherent in the concept of harm.

Harm

In arguing for the impermissibility of infant male circumcision, van Howe emphasises the harm which is caused by this practice. He tells us that 'nearly all rational people would not choose to have their basic liberty to bodily integrity violated' and that 'the harm [in male circumcision] is easy to demonstrate'. In saying this, he implies that the concept of harm is both uncontroversial and objective, and that physical damage of the kind involved in circumcision is incontestably harmful. But it is not at all obvious that this is so. Many writers have drawn attention to the ways in which the concept of harm, far from being objective, may in fact be both morally and culturally determined. John Horton, for example, has queried the possibility of identifying 'paradigm cases' of harm, and has suggested that 'where there is serious disagreement about the moral quality of any activity there will also be disagreement about whether it is harmful' (Horton 1985). And similar arguments have been adduced by philosophers such as Mounce and Phillips (1969).

More generally, the point to be made here is that the concept of harm is not morally neutral and that it therefore cannot be deployed in order to decide what is morally permissible and what is not. It is, in no small part, our beliefs about what is morally wrong which determine what we think to be harmful, not the other way around, and as a result van Howe's insistence that the harm of circumcision is easy to demonstrate is both premature and under-argued. It is certainly not a claim that will find much support amongst the religious communities which favour circumcision and see its provision as a matter of parental duty.

I should emphasise here that van Howe is not alone in thinking that, in many cases, if not all, it is a simple and objective matter to decide what is harmful and what is not. This, indeed, was John Stuart Mill's hope in *On Liberty.* But the hope has been dashed many times since the publication of Mill's essay and, in multi-faith societies such as ours, the difficulty of reaching agreement about what constitutes harm is a very significant part of our problem, not something which can be 'read off' from a simple catalogue of the objective facts.

This brings me on to the third theme, which van Howe discusses in his paper: religious belief.

Religious belief

In Section 9 of his paper, van Howe turns to the question of whether and why Rawls's political liberalism would permit infant male circumcision in cases where it was a requirement for some religious believers – Muslims and Jews, for example. In discussing this question, he rejects Viens' appeal to the importance of religious liberty and focuses instead on Rawls's requirement that decisions about justice not be dependent upon specific comprehensive (including religious) conceptions of the good. Of course, both considerations are important to liberalism in general, and especially important to modern political liberalism, but an emphasis on religious liberty draws us in the direction of a permissive attitude to circumcision, whereas an emphasis on the political, and free-standing, character of justice draws us in the direction of a prohibitive attitude. As before, public policy cannot simply be 'read off' from the central texts of liberalism, and indeed those texts contain arguments that are sometimes in tension with one another. So, again, the dispute between Viens and van Howe highlights tensions within modern liberalism itself.

That said, it is not clear that van Howe has fully understood either Rawls's position in *Political Liberalism* or the problems attendant upon it. He (van Howe) tells us that, according to Rawls, 'comprehensive religious and philosophical doctrines should not be specified as public reason' (by which I take him to mean that comprehensive doctrines should not be used in the justification of principles of justice), and he then goes on to quote Rawls's view on fundamentalist religious doctrines thus: 'fundamentalist religious doctrines and autocratic and dictatorial rulers will reject the ideas of public reason and deliberative democracy'. But this implies that all those who hold comprehensive religious doctrines are unreasonable, and that is not so. Nor does Rawls think that it is so. Van Howe's tendency to elide Rawls's concerns about the unreasonable with Rawls's concerns about comprehensive doctrines makes his paper less clear than it ought to be, and this is a pity in an otherwise direct and forthright paper.

Beyond all this, however, the fundamental question for political liberalism is how people with very different and conflicting conceptions of the good may nonetheless converge on principles of justice, and, especially, how they may do so in a way that is neither forced nor strategic, but principled. As Rawls puts it, 'the problem of political liberalism is: How is it possible that there may exist over time a stable and just society of free and equal citizens profoundly divided by reasonable religious, philosophical and moral doctrines?' (Rawls 1993). In attempting to answer this question, Rawls seeks consensus: he hopes that people will be able to affirm the core principles of political liberalism from within their own moral perspective, even if those principles were not initially established from that perspective, but van Howe largely ignores this aspect of the Rawlsian project, and focuses instead on demonstrating the irrationality of those who disagree with him. Van Howe seeks victory rather than consensus and, to the extent that he does so, his response to the problem of infant male circumcision is both less persuasive and less liberal than one would hope.

References

Horton, John. 1985. "Toleration, Morality and Harm." In *Aspects of Toleration*, edited by John Horton and Susan Mendus, 113–135. London: Methuen.

Phillips, D. Z., and H. O. Mounce. 1969. *Moral Practices*. London: Routledge & Kegan Paul.

Rawls, John. 1971. *A Theory of Justice (Original Edition)*. Cambridge, MA: Harvard University Press.

Rawls, John. 1993. *Political Liberalism*. New York: Columbia University Press, xxv.

Van Howe, R. 2013. "Infant Male Circumcision in the Public Square: Applying the Public Reason of John Rawls." *Global Discourse*. 3 (2): 214–229.

Viens, A. M. 2004. "Value Judgement, Harm and Religious Liberty." *Journal of Medical Ethics* 30 (3): 242.

How reasonable is intactivism?: a reply to Van Howe

Martyn Griffin

Durham University Business School, Durham, UK

This is a reply to:

Van Howe, R. 2013. "Infant male circumcision in the public square: applying the public reason of John Rawls." *Global Discourse.* 3 (2): 214–229. http://dx.doi.org/10.1080/23269995.2013.805515.

I broadly agree with the argument that Robert Van Howe (2013) makes, and find it hard to defend any practice that does irreversible harm to a child in this manner. I would place the fundamental rights of the child to bodily integrity above the rights of parental choice. Despite this, however, the recent decision by the German courts to ban circumcision for boys until they are old enough to make their own decisions has provided a practical example of how complicated this issue can be. To explain the situation briefly, which has occurred since the author wrote the original article, a 4-year-old Muslim boy was circumcised by a doctor in Cologne. Due to complications, the boy had to be taken to a hospital where the doctor was subsequently accused of doing harm to the child. The doctor was subsequently charged and tried by a court which acquitted him of the charges but ruled that circumcision for non-medical reasons was a violation of the German constitution on the basis that it undermines the bodily integrity of the child. This decision effectively made circumcision for non-medical reasons a crime. The reaction of the Jewish community in particular was one of surprise and suspicion, with Rabbi Herzfeld suggesting the ruling was 'an existential attack upon the Jewish people' (Herzfeld 2012). Rabbi Sacks even went as far to address German Chancellor Angela Merkel directly in Brussels, telling her that following this ruling the Jewish people were actively considering 'whether there is a future for Jews in Europe' (Sacks 2012). Sacks went on to dismiss the idea that circumcision is an assault on the rights of the child as according to him, if this were to be true 'teaching children to speak German, sending them to school and vaccinating them against illness are all assaults against the rights of the child since they are done without consent'. This conveniently overlooks the fact that things like vaccination, teaching in schools and learning German are things that all rational adults (who live in Germany at least) would hope to happen to them as children. As the author of the article points out, it is less clear that they would want the most sensitive part of their penis removed.

Despite this, however, I have two main problems with the argument presented by the author, problems that need to be taken more seriously so that a more nuanced approach to phasing out circumcision can take place over a number of years. It is my contention that banning it immediately in a manner of this kind is not only dangerous and unnecessarily inflammatory but it is counter-productive to the aims of those trying to change people's minds. This isn't a straightforward public health issue based on consent and harm. This, for me, would allow us to draw a simple analogy between the issue of male infant circumcision and issues like smoking in the household where the right of parental choice (to expose their children to the harmful effects of smoke) regularly trumps the right of the child to bodily integrity leading to an increased likelihood of associated health issues such as asthma and cancer. It should be clear that when such a straightforward case of harm to a child is not routinely outlawed that circumcision with its added religious, cultural and historical baggage would be even more complicated and difficult to address. Certainly more difficult than simply outlawing it and expecting groups of individuals to change their beliefs and behaviours over night or simply move elsewhere.

First, then, I would like to take issue with the author's assertion that circumcision is done on a 'whim'. Clearly not all circumcisions are performed for religious reasons, and in the United States it is performed as a matter of course in many hospitals. However, in a large proportion of cases it is performed for religious or cultural reasons, and I believe the author fails to give these issues enough respect. They may not be strong enough reasons to convince us that circumcision should continue for boys, but they may inform how we go about changing practice over time. For the Jewish community in particular this practice – to be performed within 8 days on the birth of a boy – is a central part of male identity. Similar to the religious chants or prayers that they partake in, circumcision connects these Jewish children to their ancestors stretching back for thousands of years. In fact, it is a key rite of passage to join this community. As Rabbis Hier and Cooper have suggested, 'for 3500 years, every male child has entered the Jewish people through the rite of circumcision. We are not talking about a mere custom, but a biblical principle that has defined the Jewish people from time immemorial' (AAP 2012). It is important not to underestimate how fundamental this issue is. The implications of the ruling are therefore highly significant as banning it as a practice makes it very difficult for Jews to continue to live in Germany. Given the relatively recent history of the country – Hitler described circumcision as a 'blemish' and outlawed it – simply banning the practice and forcing the Jewish community to consider whether they are welcome is a dangerous and inflammatory measure that undermines integration. Furthermore, Muslim boys for whom it is not a religious prescription to be circumcised within 8 days (they may wait longer if their parents wish), may be taken to other countries to be given the procedure in what will often amount to third world medical conditions. Ironically, in trying to protect the child, an immediate and culturally insensitive ban that does not consider all the above issues may end up being counter-productive to their well-being.

Second, it worries me slightly that words like 'intactavist' have sprung up around the discourse, highlighting those people who wish to proclaim the virtues of remaining uncircumcised. It is quite easy to imagine how this could lead to the suggestion that Jewish and Muslim men (and others who have the procedure for medical and non-medical reasons) are somehow not *intact*. They are missing a part of their manhood, in a physical sense of course but also it could be maliciously implied in a wider sense. The discourse marks these individuals out as different and incapable of fully indulging in the pleasures of sex to the degree that intact men can – despite the fact that we cannot truly compare experiences in any meaningful or measurable way. In addition to this, there are also further ramifications of this logic. It could quite easily be misappropriated by individuals and groups who would wish to undermine the Jewish or Muslim community leading to a level of dehumanization and stigmatization that could have terrible consequences. It is by no means my suggestion that the author of this paper would have such an intention but it is quite possible that this agenda could be hijacked by racist and far right groups to fulfil their repugnant aims. Clearly the solution is not to merely bury our heads in the sand and pretend that the situation simply does not exist for fear of the consequences. It does suggest, however, that as with the first of my objections outlined above, a more nuanced and sensitive approach is required to tackle this issue than is currently taking place.

Perhaps a more sensible approach to this issue, and dare I say it a more Rawlsian approach, would be to distinguish between what the state supports through its medical institutions and what communities may offer separately. America is currently taking this route, posing the question of whether their state-funded *Medicaid* should support the circumcision of male infants. In this scenario, state-funded hospitals would not offer circumcisions on any other basis than for medical reasons. Meanwhile, a small number of private clinics could continue to offer the service to religious groups so that – if they intend to raise a family – they do not feel unable to stay in the country. Of course, the issue of bodily integrity remains, but as suggested above there are other issues at stake here that need to be taken in to account when trying to phase this ancient practice out of the modern world. There are groups within the Jewish faith already practising *Brit Shalom* or 'covenant without circumcision' and it is these groups that should be the focus for change within these communities, with public education programmes helping to change minds particularly through dialogue with the Rabbis, Imams and other religious leaders. The aim should be to gradually reduce the proportion of parents within these communities who feel it is necessary to circumcise their children, so that over the next two or three generations it becomes increasingly normal for parents to look past the option. It is correct to say that if we were starting society today, determining our rules of justice and law from a blank slate, we would not find a place anywhere for this practice. However, we are not working from a blank slate, and four millennia of history and tradition must at least influence how we react and legislate around an exceptionally complicated issue of this kind.

References

AAP. 2012. "US Jews Slam German Circumcision Ruling." *The Australian*, July 6.

Herzfeld, S. 2012. "Is the Ruling in Germany Anti-Circumcision?." *Huffington Post*, July 5.

Sacks, J. 2012. "'The Europeans' Skewed View of Circumcision." *Jerusalem Post*, July 6.

Van Howe, R. 2013. "Infant Male Circumcision in the Public Square: Applying the Public Reason of John Rawls." *Global Discourse* 3 (2): 214–229.

Promoting genital autonomy by exploring commonalities between male, female, intersex, and cosmetic female genital cutting

J. Steven Svoboda[1]

Attorneys for the Rights of the Child, Berkeley, CA, USA

All forms of genital cutting – female genital cutting (FGC), intersex genital cutting, male genital cutting (MGC), and even cosmetic forms of FGC – are performed in a belief that they will improve the subject's life. Genital autonomy is a unified principle that children should be protected from genital cutting that is not medically necessary. Safeguarding genital autonomy encompasses helping societies and individuals to explore wounds common across different forms of genital cutting regarding gender, power, the quest for cultural belonging, and social and sexual control. A desire to prevent alternative sexualities helps explain the origins of MGC's medicalization starting in the nineteenth century, as well as the roots of the failed attempt to similarly medicalize FGC. The child with 'ambiguous' genitalia brings us face to face with the failure of the attempted alignment of sex and gender. Medical ethics, law, and human rights suggest a path forward toward genital autonomy.

All forms of genital cutting – female genital cutting (FGC), intersex genital cutting (IGC), male genital cutting (MGC), and even cosmetic forms of FGC (CFGC) – are performed in a belief that they will improve the subject's life. Genital autonomy is a unified principle that children should be protected from genital cutting that is not medically necessary. Safeguarding genital autonomy encompasses helping societies and individuals to explore wounds common across different forms of genital cutting regarding gender, power, the quest for cultural belonging, and social and sexual control.

A desire to prevent alternative sexualities helps explain the origins of MGC's medicalization starting in the nineteenth century, as well as the roots of the failed attempt to similarly medicalize FGC. Ritual circumcision – male or female – is a public political statement by the compliant parents of sexual and social alignment and of submission to power. The cost of nonconformity is seen as too high and so the decision is carved in the body of the necessarily nonconsenting child. Genital cutting's transformation power may promise to turn a child into an adult, a person of indeterminate sex into an unequivocal girl, or even a nonvirgin back into a virgin.

The child with 'ambiguous' genitalia brings us face to face with the failure of the attempted alignment of sex and gender. If contradictory responses to nonconsensual genital surgeries on female and male minors respectively reveal inconsistencies, the same can be said when comparing FGC and CFGC. CFGC is often performed in the developed world to conform oneself with conventional, heterosexuality based norms regarding body appearance, and is driven by a medicalized model of women's sexuality.

Medical ethics, law, and human rights suggest a path forward toward genital autonomy insofar as they protect groups that we are less inclined to safeguard. Applying these tools skillfully can assist us in making sense of what we see when we dare to glimpse into that awful darkness that reflects our own culture's strange obsessions, thereby helping us to find commonalities between different forms of genital cutting and different cultural wounds that help perpetuate genital cutting practices.

Introduction: genital autonomy defined and advocated

Genital cutting, in whatever form it may come – FGC, IGC, MGC, or even CFGC performed on adults – is performed in the belief that the procedure – no matter how physically injurious – will in some way improve the subject's life. Genital autonomy may be defined as the unified principle that all children should be protected from genital cutting that is not truly medically necessary.

Regrettably, humanity, for all our technological achievement and advancement in individual rights, may only be a short evolutionary step away from superstition, fear, and prejudice. Accordingly, genital cutting often arises as a by-product of an individual's or a society's attempt to resolve needs relating to one or more of gender, power, the quest for cultural belonging, and social and sexual control including control of alternative sexualities. Work to advance genital autonomy often encompasses helping societies and individuals to explore wounds around these issues that are common to the different forms of genital cutting.

While the terminology is of relatively recent provenance, the concept of unifying the separate movements and discussions relating to FGC (potentially including CFGC), MGC, and IGC has been around for decades. Hanny Lightfoot-Klein issued an early plea for genital autonomy, inserting a passionate chapter on male circumcision into her groundbreaking 1989 book on FGC, *Prisoners of Ritual* (Lightfoot-Klein 1989, 183–192). A decade later, Lenore T. Szuchman and Frank Muscarella traced connections between FGC, MGC, and IGC:

> Sexual pleasure is limited physically by genital mutilation. In our culture, there is general agreement that the genital cutting performed on girls in some African cultures constitutes a gross violation of the individual's right to sexual fulfillment. Some have argued that a similar violation and consequent abrogation of the individual's right to sexual fulfillment occurs routinely in the United States in the 'corrective' genital surgery performed on intersexuals and in the circumcision of male infants. (Szuchman and Muscarella 2000, xii–xiii)

Szuchman and Muscarella included in the same book an arguably even more potent endorsement of genital autonomy, an integrated article by four expert authors titled 'Genital Surgery on Children Below the Age of Consent', addressing all three principal aspects of genital autonomy: FGC, MGC, and IGC (Lightfoot-Klein et al. 2000, 440–479).

MGC and FGC: querying gender-based terminology

Consideration of two of the three primary forms of genital autonomy – FGC and MGC – has been shaped by the gender-based formulation of the debate. Szasz has noted that:

> [w]e call the removal of the foreskin of the male newborn 'routine neonatal circumcision', and the removal of parts of the female genitalia 'female genital mutilation'. Language thus prejudges the legitimacy (or illegitimacy) of the practice. (Szasz 1996, 143)

The very distinction between MGC and FGC is artificial. We do not have separate terminology for assault of males and assault of females, nor for male murder and female murder. Isabelle Gunning notes commonalities between the two practices: 'Both can be seen as unnecessary alterations of normal, healthy genitalia justified by questionable health benefits and bolstered by culturally, socially, or religiously defined notions of aesthetics and clearly delineated binary ideas of gender' (Gunning 1999, 655–656).

The separate categories came about due to the different development in the West of MGC and FGC – though perhaps, as we shall see, the paths were not as different as one may think. Janice Boddy suggests a possible explanation for the widely disparate views: 'intuitively, men and boys are not "natural" victims' (Boddy 2007, 59). It follows that whereas women's acquiescence in FGC is viewed as evidence of denial and repression, men's silence about circumcision is viewed as evidence that MGC is harmless and/or of men's bravery and machismo.

Those who have attempted to break the silence on the differential treatment of these two issues have not always found the road a smooth one. When the Canadian ethicist Margaret Somerville began speaking in opposition to circumcision of newborn males, she found herself denounced by feminists who accused her of:

> detracting from the horror of female genital mutilation and weakening the case against it by speaking about it and infant male circumcision in the same context and point out that the same ethical and legal principles applied to both. (Somerville 2000, 211)

Anthropologist Kirsten Bell received similar reactions when she started to trace commonalities between FGC and MGC (Bell 2005, 131).

In a study by Reed Riner (1989) of 144 preindustrial cultures, genital modification was performed in 23. These 23, Riner found, were distinguished from the other 121 cultures by a 'particular combination of traits – patrilineal descent, patrilocal residence, polygamy, the presence of strong fraternal interest groups, internal warfare, male individuality, and control over women and children'. Of the 23, some cultures modified the genitals of both boys and girls, or boys but not girls, but not a single culture modified girls and not boys. 'This suggests', Riner comments, 'that female genital modification is somehow dependent on the cultural presence of male genital modification, and that if we explain the latter we have, for the most part, explained the former' (Riner 1989). Clearly a powerful process of association is at work: an association of two genital modifications that are habitually conceived of as radically different phenomena.

Intersex surgeries interject an illuminating third perspective, intriguingly – and troublingly – querying the boundary between the asserted dichotomy, raising potentially troubling questions that culture tries to quash through medicalized (though not truly medical) procedures. For those individuals born with genitalia that do not fit cultural desires or that raise discomfort, genital cutting is often the recommended course of action. Families are encouraged by the community at large to physically transform their child, even if (or perhaps because) conformity exacts serious physical, sexual, and psychological tolls on the individuals.

The root problem with our grasping the parallels between, on the one hand, FGC, and on the other hand, MGC or IGC, seems to be our inability to understand that, as Henrietta

Moore wryly puts it, 'The West, it turns out, has culture just like everyone else' (Moore 2007, 311). African women, or so the unconscious assumption all too often runs, are mired in culture; 'we' hold the truth (Boddy 2007, 57). Yet it is not only *other* cultures that may fall prey to gender and sexual stereotypes. And our failure to grasp this simple truth is precisely a blind spot that most persistently sticks in the throat of non-Western women.

It is understandable that Western observers have trouble objectively analysing the West's own practice, male genital cutting. Throughout the world, as Richard Shweder has written, people recoil and say 'yuck' to other cultures' body mutilation practices while justifying their own practices and saying 'yuck' to cultures that have *not* adopted their own particular customs (Shweder 2002, 222, 225).

Medicalization to the rescue?

One of the most powerful forces in what we might call the 'yummifying' of genital cutting has been the process of increased medicalization of our lives. With the historical development of the medical institution, and with the shift of the epistemological paradigm from religion to science, physicians greatly elevated their social status and assumed greatly enhanced power over the human body.

In the nineteenth century, at least portions of the medical community came to perceive a medical need to circumcise both boys and girls. The first known medicalized genital surgery occurred in 1822 in Berlin. No physician practicing at the end of the nineteenth century would have disagreed that masturbation, unless stopped at a young age, had all sorts of dire consequences, including blindness and insanity (Gollaher 2000). The doctors knew the obvious, that the foreskin enhanced male erotic response. Accordingly, doctors focused on demonizing the foreskin to further their campaign to control childhood sexual activity (see Darby 2005, 93). Doctors and society feared a danger of knowledge of masturbation spreading virally through boys' schools as one boy initiated another into this intimate act, so that by preventing masturbation, circumcision would also stop at least one of the most fearsome alternative forms of sexuality, sexual intimacy between males (see Lyttelton 1887).

One early author conjured up horrific images of masturbation and other forms of alternative sexuality (sodomy) terrorizing patients, and then presents the salvation, circumcision:

> Hand in hand with its boon companion, sodomy, it [masturbation] stalks through every [mental] ward, entangling its victims more hopelessly with each passing night... In all cases, taken as they come, circumcision is undoubtedly the physician's closest friend and ally, offering as it does a certain means of alleviation and pronounced benefit, granting as it does immunity from after-reproach. (Spratling 1895, 442–443)

This medicalization of children's sexuality seemingly struck a chord with parents by providing them with an explanation of the origin of their children's undesirable behaviors. Doctors promoted circumcision as a general means of social and sexual control capable of promoting improved health, enhanced work capabilities, longevity, and protection from tantrums and diseases. Genital surgeries gave parents a tool to control their children's sexuality and gave doctors a chance to emphasize their authority over children and women's bodies (Abd el Salam 2003).

It is important to remember, as mentioned earlier, that this antisex advocacy was not at all limited to males. At the birth of the medicalization of MGC, many doctors also forcefully advocated for the parallel use of FGC, based on more or less identical reasons – ostensible prevention of masturbation and other alternative sexualities, including homosexuality, ostensible cure of numerous diseases, and – in what was at the time partly synonymous – promotion of moral rectitude.

A 14-year-old 'idiotic' patient was said to have been cured of her 'excessive masturbation and nymphomania' after being 'declitorized' (Shorter 1992, 82). Early advocates of genital cutting wrote about MGC and FGC in the same breath, as in Belle Eskridge's 1918 article in the *Texas State Journal of Medicine*, 'Why Not Circumcise the Girl as Well as the Boy?' (Eskridge 1918) or Kistler's article in JAMA in 1910, 'Rapid Bloodless Circumcision of Male and Female and Its Technic'. Kistler writes, 'Many females need circumcision, and the operation is more easily performed than in the male' (Kistler 1910, 1782). Although several European authorities had recommended clitoridectomy to treat nymphomania (Shorter 1992, 82), they had few English followers. One was Samuel Ashwell, who wrote in 1845 that 'an enlarged clitoris' was sometimes marked 'by exquisite sensibility of its mucous membrane', which often 'gives rise to sexual passion and subdues every feeling of modesty'. The result was headaches, attacks of hysteria, and loss of mental discipline, and Ashwell recommended extirpation of the organ in these instances (Ashwell 1845, 708)

Darby stresses the similarity in the historical views of the two practices, noting that we may have come very close to a present-day United States in which both FGC and MGC are routinely practiced:

> Comparisons between the male and female anatomies were central to the debate over clitoridectomy, but it was widely assumed that the foreskin and clitoris had similar a function [sic] and played the same vital role in masturbation.... Sander Gilman... comments that "circumcision and clitoridectomy were seen as analogous medical procedures". It is remarkable how close the British medical profession came to endorsing clitoridectomy. (Darby 2005, 144)

Probably this fate was avoided only due to the fact that authorities tended to be less concerned about the distaff side as they supposedly pleasured themselves at much lower frequency.

Medicalization can be understood as medicocultural disciplining of bodies whose appearance departs from social and cultural desires. Surgical normalization – whatever the letter may be preceding 'GC' – has been one method of reconfiguring such 'deviant' bodies (see, e.g., Karkazis 2008, 10). When such procedures become accepted, physicians can shift responsibility for making the decision from themselves to the parents. One conundrum posed by medicalization of genital cutting of infants is the requirement of informed consent for all medical procedures. It is questionable whether parents have the legal right to consent to surgery on their infants that is irreversible, fundamentally cosmetic, and often medically unnecessary (Lareau 2003, 130–131; see also Ford 2001; see also Svoboda 2012).

In recent decades, childbirth has been increasingly medicalized, and that process has helped reinforce the medicalization of MGC. Of course, the medicalization has continued into recent times with California legislators having passed into law Assembly Bill 768, which declares that male circumcision has 'health and affiliative benefits' and thereby purports to establish a parental right to circumcise. Medicalization of MGC is of course in full swing in Africa as an asserted protection against AIDS, with the enthusiastic endorsement of the World Health Organization (WHO 2006), under what certain critics (see, e.g., Garenne 2006) consider an imperialistic impetus propelled by developed world dollars.

Medicalization does have at least some theoretical benefits, in that a hospital procedure carries reduced risks relative to a procedure by nonmedically trained practitioners. Nevertheless, a major concern raised against any form of harm-reducing medicalization is that cutting will – given the stamp of approval of the medical establishment – become entrenched, which will prevent its eventual eradication.

Again, the parallels with FGC are closer than some may believe. Medicalization of FGC in the United States ended more recently than is commonly realized, as FGC was recommended in US medical journals (Wollman 1973) and written about in *Cosmopolitan* magazine well into the 1970s (Isenberg and Elting 1976), thereby incidentally laying the groundwork for today's cosmetic FGC.

Roots of FGC, MGC, and IGC in quest for social control and sexual control

Genital cutting – whether it be FGC, MGC, IGC, or CFGC – often arises in response to issues partaking of one or more of gender, power, the desire to achieve cultural belonging, and social and sexual control including control of alternative sexualities.

Gender is one potent axis along which both FGC and MGC are commonly explained and justified. Numerous cultures, including the Dogon and Bambara of Mali, the Kono of Sierra Leone, and in Somalia, believe that the human body has soft female and hard male components, and that FGC removes the hard parts from the girls and MGC takes the soft parts from the boys to give both an unambiguous sex (Brain 1979, 87; Montagu 1995, 13; van der Kwaak 1992). Among the Kono, '[r]emoval of the external glans and hood is said to activate women's 'penis *within* the vagina' (Shweder 2009, 14). One Egyptian author notes:

> As a young boy grows up and finally is admitted into the masculine society he has to shed his feminine properties. This is accomplished by the removal of the prepuce, the feminine portion of his original sexual state. The same is true with a young girl, who upon entering the feminine society is delivered from her masculine properties by having her clitoris or her clitoris and labia excised. Only thus circumcised can the girl claim to be fully a woman and thus capable of the sexual life. (Shaalan 1982)

Also evident here is a normative sexuality and hidden heterosexism, an attachment to mainstream sexual practices and an aversion to alternative sexualities. Pollack writes that male circumcision partakes of issues of identity, gender, and power, commenting, 'In every circumcising society, MGC functions to fulfill multiple unspoken social, political-tribal, and sexual needs' (Pollack 2011). MGC and FGC always entail a larger individual performing a harmful and hurtful procedure to a smaller individual. IGC also supplies a piece in the puzzle that society is evidently trying to solve relating to gender. Through IGC, difference is literally inscribed on the bodies of women and men whose 'natural' bodies are not sufficiently different for socially appropriate reproduction. Thus, all three forms of genital cutting are closely related to issues of power and domination.

Paige and Paige claim that male circumcision originally functioned as a vehicle for attempting to achieve by means of ritual, what could not be accomplished by means of political arrangement: that is, the defusing of possible competitive claims by male progeny for the same limited resources (Paige and Paige 1981, 166). In preindustrial societies, in which survival was predicated on secure allegiance to clan and tribe, the father proved his loyalty to his tribe by subjecting his son's potential for procreation to the knife (Glick 2005, 18; Paige and Paige 1981, 151). Accordingly, circumcision was not a private ceremony or surgery but rather a social and political statement of alignment and loyalty. Pollack notes the nominally incidental outcome of 'a re-assertion and institutionalization of a power structure based on gender' (Pollack 2011). MGC represents a permanent, dramatic, bloody, public ritual of submission of the individual to the group, of the father to his 'fathers'. It represents a taming, a harnessing, done for the ostensible sake of the group's survival, but done without regard to effects on the individual or, indeed, the long-term effects on the group.

Genital cutting serves as a means of social and sexual control of children. One frequently cited justification for FGC is that it is a means to contain women's sexuality within socially approved bounds, focusing it on the social goals of marriage, fertility, and reproduction (Moore 2007, 321–322). Both FGC and MGC were intended to help incorporate boys and girls into adult societies of sexuality, reproduction, and family. Even where performed on infants and thus necessarily not a rite of passage for the infant himself, secular MGC doubtless may be motivated by an inchoate desire to formally induct them into the community and to help them along in life. Men are performers, initiators, and often the most ardent supporters of MGC, and women are performers, initiators, and often the most ardent supporters of FGC (Boddy 1982, 686–687). Interestingly, some of the leading advocates of CFGC are portraying it as a form of liberation demanded by women:

> Women should be empowered by knowledge of the modern day advances in vaginal surgery, including rejuvenation techniques and cosmetic enhancement. Knowing what is available, if so desired, is itself a form of liberation. Males are not the motivating force behind these new techniques, as many proclaim. Women are the ones pushing for this liberation. (Apesos et al. 2008, vi)

Similar to MGC, FGC often is practiced to facilitate social control. Elena Jirovsky found that in Burkina Faso FGC occurs to channel female sexuality, not to negate it, but as a means of ensuring morally acceptable behavior (Jirovsky 2010, 84). Analogously, Bettina Shell-Duncan et al. recently determined that in Senegambia, 'being circumcised serves as a signal to other circumcised women that a girl or woman has been trained to respect the authority of her circumcised elders and is worthy of inclusion in their social network' (Shell-Duncan et al. 2011, 1275). Echoing Paige's work regarding MGC as a ritualized indication of loyalty and submission, Shell-Duncan et al. write that circumcision demonstrates a young woman's self-control over her sexuality and thus over her life:

> in order to gain entry into women's networks, young women offer their deference or obedience to older women in the network, enhancing the leader's power and standing in the community… female circumcision serves as a signal that girls have been taught the art of subordination to their future husband, husband's brothers, and most importantly, to their mothers in-law. (Shell-Duncan et al. 2011, 1281)

Along the same lines, El Guindi writes that FGC is meant to control sexuality only temporarily and for the purpose of social cohesion: '[female] circumcision is intended to control the sexual energy of a virgin until marriage. It is not considered a mechanism for the permanent reduction of the woman's sexuality' (El Guindi 2006, 37). Furthermore, striking parallels may be observed in the evolving rationales for both female and male circumcision, rooted in a combination of restrictive sexual mores, religious rituals, and medical justifications (DeLaet 2009, 407).

As shown by the renowned anti-FGC activist, Hanny Lightfoot-Klein, parallel justifications are offered for FGC and MGC; these include claimed health benefits, absence of 'bad' genital odors, enhancement of physical beauty, greater attractiveness and acceptability of the sex organs, incorrect medical reasons, minimization of damage and pain, hygiene, preventing future problems, mistaken theories that it improves sex, or is universal, and its use as a rite of initiation into adulthood (Lightfoot-Klein 1997, 131–135). Others include looking like other children or like the child's parents, fear of promiscuity, and acceptance of altered genitalia as more attractive to the opposite sex (Hernlund and Shell-Duncan 2007, 18–19).

Intersex surgeries: responses to a social emergency or medicalized discipline?

By the middle of the twentieth century, intersex births had come to be labeled a medical and social emergency. Some medical authors addressing intersex surgeries explicitly label the situation as an emergency (Canty 1977; Lobe et al. 1987, 651; Farkas, Chertin, and Hadas-Halpren 2001, 2343), as did the American Academy of Pediatrics (AAP) (American Academy of Pediatrics 2000, 138), while others suggest that a 'lifetime of social tragedy can follow for the patient and family if the infant is not properly managed' (Donahoe, Crawford, and Hendren 1977, 1053). Ford adroitly observes, '[I]t is the parents and doctors of intersexed infants who are experiencing a medical emergency, not the intersexed infant' (Ford 2001, 477). Emphasizing thorough but swift clinical workups to determine the etiology, clinicians determine a sex for these infants, and surgeons then modify the infant's body, especially the genitals, to conform to the assigned sex (Karkazis 2008, 204, 207). Similarly, for tribal MGC, Paige and Paige (1981, 149) note that 'the boy who is circumcised is not himself the object of the ceremony, which is, in fact, conducted to impress others'.

With IGC, sexual and gender identity is also culturally created through genital cutting. Those outlaws who fail to conform their sex and gender to one of the two permitted options must be – or under the new more enlightened regime, may be – subjected to medicalized discipline. Gunning has noted the striking parallels between FGC and IGC:

> While these [intersex] surgeries are performed on a smaller segment of the population, some of their functions are similar to those of the more common forms of [FGC]. In both cases, the dominant patriarchal culture constructs certain ideals based upon the notion that people are 'naturally' divided into only two distinct genders.... For those individuals born with genitalia that do not fit these rigidly defined categories, surgery or mutilation is the recommended course of action. Families are again encouraged by the community at large, including its most respected members, to physically transform their child, even if conformity exacts serious physical, sexual, and psychological tolls on the individuals.... In both cases, the parents decide that the cost of nonconformity for the child, for themselves, and for their families is too great, and decide for their children. (Gunning 1999, 663–664)

Gunning refers, of course, to the parents' decision to, as it were, carve their decision in their children's body. The motivation seems to be socio-cultural rather than medical, revealing less about *intersexuality* than about a social and medical *discomfort with intersexuality.* As one of the first books devoted to intersexuality tersely summarizes matters, 'In our society there are males and females and that is all. A person must live as one or the other' (Dewhurst and Gordon 1969, 304).

With apologies for the double pun, Cheryl Chase (now Bo Laurent) cuts to the chase:

> The surgeries are incredibly sexist. They're based on the idea that men have sex; women are penetrated by men and have babies. What you produce [through intersex surgery] is somebody who has a body that is vaguely female, is infertile, doesn't menstruate, probably doesn't have any sexual function, might have genital pain, and has been lied to and shamed. That is supposed to be less painful than having a small dick? (Hegarty 2000, 124)

In a strange twist on the Dogon and Bambara, employing heterosexist norms, femaleness is defined as the absence of maleness (Hegarty 2000, 124–125).

Some surgeons performing surgery on intersex individuals have candidly acknowledged having made 'serious mistake[s]' and 'serious errors' (Gross and Meeker 1955, 315, 320). For well over a decade, Diamond and others have been eloquently and in closely reasoned papers calling for a moratorium on cosmetic sex assignment surgeries performed without the patient's consent (Diamond and Sigmundson 1997, 1047; Diamond 1999, 1025–1026). In recent years, these arguments have started to bear fruit as 'a slower and more judicious approach' has emerged to sex assignment surgery (Diamond and Beh 2008, 4). Nevertheless, 'despite the absence of any evidence linking cosmetic genital surgery with psychological well-being and medical benefit, these surgeries are still being performed' (Greenberg 2012, 21).

Shockingly, at least two studies have been published, the second a scant five years ago, announcing without a trace of ethical justification or apology studies done on infants to test clitoral sensitivity after intersex surgery (Gearhart, Burnett, and Owen 1995; Yang, Felsen, and Poppas 2007).

The FGC-MGC dichotomy in perspective

As we have seen, many of those who deplore operations on women as FGC have no objection to similar surgery on boys. In the traditional African societies that practice these forms of initiations, however, FGC has cultural significance similar to the meanings ascribed to MGC of boys (Beidelman 1997; Setel 1999, 27–50).

Activists opposed to FGC and/or to MGC can greatly enhance their effectiveness by collaborating together. Refusal to confront male circumcision actually makes the task of eradicating female circumcision more difficult. As we have seen, the same arguments used to buttress modification of male genitals in one part of the world support female genital modification in another part. Sami Aldeeb Abu-Sahlieh writes:

> Female circumcision will never stop as long as male circumcision is going on. How do you expect to convince an African father to leave his daughter uncircumcised as long as you let him do it to his son? (Abu-Sahlieh 1994, 612)

Supporters of female circumcision in cultures that still practice it are quick to identify the double standard in the attitude of Western agencies that seek to eradicate female circumcision while tolerating, or even promoting, male circumcision. They point out that 'American parents circumcise their newborns so that the sons will look like the fathers… What, they ask, gives Americans the right to apply a different standard to African women?' (Gollaher 2000, 200)

The AAP opposes all forms of female circumcision as examples of genital mutilation that members are advised they should refuse to perform and should actively discourage (American Academy of Pediatrics Committee on Bioethics 1998). A brief egregious foray that attempted to condone clitoral 'pricks' (American Academy of Pediatrics Committee on Bioethics 2010, 1092) was hastily reversed (Wyckoff 2010), highlighting the disparity. This position, short-lived though it was, sharply contrasts with the AAP's willingness to countenance the equivalent procedure on boys despite an admitted lack of medical justification, which one might reasonably conclude would forbid a medical organization from permitting the practice (American Academy of Pediatrics 1999). A new statement is reportedly imminent. One incisive authorial pair noted the instability of the double standard:

> Feminists' insistence on the legal prohibition of symbolic genital nicks that remove no tissue may be more easily sustainable if male operations 'involving much more removal of tissue and no consent' are no longer permitted to proceed without protest. (Hernlund and Shell-Duncan 2007, 23–24)

Along similar lines, but bringing in CFGC as another point of comparison with MGC and FGC, and concluding that the three practices are treated inconsistently, Johnsdotter adds that a clitoral prick:

> is far less invasive than what is done to male infants at Swedish hospitals during male circumcision and what is permitted on young women who go through genital plastic surgery. In a strictly medical sense, then there is no reasonable motive to forbid pricking of girls' genitalia while permitting male circumcision, genital plastic surgery, and genital piercing for aesthetic or erotic reasons. (Johnsdotter 2007, 126)

Despite the legal tolerance of MGC, no medical association that has issued a policy on MGC has found sufficient 'potential benefits' to justify the procedure. The British Medical Association (2006) points out that there is rarely any clinical need for circumcision, and that 'parental preference alone is not sufficient justification for performing a surgical procedure on a child'. Swedish (Guiborg 2012) and Dutch (van Dijk, Wigersma, and de Jong 2011) medical associations have recently issued calls for the cessation of the practice.

Given all the harms and risks, it can be hard to understand these practices' persistence, unless one appreciates the incredible transformational power that has been culturally attributed to genital cutting. One nineteenth-century physician's medical journal article stated in all seriousness that, 'Fully three-fourths of all male babies have abnormal prepuces' (Brown 1896–97, 300). While we might smile at the particular form this fantastic claim took, such a redefinition of normality is inherent in the process of genital cutting, and, indeed, is often one of its main goals. Genital cutting promises to turn a boy into a man, a girl into a woman, a person of indeterminate sex into an unequivocal girl (or, less often, an unequivocal boy), or even a nonvirgin back into a virgin. Regarding the final possibility, the Sudanese have an apparently unique twist on things in that virginity is literally recreatable through genital cutting:

> [I]n Sudan, virgins are made, not born. The concept of virginity is an anomaly to the Western world.... Virginity in Sudan can be thought of as a social category, in the sense that the physiological manifestation can be socially controlled. Pharaonic circumcision [infibulation] actually transforms a girl or woman (whether or not she is a virgin by the Western definition) into a Sudanese virgin. (Hayes 1975, 622)

Lightfoot-Klein notes, 'Women have themselves resutured to pinhole size in order to be "like virgins once more"' (Lightfoot Klein 1989, 100). This surgery, as is common with all forms of genital cutting, is done for society's benefit, not for the good of the patient herself:

> *Q:* So no one is really concerned over the physical or psychological trauma to which the child is subjected.
> A: 'No, they are not worried about that at all. They do not even think about that. They think only of the virginity, not the child itself'. (Lightfoot-Klein 1989, 158)

Katrina Roen writes about intersex surgery using words that allude to fear of alternative sexualities while also applying to other forms of genital cutting:

> The child's scars and lost genital tissue are the physical manifestation of the adults' fear of atypicality. Here, the adults are imagining a particular kind of embodied subject and surgically molding the child's body in the hope that the child will become that subject that the adults imagine. (Roen 2009, 22)

CFGC as an enforcer of social norms among consenting adults

Intersex surgery, like MGC and FGC, is primarily done for the benefit of the parents. One relatively recent study indicated, somewhat surprisingly, that parents would support genital surgery on their intersex infants 'even at the risk of reducing genital sensitivity'. (Dayner, Lee, and Houk 2004, 1762). Raising a child with a gender-atypical anatomy is still usually seen as untenable in North America. Surgery locates the problem in the child's genitals, not in social conceptualizations of what counts as sex (Karkazis 2008, 137). Intersex surgeries were undertaken to 'treat' parental and social anxiety about gender ambiguity, rather than to restore 'health' to their child (Murray 2009, 274). Nancy Ehrenreich and Mark Barr observe, 'Despite their good intentions, medical practitioners performing intersex surgeries, like their counterparts who perform female circumcisions, do not provide medically necessary treatment but rather enforce (perhaps unwittingly) a system of culturally specific gender norms'. The child with 'ambiguous' genitalia brings us face to face with the failure of our attempted alignment of sex and gender and our opposition of male and female (Ehrenreich and Barr 2005, 104–105).

A similar analysis could be applied to CFGC, which like other forms of genital cutting carries risks of complications (see, e.g., SteadyHealth 2011) and is performed without clear pathology and without an evidence base supporting its performance (Braun and Tiefer 2009). CFGC procedures include labia minora reduction, labia majora remodeling, pubic liposuction and lifts, and clitoral reduction, some of which resemble quite closely – in results, if not in the context of the surgeries – genital cutting procedures done 'traditionally' in African societies. Often the procedures are performed in a quest by the woman undergoing the knife to sculpt her body to match an 'ideal' set forth in pornography or other sources of normative sexuality (Crouch et al. 2011, 1508). One of the leading practitioners, David Matlock, M.D., in a chapter of his book titled *Centerfold Material*, relates, 'Many women arrive at my office with copies of *Playboy* and *Penthouse* in hand. They point to the models and tell me that they want their vaginas to look like those' (Matlock 2004, 64).

In a fascinating twist on the myths regarding gender dimorphism often driving FGC and MGC, labioplasty 'identifies as pathological a body that blurs the boundaries between distinctly "female" or distinctly "male" – "too long" labia render the vulva open to a male reading' (Braun and Tiefer 2009). One subject feels her inner labial lips are so long that '[i]t looked like I had a small penis dangling down' while another 'was so worried I thought I might not actually be fully female' (Braun and Tiefer 2009).

Observers have decried the evident manipulation 'of the media and public opinion to create markets for a *medicalised* view of sexual problems' (Braun and Tiefer 2009). The medicalization of cosmetic FGC is facilitated through a vaguely defined condition created called 'hypertrophy of the labia minora' (Radman 1976), in close analogy with how false diagnoses of 'phimosis' and 'redundant foreskin' are used to justify neonatal male circumcision, despite the fact that the foreskin does not separate from the glans till the child is older and the foreskin naturally folds over itself. As with male circumcision, an American professional body has issued a somewhat ambivalent statement, on the one hand, admitting that the procedures 'are not medically indicated', while, on the other hand, not coming out and squarely recommending against them (American College of Obstetricians and Gynecologists 2007).

Paradoxically, the language and images describing such procedures is often an alternately sexualized and puritanical language, employing images of women using surgery to return to an ostensibly purer, freer, more natural form for their bodies. For example, one of the leading advertisers nationwide in the United States for labioplasty, Tri Valley Plastic Surgery in California, prominently features on its website stunningly suggestive, glossy photographs of beautiful women (Tri Valley Plastic Surgery 2012). Another website typically mixes the sexual with the ending promise of a return to a 'presexual' state:

> Sometimes how a woman 'perceives' how she looks in the vaginal region can mean devastating effects on her life. It can threaten her self-esteem, reduce her sexual desire and excitement, ruin her love life, or cause vaginal discomfort. That's why many women are now seeking cosmetic vaginal surgery to recreate sexual excitement, restore self-esteem and rejuvenate their love lives. [The surgery] returns the ruptured hymen to a pre-sexual state. (Cosmetic Surgery, P.A. 2012)

Numerous other observers have noted the apparent attempt of labia reduction 'to return the vulva to a pre-pubescent state' (e.g., Braun and Tiefer 2009), or so that one's 'fiancé says that sex with her is like being with a virgin' (Matlock 2004, 48), both echoing the Sudanese view that infibulation can recapture virginity.

A number of observers point to the ironies of such widely varying valuations of related procedures. As if we did not already have enough double standards to deal with, African women perceive the legality of labioplasty as a 'double standard' in light of aggressive campaigns against any genital modifications, however minor, among women of African origin (Hernlund and Shell-Duncan 2007, 19). Ford comments that 'Beyond the geographic location of the surgery performed, there seems little functional difference between what is done by surgeons here and what they condemn elsewhere' (Ford 2001, 485).

Sheldon and Wilkinson conclude, 'there seems to be no relevant difference between all those practices prohibited together under the label of female genital mutilation and all those broadly tolerated as cosmetic surgery' (Sheldon and Wilkinson 1998, 274). They find that FGC and CFGC are not necessarily fundamentally different but rather both practices appear to be situated on a continuum of body modification practices.

Medical ethics, law, and human rights: Can we back into protecting children?

Medical ethics, law, and human rights may offer a solution to the quest for unified genital autonomy, even if inadvertently so. Among the protections conferred by these three domains are safeguards against genital mutilations that are not medically justified.

Ethical concerns support genital autonomy. Denniston has shown that circumcision violates all nine ethical principles of the American Medical Association (Denniston 1996).[2] As Bell comments, from an ethical perspective, FGC and MGC look very similar, as 'each operation involves an unnecessary bodily violation that entails the removal of healthy tissue without the informed consent of the person involved' (Bell 2005, 130). Even in the case of CFGC, which is of course performed on consenting adults, ethical issues may arise (Kelly and Foster 2012).

Regardless of whether FGC, MGC, or IGC is performed, the needs of the genitally modified infant are not addressed by the procedures. Rather, genital cutting treats the child as a means to society's ends rather than an end in himself or herself, violating Kantian ethics.

The instabilities between the different practices are clear. FGC is strongly disfavored worldwide with numerous national laws prohibiting the practice. IGC is falling into disfavor but is still legally and medically tolerated, with some limitations. Sweden and South Africa have regulated MGC, though these countries' laws have not substantially curtailed neonatal circumcision. Recently, a German court drew international attention for its decision that infant circumcision – either performed on a religious basis or otherwise – constitutes an assault that violated the child's rights. In response, a resolution was passed by one house of the German legislature. Otherwise, the practice is legal worldwide. The law in the United Kingdom, the United States, and Australia forbids CFGC (see, e.g., Crouch et al. 2011, 1509–1510; see, e.g., Berer 2010, 107, 108), yet the law is never applied to them (see, e.g., Kelly and Foster 2012, 391). Johnsdotter and Essen ask:

> How can it be that extensive genital modifications, including reduction of labial and clitoral tissue, are considered acceptable and perfectly legal in many European countries, while those same societies have legislation making female genital cutting illegal, and the World Health Organization bans even the 'pricking' of the female genitals? (Johnsdotter and Essen 2010, 29)

With regard to both IGC and MGC, the legal world is starting to catch up with activists and changing societal perceptions. In 1999, the Constitutional Court of Colombia significantly restricted parents' and doctors' abilities to perform genital cutting on intersexed children, forcing the child's best interests to be prioritized over parental fears and social concerns. In *Boldt v. Boldt*, the Oregon custody case filed in 2004, which quickly became the most famous MGC-related legal case ever, a recently converted Jewish father had been seeking the circumcision of his son Misha against the wishes of the boy's mother. The Oregon Supreme Court returned the case to the trial court for further proceedings including a determination of the boy's wishes in the matter. At the remand hearing, held five years later in April 2009, the then 14-year-old boy testified privately to the judge that he did not want to be circumcised, testimony that the judge accepted on the record.

Numerous authors have critiqued the gender-based double standard in legal and human rights responses to MGC and FGC (see, e.g., DeLaet 2009, 423). Hellsten has argued:

> male genital mutilation should not be considered in isolation from… female genital mutilation. From a human rights perspective, both male and female genital mutilation, *particularly* when performed on infants or defenceless small children… can be clearly condemned as a violation of children's rights. (Hellsten 2004, 248–249)

And the whole reason intersex exists as a category is because these bodies violate *cultural* rules about gender.

Although MGC is currently illegal under existing laws and human rights treaties, Western-biased cultural blindness – the flip side of cultural relativism – has prevented widespread official acknowledgment of this (Smith 1998). Cultural relativism is a nominally egalitarian doctrine, like equal protection and genital autonomy, calling on us to treat familiar and unfamiliar cultures with equal consideration and acceptance, yet somehow our impulses lead us to preferentially apply it to certain groups and not so rigidly to others (Ehrenreich and Barr 2005).

El Guindi notes that the feminist 'agenda is narrowly focused on women in Africa and the Middle East, who can be presented as inferior, less advanced, or more oppressed than Western women' and who ostensibly 'must be saved by Western missionaries and feminists' (El Guindi 2006, 42). Claire Robertson deftly observes that all too often Westerns find themselves operating from a 'smug consensus that considers the United States to be an enlightened place that has long abandoned "terrible, cruel" practices, unlike [African] countries' (Robertson 2002, 79).

As Diana Tietjens Meyers sums up matters, 'The misconception that most incenses non-Western women is the "othering" of the very idea of culture – that is, the supposition that culture itself is a non-Western phenomenon and that Westerners are not themselves enculturated' (Meyers 2000, 474). Along similar lines, Claire Robertson decries the:

> American assumption of a superior U.S. civilization and African barbarity. It is also the pervasiveness of these assumptions that explains a set of U.S. laws that criminalizes genital operations done by Africans or for Africans but not those done by North Americans, even if the results are the same or similar. (Robertson 2002, 77)

Ehrenreich makes a similar point regarding IGC. 'The Western medical science upon which the "need" for such [intersex] surgeries is based is not objective, neutral, or universally true but rather reflects patriarchal and heteronormative cultural influences' (Ehrenreich and Barr 2005, 77).

Two commentators have argued that given the American law against FGC, MGC must also be illegal under the US constitutional principle of equal protection (Povenmire 1998; Bond 1999).

Kirsten Bell contends that the international scrutiny of FGC 'must be accompanied by a similar willingness to scrutinize male circumcision and recognition that perceptions of one are fundamentally implicated in understandings of the other'. (Bell 2005, 140). A similar argument is put forth by R. Charli Carpenter, who criticizes the double standard inherent in the United Nations' approach to 'harmful traditional practices', which focuses exclusively on women and girls and ignores 'the most obvious one of all – the genital mutilation of infant boys, euphemistically known as... circumcision' (Carpenter 2004, 309). Jacqueline Smith (1998) asserts that the relative degrees of harm arising from FGC and MGC are irrelevant, and that circumcision of male minors is as much a human rights violation as any form of FGC. 'By condemning one practice and not the other', she writes, 'another basic human right, namely the right to freedom from discrimination, is at stake. Regardless of whether a child is a boy or a girl, neither should be subject to a harmful traditional practice' (Smith 1998, 498).

While the United Nations has already endorsed in official documents the principle that MGC qualifies as a human rights violation under certain circumstances (United Nations 1994a, 1994b), it is only in the current millennium that male circumcision has been raised at the United Nations as a general human rights issue (Svoboda 2002), and to date no serious discussion of the topic has occurred, let alone any action (Svoboda 2004).

As with the inadvertent use of the Voting Rights Act to support women's suffrage, at first equal protection of males from MGC may arise as an accidental yet necessary result of our structure of human rights and legal doctrines. In short, we may back into conferring legal and human rights protections on males, but the rights will apply nevertheless.

Conclusion

We must remember, as Dreger reminds us (Dreger 1999, 18), that *every* gender assignment is necessarily preliminary, whether the child being assigned a gender is intersexed or nonintersexed. We need more enlightened doctors and citizens who say, as one did, 'If the [genetically XY] child grows up, and she's happy being a girl, we can do the [vaginal] surgery then. The difference is she is a part of the decision' (Karkazis 2008, 161). Humility helps, and also, as Vicki Kirby trenchantly wrote a full quarter-century ago, instead of the self-congratulatory and clichéd lamentations about third world clitoridectomy, 'we should dare to glimpse into that awful darkness which "reflects" our own culture's strange obsessions' (Kirby 1987, 52).

Such an objective approach may help us to expunge any potential taint of colonialism or favoritism toward the developed world that may arise from differential interpretations of various incarnations of genital cutting. This framework can facilitate finding commonalities between different forms of genital cutting and the different cultural wounds that can help perpetuate genital cutting practices.

Notes

1. An earlier and subsatantially different version of this article was presented on 1 September 2011 at a conference entitled 'Law, Human Rights, and Non-Therapeutic Interventions on Children' held at the University of Keele, UK.
2. Denniston addressed the then applicable seven AMA principles, but his analysis can be applied to all nine current AMA principles.

References

Abd el Salam, S. 2003. "Genital Mutilations: History and Suggestions for Change." *NORM-UK*. Accessed February 25, 2012 http://www.norm-uk.org/page.html?action=showitem&item=885

Abu-Sahlieh, A. 1994. "To Mutilate in the Name of Jehovah or Allah: Legitimization of Male and Female Circumcision." *Medicine and Law* 13: 575–622.

American Academy of Pediatrics Committee on Bioethics. 1998. "Female Genital Mutilation." *Pediatrics* 102: 153–156.

American Academy of Pediatrics Committee on Bioethics. 2010. "Policy Statement – Ritual Genital Cutting of Female Minors." *Pediatrics* 125: 1088–1093.

American Academy of Pediatrics Committee on Genetics and Section on Endocrinology and Urology. 2000. "Evaluation of the Newborn with Developmental Anomalies of the External Genitalia." *Pediatrics* 106: 138–142.

American Academy of Pediatrics Task Force on Circumcision. 1999. "Circumcision Policy Statement." *Pediatrics* 103: 686–693.

American College of Obstetricians and Gynecologists. 2007. "ACOG Committee Opinion No. 378: Vaginal 'Rejuvenation' and Cosmetic Vaginal Procedures." *Obstetrics and Gynecology* 110: 737–738.

Apesos, J., R. Jackson, J. R. Miklos, and R. D. Moore. 2008. *Vagina Makeover & Rejuvenation*. Cape Town: MWP Media.

Ashwell, S. 1845. *A Practical Treatise on the Diseases Peculiar to Women*. Philadelphia, PA: Lea and Blanchard.

Beidelman, T. O. 1997. *The Cool Knife: Imagery of Gender, Sexuality and Moral Education in Kaguru Initiation Ritual*. Washington, DC: Smithsonian Institution Press.

Bell, K. 2005. "Genital Cutting and Western Discourses on Sexuality." *Medical Anthropology Quarterly* 19: 125–148.

Berer, M. 2010. "Labia Reduction for Nontherapeutic Reasons vs. Female Genital Mutilation: Contradictions in Law and Practice in Britain." *Reproductive Health Matters* 18: 106–110.

Boddy, J. 1982. "Womb as Oasis: The Symbolic Content of Pharaonic Circumcision in Rural Northern Sudan." *American Ethnologist* 9: 682–98.

Boddy, J. 2007. "Gender Crusades: The Female Circumcision Controversy in Cultural Perspective." In *Transcultural Bodies: Female Genital Cutting in Global Context*, edited by Y. Hernlund and B. Shell-Duncan, 46–66. New Brunswick, NJ: Rutgers University Press.

Bond, S. L. 1999. "State Laws Criminalizing Female Circumcision: A Violation of the Equal Protection Clause of the Fourteenth Amendment." *John Marshall Law Review* 32: 353–380.

Brain, R. 1979. *The Decorated Body*. New York: Harper & Row.

Braun, V., and Tiefer, L. 2009. "The 'Designer Vagina' and the Pathologisation of Female Genital Diversity: Interventions for Change." *Radical Psychology* 8. Accessed February 28, 2012. www.radicalpsychology.org/vol8-1/brauntiefer.html

British Medical Association. 2006. "The Law and Ethics of Male Circumcision: Guidance for Doctors." *British Medical Association.* Accessed February 22, 2012. www.bma.org.uk/ap.nsf/Content/malecircumcision2006

Brown, S. G. A. 1896–97. "The Mosaic Rite of Circumcision: A Plea for Its Performance during Childhood." *Journal of Orificial Surgery* 5: 299–304.

Canty, T. G. 1977. "The Child with Ambiguous Genitalia: A Neonatal Surgical Emergency." *Annals of Surgery* 186: 272–281.

Carpenter, R. C. 2004. "A Response to Bronwyn Winter, Denise Thompson and Sheila Jeffreys." *International Feminist Journal of Politics* 6: 308–313.

Cosmetic Surgery, P. A. 2012. "Cosmetic Surgery of the Female Genitalia." *Cosmetic Surgery.* Accessed February 25, 2012. www.cosmeticsurgery2.com/cs1-female.htm

Crouch, N. S., R. Deans, L. Michala, L. M. Liao, and S. M. Creighton. 2011. "Clinical Characteristics of Well Women Seeking Labial Reduction Surgery: A Prospective Study." *International Journal of Obstetrics and Gynaecology* 118: 1507–1510.

Darby, R. 2005. *A Surgical Temptation: The Demonization of the Foreskin and the Rise of Circumcision in Britain*. Chicago, IL: University of Chicago Press.

Dayner, J. E., P. A. Lee, and C. P. Houk. 2004. "Medical Treatment of Intersex: Parental Perspective." *Journal of Urology* 172: 1762–1765.

DeLaet, D. L. 2009. "Framing Male Circumcision as a Human Rights Issue? Contributions to the Debate over the Universality of Human Rights." *Journal of Human Rights* 8: 405–426.

Denniston, G. 1996. "Circumcision and the Code of Ethics." *Humane Health Care International* 12: 78–80.

Dewhurst, C. J., and R. R. Gordon. 1969. *The Intersexual Disorders*. London: Bailliere Tindall & Cassell.

Diamond, M. 1999. "Pediatric Management of Ambiguous and Traumatized Genitalia." *Journal of Urology* 162: 1021–1028.

Diamond, M., and H. G. Beh. 2008. "Changes in the Management of Children with Intersex Conditions." *Nature Clinical Practice Endocrinology & Metabolism* 4: 4–5.

Diamond, M., and H. K. Sigmundson. 1997. "Management of Intersexuality: Guidelines for Dealing with Persons with Ambiguous Genitalia." *Archives of Pediatric and Adolescent Medicine* 151: 1046–1050.

Donahoe, P. K., J. D. Crawford, and W. H. Hendren. 1977. "Management of Neonates and Children with Male Pseudohermaphroditism." *Journal of Pediatric Surgery* 12: 1045–1057.

Dreger, Alice. 1999. *Intersex in the Age of Ethics*. Frederick, MD: University Publishing Group.

Ehrenreich, N., and M. Barr. 2005 "Intersex Surgery, Female Genital Cutting, and the Selective Condemnation of 'Cultural Practices.'" *Harvard Civil Liberties – Civil Rights Law Review* 40: 71–140.

El Guindi, F. 2006. "Had *This* Been Your Face, Would You Leave It As Is? – Female Circumcision Among the Nubians of Egypt." In *Female Circumcision: Multicultural Perspectives*, edited by R. M. Abusharaf. Philadelphia: University of Pennsylvania Press.

Eskridge, B. C. 1918. "Why Not Circumcise the Girl as well as the Boy?" *Texas State Journal of Medicine* 14: 17–19.

Farkas, A., B. Chertin, and I. Hadas-Halpren. 2001. "1-stage Feminizing Genitoplasty: 8 Years of Experience with 49 Cases." *Journal of Urology* 165: 2341–2346.

Ford, K-K. 2001. '"First, Do No Harm' – The Fiction of Legal Parental Consent to Genital-Normalizing Surgery on Intersexed Infants." *Yale Law and Policy Review* 19: 469–488.

Garenne, M. 2006. "Male Circumcision and HIV Control in Africa." *PLoS Medicine* 1: 143–144.

Glick, L. B. 2005. *Marked In Your Flesh: Circumcision from Ancient Judea to Modern America*. Oxford: Oxford University Press.

Gollaher, D. L. 2000. *Circumcision: The World's Most Controversial Surgery*. New York: Basic Books.

Greenberg, J. A. 2012. *Intersexuality and the Law: Why Sex Matters*. New York: New York University Press.

Gross, R. E., and I. A. Meeker, Jr. 1955. "Abnormalities of Sexual Development: Observations from 75 Cases." *Pediatrics* 16: 303–324.

Guibourg, C. 2012. "Swedish Docs in Circumcision Protest." *The Local*, 19 February 2012. Accessed February 25, 2012. http://m.thelocal.se/39200/20120219/

Gunning, I. 1999. "Women and Traditional Practices: Female Genital Surgery." In *Women and International Human Rights Law*, Vol. 1, edited by K. D. Askin and D. M. Koenig, 651–682, New York: Transnational Publishers.

Hayes, R. O. 1975. "Female Genital Mutilation, Fertility Control, Women's Roles, and the Patrilineage in Modern Sudan: A Functional Analysis." *American Ethnologist* 2: 617–633.

Hegarty, P. 2000. "Intersex Activism, Feminism and Psychology: Opening a Dialogue on Theory, Research and Clinical Practice." *Feminism & Psychology* 10: 117–132.

Hellsten, S. 2004. "Rationalising Circumcision: From Tradition to Fashion, from Public Health to Individual Freedom." *Journal of Medical Ethics* 30: 248–253.

Hernlund, Y., and B. Shell-Duncan. 2007. "Transcultural Positions: Negotiating Rights and Culture." In *Transcultural Bodies: Female Genital Cutting in Global Context*, edited by Y. Hernlund and B. Shell-Duncan, 1–45. New Brunswick, NJ: Rutgers University Press.

Isenberg, S., and L. M. Elting.1976. "A Guide to Sexual Surgery." *Cosmopolitan* 181: 104–164.

Jirovsky, E. 2010. "Views of Women and Men in Bobo-Dioulasso, Burkina Faso, on Three Forms of Female Genital Modification." *Reproductive Health Matters* 18: 84–93.

Johnsdotter, S. 2007. "Persistence of Tradition or Reassessment of Cultural Practices in Exile?: Discourses on Female Circumcision Among and About Swedish Somalis." In *Transcultural Bodies: Female Genital Cutting in Global Context*, edited by Y. Hernlund and B. Shell-Duncan, 107–135. New Brunswick, NJ: Rutgers University Press.

Johnsdotter, S., and B. Essen. 2010. "Gender and Ethnicity: The Politics of Genital Modifications." *Reproductive Health Matters* 18: 29–37.

Karkazis, K. 2008. *Fixing Sex: Intersex, Medical Authority, and Lived Experience*. Durham, NC: Duke University Press.

Kelly, B., and C. Foster. 2012. "Should Female Genital Cosmetic Surgery and Genital Piercing Be Regarded Ethically and Legally as Female Genital Mutilation?" *International Journal of Obstetrics and Gynaecology* 119: 389–392.

Kirby, V. 1987. "On the Cutting Edge: Feminism and Clitoridectomy." *Australian Feminist Studies* 5: 35–55.

Kistler, S. L. 1910. "Rapid Bloodless Circumcision of Male and Female and Its Technic." *Journal of the American Medical Association* 54: 1782–1783.

Lareau, A. C. 2003. "Who Decides? – Genital-Normalizing Surgery on Intersex Infants." *Georgetown Law Journal* 92: 129–151.

Lightfoot-Klein, H. 1989. *Prisoners of Ritual: An Odyssey into Female Genital Circumcision in Africa*. Binghamton, NY: Harrington Park Press.

Lightfoot-Klein, H. 1997. "Similarities in Attitudes and Misconceptions about Male and Female Sexual Mutilations." In *Sexual Mutilations: A Human Tragedy*, edited by G. Denniston and M. Milos, 131–135. New York: Plenum Press.

Lightfoot-Klein, H., C. Chase, T. Hammond, and R. Goldman. 2000. "Genital Surgery on Children Below the Age of Consent." In *Psychological Perspectives on Human Sexuality*, edited by L. T. Szuchman, and F. Muscarella, 440–479. New York: John Wiley & Sons.

Lobe, T. E., D. L. Woodall, G. E. Richards, A. Cavallo, and W. J. Meyer. 1987. "The Complications of Surgery for Intersex: Changing Patterns Over Two Decades." *Journal of Pediatric Surgery* 22: 651–652.

Lyttelton, E. 1887. *The Causes and Prevention of Immorality in Schools*. London: privately printed.

Matlock, D. 2004. *Sex by Design*. Los Angeles, CA: Demiurgus Publications.

Meyers, D. T. 2000. "Feminism and Women's Autonomy: The Challenge of Female Genital Cutting." *Metaphilosophy* 31: 469–491.

Montagu, A. 1995. "Mutilated Humanity." *Humanist* 55: 12–15.

Moore, H. 2007. "The Failure of Pluralism?." In *Transcultural Bodies: Female Genital Cutting in Global Context*, edited by Y. Hernlund and B. Shell-Duncan, 311–330. New Brunswick, NJ: Rutgers University Press.

Murray, S. 2009. "Within or Beyond the Binary Boundary?" *Australian Feminist Studies* 24: 265–274.

Paige, K. E., and J. M. Paige, 1981. *The Politics of Reproductive Ritual*. Berkeley, CA: University of California Press.

Pollack, M. 2011. "Circumcision: Identity, Gender, and Power." *Attorneys for the Rights of the Child Newsletter* 25. Accessed February 25, 2012. http://www.arclaw.org/newsletter/vol-9/no-1/jewish-perspectives/circumcision-Identity-Gender-and-Power

Povenmire R. 1998. "Do Parents Have the Legal Authority to Consent to the Surgical Amputation of Normal, Healthy Tissue from their Infant Children?" *Journal of Gender Social Policy & Law* 7: 7–123.

Radman, H. M. M. F. 1976. "Hypertrophy of the Labia Minora." *Obstetrics and Gynecology* 48: 78s–80s.

Riner, R. D. 1989. "Circumcision: A Riddle of American Culture." presented at *First International Symposium on Circumcision*, Anaheim, CA, March 1–2. Accessed February 23, 2012. http://www.nocirc.org/symposia/first/riner.html

Robertson, C. C. 2002. "Getting Beyond the Ew! Factor: Rethinking US Approaches to African Female Genital Cutting." In *Genital Cutting and Transnational Sisterhood: Disputing U.S. Polemics*, edited by S. M. James and C. C. Robertson, 54–86. Chicago: University of Illinois Press.

Roen, K. 2009. "Clinical Intervention and Embodied Subjectivity: Atypically Sexed Children and Their Parents." In *Critical Intersex*, edited by M. Holmes, 15–40. London: Ashgate.

Setel, P. W. 1999. *A Plague of Paradoxes: AIDS, Culture and Demography in Northern Tanzania*. Chicago, IL: University of Chicago Press.

Shaalan M. 1982. *Clitoral Envy: A Psychodynamic Construct Instrumental in Female Circumcision*. Alexandria: WHO Regional Office for the Eastern Mediterranean.

Sheldon, S., and S. Wilkinson. 1998. "Female Genital Mutilation and Cosmetic Surgery: Regulating Non-Therapeutic Body Modification." *Bioethics* 12: 263–285.

Shell-Duncan, B., K. Wander, Y. Hernlund, and A. Moreau. 2011. "Dynamics of Change in the Practice of Female Genital Cutting in Senegambia: Testing Predictions of Social Convention Theory." *Social Science & Medicine* 73: 1275–1283.

Shorter, E. 1992. *From Paralysis to Fatigue: A History of Psychosomatic Illness in the Modern Era*. New York: The Free Press.

Shweder, R. A. 2002. "'What About Female Genital Mutilation?' and Why Understanding Culture Matters in the First Place." In *Engaging Cultural Differences*, edited by R. A. Shweder, H. R. Markus, and M. Minow, 209–232. New York: Russell Sage Foundation.

Shweder, R. A. 2009. "Disputing the Myth of the Sexual Dysfunction of Circumcised Women: An Interview with Fuambai S. Ahmadu." *Anthropology Today* 25: 14–17.

Smith, J. 1998. "Male Circumcision and the Rights of the Child." In *To Baehr in Our Minds: Essays in Human Rights from the Heart of the Netherlands*, edited by M. Bulterman, A. Hendricks, and J. Smith, 465–498. Utrecht: Institute of Human Rights.

Somerville, M. 2000. *The Ethical Canary: Science, Society and the Human Spirit*. Toronto, ON: Viking.

Spratling, E. 1895. "Masturbation in the Adult." *Medical Record* 48: 442–443.

SteadyHealth. 2011. "Labiaplasty Nightmare – Reproductive Organs & Vaginal Problems Discussion." *SteadyHealth*. Accessed February 28, 2012. http://www.steadyhealth.com/Labiaplasty_Nightmare_t112049.html

Svoboda, J. S. 2002. "Male Circumcision." *United Nations*. Accessed February 23, 2012. http://www.unhchr.ch/Huridocda/Huridoca.nsf/(Symbol)/E.CN.4.Sub.2.2002.NGO.1.En?Opendocument. United Nations Document No. E/CN.4/Sub.2/2002/1

Svoboda, J. S. 2004. "Educating the United Nations about Male Circumcision." In *Flesh and Blood: Perspectives on the Problem of Circumcision in Contemporary Society*, edited by G. C. Denniston, M. F. Milos, and F. M. Hodges, 89–108. New York: Kluwer Academic/Plenum Publishers.

Svoboda, J. S. 2012. "Tortured Bodies, Tortured Doctrines: Informed Consent as a Legal Fiction Inapplicable to Male Circumcision." In *The Rights of the Child: Ensuring Every Child's Fundamental Right to Body Ownership and Protection from Medical, Cultural, and Religious Infringements*, edited by G. C. Denniston, M. F. Milos, and F. M. Hodges, 1–28. New York: Springer.

Szasz, T. 1996. "Routine Neonatal Circumcision: Symbol of the Birth of the Therapeutic State." *Journal of Medicine and Philosophy* 21: 137–148.

Szuchman, L. T., and Muscarella, F., eds. 2000. *Psychological Perspectives on Human Sexuality*. New York: John Wiley & Sons.

Tri Valley Plastic Surgery. 2012. "Welcome to Tri Valley Plastic Surgery." *Tri Valley Plastic Surgery*. Accessed February 25, 2012. www.trivalleyplasticsurgery.com

United Nations. 1994a. Commission of Experts. "Final report". UN doc. no. S/1994/674.

United Nations. 1994b. *Convention on the Rights of the Child: Initial Reports of States Parties due in 1994: Lesotho*. UN doc. no. CRC/C/11/Add.20.

van der Kwaak, A. 1992. "Female Circumcision and Gender Identity: A Questionable Alliance?" *Social Science and Medicine* 35: 777–787.

Van Dijk, G., L. Wigersma, and T. de Jong. 2011. "Royal Dutch Medical Association Launches Anti-Circumcision Campaign." *Intact News*. Accessed February 25, 2012. http://intactnews.org/node/128/1316026077/royal-dutch-medical-association-launches-anti-circumcision-campaign

Wollman, L. 1973. "Female Circumcision." *Journal of the American Society of Psychosomatic and Dental Medicine* 20: 3–4, 130–131.

World Health Organization. 2006. *Manual for Male Circumcision Under Local Anaesthesia* (version 2.2). Geneva: World Health Organization.

Wyckoff, S. A. 2010. "Culture Shock: AAP Opposes Ritual Genital Cutting of Female Minors, Recommends Cultural Sensitivity." *AAP News* 31: 31.

Discourses on sexual pleasure after genital modifications: the fallacy of genital determinism (a response to J. Steven Svoboda)

Sara Johnsdotter

Faculty of Health and Society, Malmö University, Sweden

This is a reply to:

Svoboda, J. Steven 2013. "Promoting genital autonomy by exploring commonalities between male, female, intersex, and cosmetic female genital cutting." *Global Discourse.* 3 (2): 237–255. http://dx.doi.org/10.1080/23269995.2013.804757

Introduction

In his compelling paper, 'Promoting Genital Autonomy by Exploring Commonalities Between Male, Female, Intersex, and Cosmetic Female Genital Cutting', J. Steven Svoboda (2013) explores commonalities between various forms of genital modifications and shows how the West responds inconsistently from a human rights perspective, failing to grant every child the same right to a genital integrity. Svoboda arrives at the conclusion that circumcision of male infants on religious or traditional grounds ought, like female circumcision, to be legally banned. Such a juxtaposition between female and male genital cuttings[1] could also lead to the conclusion that societies ought to make (certain forms of) female genital alterations in girls lawful, as has been put forth by the American anthropologist Richard A. Shweder (2002, 2013). Irrespective of the stance, such analysis of commonalities between different forms of genital modifications – taking gender or ethnic equity as a starting point – is a fruitful approach to uncovering cultural blind spots. This is particularly productive when surgery in intersexed children is included in the analysis, as Svoboda demonstrates.

In his article, Svoboda touches upon sexual effects of genital modifications, and I would like to take the opportunity to elaborate on this question. This is not a critique of Svoboda's views. He is critical of the 'medicalized model of women's sexuality' and in an earlier co-authored paper (Darby and Svoboda 2007) it is emphasized that 'sexual pleasure is a highly subjective response, and it is difficult to arrive at quantitative data on this issue' (310). Yet I would like to discuss these issues in some more detail, since it seems to be in this field – genital modifications and sexual pleasure – that some of the future disputes will unfold.

My argument is that there are no scientific truths about sexual pleasure after genital modifications – only cultural constructions disguised as a medical science. Also, I intend to demonstrate with a few examples how these medical statements about effects on sexual pleasure are associated with politics. I conclude by arguing that current discussions on the sexual effects of genital modifications are reductionist due to widespread assumptions about the role of genitalia in sexuality – what might be characterized as 'genital determinism'.

Discourses on sexual effects of genital modifications

Effects on ability to feel sexual pleasure after genital modifications have been discussed in all the contexts presented by Svoboda: in relation to circumcision of boys and girls, surgery of intersexed children and cosmetic genital surgery in adult women.

Cosmetic genital surgery in women includes, for example, removal or reduction of the inner labia, vaginal tightening, liposuction of the *mons veneris* (fatty tissue over the pubic bone – these are performed in order to create a sense of proportion when the inner labia have been shortened), clitoral reduction and clitoral repositioning (see e.g. Braun 2005; Renganathan, Cartwright, and Cardozo 2009; Kelly and Foster 2012). These modifications are often framed in positive terms, as a means of improving the sexual pleasure. Australian gender scholar Virginia Braun concludes after a media analysis and interviews with surgeons:

> While *impeded* sexual possibilities and pleasures were central in media and surgeon accounts of why women might choose to have [female genital cosmetic surgery], *increased* sexual pleasure as an outcome of surgery was the main area in which sexual pleasure was discussed. (Braun 2005, 412; emphasis in original)

A case recently debated concerns a 33-year-old British woman who went through clitoridectomy for aesthetic reasons, with the physicians involved in the case testifying that her sexual life, including her scores for sexual satisfaction, was enhanced after the surgery; 'Her libido and sexual relationship with her husband had significantly improved' (Veale and Daniels 2012, 728; the case debated in later issues of the journal, *Archives of Sexual Behavior*).

In contrast, medical statements – made by both activists opposing 'female genital mutilation' and medical scholars – about negative effects on sexual pleasure after female circumcision are a commonplace. A statement by obstetricians:

> The operation destroys much or all of the vulvar nerve endings, and seems likely to delay or prevent arousal and subsequent orgasm. [...] Even the mildest form of circumcision removes the part of a woman's body containing nerves of vital importance to sexual pleasure and fulfillment. (Elchalal et al. 1997, 106)

This is in line with the public discourse on 'female genital mutilation' where there is a widespread assumption that female circumcision is detrimental to the ability to enjoy sex (noted by e.g. Darby and Svoboda 2007; Dustin 2010; Johnsdotter and Essén 2010; Wade 2012). In reality, no research supports such assumptions, and studies show that differences in sexual function between cut and uncut women are small or non-existent (for overviews, see e.g. Obermeyer 2005; Berg and Denison 2012).

Yet another example of medical statements, which undermines what we can expect after having been informed in the discourse on 'female genital mutilation' about alleged destroyed ability to feel sexual pleasure, concerns descriptions of sexual function after surgery on intersexed children. In earlier texts on clitoriplasty in intersexed children, amputation and clitoridectomy are discussed rather prosaically, as in this case by a couple of American urologists:

> It is evident from reviewing the literature and from our experience that the size of the hypertrophied clitoris is the major factor in deciding whether to amputate or relocate it. If a large clitoris is recessed or relocated, it is possible for the patient to present with a turgid and painful mass during sexual excitation in later life. Hence, total clitoridectomy would be the procedure of choice in this situation. (Ansell and Rajfer 1981, 683)

In their view, 'any procedure that is utilized in the surgical reconstruction of the patient with ambiguous genitalia should create normal-appearing and functional external genitalia' (1981, 681). In recent years, surgeons are no longer so confident. For example, the British surgeon C.R.J. Woodhouse observes in a medical article that:

> All the evidence shows the great importance of the clitoris in achieving orgasm. After vaginal reconstruction about half of women will be able to achieve orgasm, but almost always with clitoral stimulation. With a natural vagina treated by regular dilatation all women can achieve orgasm, but *if the clitoris has been amputated only 71% can do so*. (Woodhouse 2004, 58, my emphasis)

Obviously, after decades of clitoral amputation in intersexed children in the West (see e.g. Karkazis 2008), the initial expectation seems to be that amputation of the clitoris did not affect ability to orgasm. It appears that attitudes toward clitoral surgery in children diagnosed with DSD (*Disorders of Sex Development*) are undergoing drastic changes – Woodhouse continues the paragraph above by saying, 'This emphasizes the need to preserve the clitoris' (2004, 58; see also e.g. Maharaj et al. 2005; Hughes et al. 2006; discussing later recommendations to be careful with clitoral tissue in intersex surgery).[2] But the quote above shows the drastically different starting points when it comes to depicting the role of the clitoris in, on the one hand, a medical discourse on (western) children that go through clitoral modifications within the scope of biomedicine and, on the other hand, those who go through it in the context of African cultural traditions.[3]

There seems to be no objective or value-free mode of describing the sexual function of the various parts of female genitalia. Similar conflicting views present themselves when it comes to the male genitalia after modification. While the common view is that the foreskin of the penis is 'just a flap of skin' (critically quoted by ethicist Evans 2011, 442) and that its removal has no negative effects on sexual function (e.g. Morris, Waskett, and Gray 2012; Krieger et al. 2008), other researchers advocate the opposite view and describe the foreskin as the most sensitive part of the penis (Darby and Svoboda 2007; Johnson 2010; Bronselaer et al. 2013). Darby and Svoboda argue that the widespread comparison of the penile glans to the clitoral glans (leading to conclusions such as 'the mildest form, clitoridectomy, is anatomically equivalent to amputation of the penis', Toubia 1994, 712) is erroneous and that the correct analogy in physiological terms would be *foreskin-clitoris* (Darby and Svoboda 2007, 309–310).

Sexual pleasure after genital modifications – a vexed issue in academia

Two academic battles concerning sexual pleasure are currently taking place in the research fields of male and female circumcisions. The background is described by Svoboda (2013) in his article: there is a general acceptance of male circumcision in western contexts, while all forms of female circumcision are banned and frequently labelled barbarian. As aptly observed by Darby and Svoboda, 'we now find the WHO conducting two quite separate research projects: one to find evidence for the harm of [female circumcision], another to find evidence for the benefits of [male circumcision]' (2007, 312).

Regarding female circumcision and sexual pleasure, there has for a long time been a void of reliable studies to support widespread assumptions about lost ability to enjoy sex as a result of genital modification. In a review of available studies in 2005, Carla Makhlouf Obermeyer concluded that 'Concerning sexuality, most of the existing studies suffer from conceptual and methodological shortcomings, and the available evidence does not support the hypotheses that circumcision destroys sexual function or precludes enjoyment of sexual relations' (2005, 443). Since this publication in 2005, no meta-analysis was conducted until the Norwegian quantitative public health researcher Berg and colleagues (2010) published their report in 2010.

Unfortunately, out of the fifteen studies in their survey, only two were deemed to be of high quality. Ten of the fifteen studies were deemed by Berg et al. themselves to be of 'low quality', a fact that did not prevent them from extrapolating results from them. The authors admit to the limitations associated with an analysis of studies of such low quality, but insist in their conclusions about reduced sexual satisfaction and desire (2010, 6).[4] A correlation worth noting in the literature on the health effects of female genital cutting is that the higher the quality of the study, the more likely it is that no statistically significant difference will be found between circumcised and uncircumcised women (e.g. Obermeyer 2005).

The political impetus to exaggerate negative effects on sexuality after female circumcision was recently criticized by a group of academicians in a policy advisory published by the *Hastings Centre Report*, 'Seven Things to Know About Female Genital Surgeries in Africa' (The Public Policy Advisory Network on Female Genital Surgeries in Africa, 2012; I was one of fifteen co-signatories). Among other things, we stated that 'a high percentage of women who have had genital surgery have rich sexual lives, including desire, arousal, orgasm and satisfaction, and their frequency of sexual activity is not reduced' (22), which is in accordance not only with studies deemed to be of good quality but also, actually, with the data in the Berg et al. survey. In a commentary, the American gynaecologist Nawal Nour objected to this statement, claiming that 'high percentage' ought to have been changed to 'some.' She found the summary of sexual effects in the advisory 'implausible' and implied it was exaggerated (Nour 2012, 31). Dr. Nour supported her objection by referring to the meta-analysis conducted by Berg and colleagues.

Indeed, the Berg et al. survey seems to fill this void experienced by activists searching for arguments to justify a condemnation of 'female genital mutilation'. The survey, disregarding the risks involved in 'garbage in, garbage out' calculations, ends in conclusions that *sound* reliable – and alarming. The WHO, key actor in this field, embraces this meta-analysis and reproduces the results and conclusions without any reservations as to the quality of the studies included:

> Sexual problems are also more common among women who have undergone FGM. They are 1.5 times more likely to experience pain during sexual intercourse, have significantly less sexual satisfaction and are twice as likely to report a lack of sexual desire. (reference to Berg et al. 2010; WHO 2012, 3)

In contrast, the given point of departure as to male circumcision is generally that such a modification does not affect men's ability to enjoy sex in any negative way. Using the search string 'circumcision sexuality pleasure' in the WHO publications database,[5] the only hit concerning effects on sexual pleasure after male circumcision is in a manual for performing circumcision, including suggestions on how to raise some issues in education about reproductive health and male circumcision:

> Do any of you have any questions or concerns about male circumcision? I [a hypothetical instructor] know that there are many myths about male circumcision that circulate. For example, some people think that circumcision can cause impotence (failure of erection) or reduce sexual pleasure. Others think that circumcision will cure impotence. Let me assure you that none of these is true. (WHO, UNAIDS, and JHPIEGO 2009, 38)

In 2011 a group of Danish epidemiologists published an article in *International Journal of Epidemiology* based on data from a national health survey in Denmark, showing an association between male circumcision and frequent orgasm difficulties, and also pointing to female partners of circumcised men having an increased risk of not feeling sexually fulfilled (Frisch et al. 2011).[6] In a letter to the editor in a later issue, Morris, Waskett, and Gray (2012) criticised the study and the conclusions drawn. In a response to this critique, Frisch defended their research and seized the opportunity to disclose some intrigue going on behind the scenes: Morris had been one of the reviewers of the submitted manuscript, and during the peer review process he had alarmed his peer group through an email list, encouraging people to send critical letters to the editors of the journal (Frisch 2012). Besides demonstrating a specific academic's ardent commitment and work methods, the conflict possibly reflects how contentious the issue of sexual pleasure in relation to a male circumcision is.[7]

As the American anthropologist Kirsten Bell (2005) has so convincingly argued (her work is also discussed by Svoboda), the descriptions of negative or positive effects with regard to sexual pleasure of female and male circumcision have everything to do with how we construct sexuality in the first place. Notions about (too) strong a male libido will result in conclusions that the male circumcision and reduced sensitivity are advantageous (examples given by Frisch 2011, 1377), while there will be assumptions that '[a] woman's sexual instincts, being fundamentally more delicate, will be crippled by any form of genital surgery' (Bell 2005, 136). Investigating the constructions of sexuality in other cultural contexts and relating them to notions of effects on sexuality after circumcision in those places may be illuminating. For example, anthropologist Maria Malmström (2009) has discussed, after fieldwork in Cairo, how the male libido is seen as weaker than its female counterpart. Female circumcision is not expected to erase the possibility to feel sexual pleasure or orgasm (and many women talk about sexual pleasure), but is regarded as a means to equalize that difference and create a balance (Malmström 2009).

Culture and sexual pleasure: the fallacy of genital determinism

After reviewing the literature on sexual pleasure after male and female circumcisions, is it possible to draw any general conclusions? Such an overview would render a picture more or less along these lines:

Most women who have been circumcised seem to have gratifying sexual lives.[8] *Some women testify that circumcision had negative effects on their sexual well-being,*[9] *and some opt for reconstructive genital surgery.*[10] *Most men who have been circumcised seem to have gratifying sexual lives.*[11] *Some men testify that circumcision had negative effects on their sexual well-being,*[12] *and some opt for reconstructive genital surgery.*[13]

Effects on sexual pleasure have been one of many themes discussed in relation to circumcision practices – it is a given consequence of the fact that genitalia play a central role in sexual activities. To arrive, however, at the conclusion that the state of the genitalia *determines* the quality of sexual activities or experiences is probably a mistake. Yet, it is precisely this fallacy that characterizes many academic contributions to the field.

In discussions about sexuality in relation to circumcision, one often finds a kind of lip service, where it is declared that sexuality is multifaceted: 'We recognize that sexual pleasure and satisfaction are multidimensional, depending, for example, also on affection and the time the partner takes to please the woman. However, the physiological viewpoint…' (Berg and Denison 2012, 50). Few authors discuss, in depth, the implications of a sexual-pleasure research approach that moves beyond the state of the genitalia (among the exceptions are Obermeyer 2005 and Esho et al. 2010).

Sexual scripting theory, introduced by the social scientists John H. Gagnon and William Simon in the 1970s, highlights the social dimensions of lived sexuality (e.g. Gagnon and Simon 1973). This framework, which demonstrates how sexuality is embedded in social and cultural contexts and how people learn how to enact their sexuality in relation to socially and culturally based norms, may be helpful in understanding how radically differently we construct, for example, the male and female sexualities. Two quotes from the literature on sexuality in groups where most of the girls and women are circumcised, Sudan and Kikuyu in Kenya, can serve as illustration of sexual scripting:

> Custom decrees that a Sudanese woman remain totally passive during the sex act. She must act like a 'block of wood' and participate in no way whatsoever. Sudanese men confirm that in nearly all cases she does just that. Sexual pleasure is considered to be entirely a male prerogative, and if it is felt by women, it is felt in secret. Nearly all women interviewed reported that showing sexual interest and pleasure openly is 'extremely shameful.' […] Sexually, the woman must exhibit an unnatural immobility. She is not required to be sexually active, 'like an animal.' Only passive behaviour will enable her to fulfill the demand for modesty imposed on her. If the woman has an orgasm, she tries to not show it, and if she is unable to control her reaction, she denies that it was brought on by sexual ecstasy. (Lightfoot-Klein 1989, 89)
>
> *Ssenga* [father's sister] teaches the girl specific utterances and techniques appropriate during an intercourse. Traditionally, women are taught to not only desire sex but to also lead an active sex life. A woman is expected to reach orgasm several times before the man and respond throughout intercourse with vigorous body movement. A man is evaluated by women according to the length of time coitus is maintained before his orgasm (about thirty minutes is typical). A too-rapid male ejaculation is likely to evoke female anger and comparison with, for example, a 'hen' (*enkoko*) who, of course, has rapid coitus. A second erection soon after orgasm is also expected of men. (Kilbride and Kilbride 1990, in Njambi 2004, 297)

In the Berg et al. meta-analysis, we are told that no significant difference between cut and uncut women has been found 'with respect to whether they initiated sex' (2012, 48). One wonders: is it not more reasonable to believe that variation has more to do with culture-based sexual scripts than with whether or not cutting of the genitals has taken place?

If one keeps this cultural variation in mind, the variables used in existing quantitative studies on sexual effects of female circumcision appear quite absurd. There is a reason to question what kind of information we have at hand when data are collected on 'frequency of intercourse' and comparisons are made between cut and uncut women.[14] Concepts such as 'sexual desire', 'libido', 'sexual satisfaction' and 'sexual problems' are employed with little or no theorizing (see also Obermeyer 2005 for critical discussion). Is it even possible to quantitatively measure 'sexual outcome', and – if it were possible – how could such a concept be operationalized in a way that takes cultural variation into consideration?

Apart from methodological flaws like these, these studies build upon faulty theoretical assumptions about the role of genitalia in sexuality. Possibly, western researchers in this field are captivated by typically western constructions of sexuality, which tend to over-emphasize the role of anatomy and physiology in framing and describing sexual activities. In the words of Australian sociologist Juliet Richters: 'as if having sex were a physiological process like digestion rather than a social interaction like having dinner' (2009, 232; see also Tiefer 2004).

I believe that it is a fallacy to see instantiations of anatomy and physiology as universal entities, as if only embedded in cultural contexts to be swiftly peeled off at investigating sexual pleasure in putatively objective ways (sexual pleasure as ahistorical and beyond culture, or beneath a cultural surface). Social and cultural dimensions are integral to lived sexuality. Findings from the emergent research field of the 'anthropology of sensations' demonstrate how sensations are culturally learned – to grow up in a certain society entails learning to 'read' one's body in specific ways: 'Sensory meaning is never a question of physiology; it is always mediated by culture, in the sense of the ways of life, language, ritual practices, beliefs and aesthetics of a group, community, or society' (Hinton et al. 2008). Sensation schemas will impact how we perceive bodily signals, whether we notice them at all, and what kind of meanings we ascribe to them. This is also true for sexual activities: we need to 'decode' bodily sensations and relate them to culturally and socially created erotic meanings in order to experience sexual pleasure (Cameron and Kulick 2003; Tiefer 2004).

Such complexity is difficult to capture in quantitative studies, as pointed out by Darby and Svoboda (2007: 310). The subjective experience, completely dependent upon cultural and social context, is difficult to measure:

> Arguments about circumcision reveal something of the limitations of evidence-based medicine. They can tell us how many circumcisions are necessary to prevent one case of penile cancer (about 1000), but they cannot engage with the subjective experiences of the sexual body. (Richters 2009, 229)

My point here is that the current academic focus on the role of genitalia in understanding sexual pleasure is a dead end. While genitalia usually are central to sexual activity,[15] and can be seen as a prerequisite for sexual intercourse, it is a misapprehension to see the state of them (cut or uncut) as determinative of the individual's experience of the sexual encounter. Consequently, ongoing debates on enhancing or detrimental effects of circumcision practices often miss the point, since they are based in too narrow a theoretical framework of sexual pleasure.

Notes

1. See e.g. Shweder (2002, 2013); Bell (2005); Darby and Svoboda (2007); Solomon and Noll (2007); DeLaet (2009); Fox and Thomson (2009); and Johnson (2010) for similar analyses.
2. When terms such as 'clitoridectomy' and 'amputation' are used, what is referred to is cutting of the external structures of the clitoris. This organ, however, stretches far into the body (O'Connell et al. 2005).
3. In a discussion where intersex surgery is juxtaposed with female circumcision, the American law scholars Nancy Ehrenreich and Mark Barr contend that 'intersex genital surgeries are medically unnecessary, are far more complicated than African genital cutting, and often have equally, if not more, serious physical and psychological consequences for their recipients' (2005, 74).
4. It is instructive to have a closer look at the actual raw data in the studies used to support the conclusions about statistically significant increased risk. The two studies showing that 'women

with FGM/C experience significantly less sexual satisfaction' are Alsibiani and Rouzi (2010) and Thabet and Thabet (2003), described by Berg et al. as follows: 'the quality of the evidence was "very low"' (Berg et al. 2010, 44). Alsibiani and Rouzi used the instrument *Female Sexual Function Index* and found that circumcised women scored 2.1 points lower on a scale of possible range from 2 to 36. Osinowo and Taiwo (2003), another study of 'low quality' and yet included in the meta-analysis, used another instrument (*Golombok-Rust Inventory of Sexual Satisfaction*) where circumcised women scored 17.5 points lower on a scale with a range between 56 and 280. Also included in the evidence presented by Berg et al. is a study (also 'low quality') showing that 69.5% of the circumcised women reported sexual problems, while only 63.7% of the uncircumcised did so. Figures like these are the strongest evidence presented of the alleged detrimental effects of female genital cutting on sexuality.

5. Accessible from: http://www.who.int/publications/en/
6. The hypothesis behind the figures, showing increased risk of pain and sexual frustration among female partners, goes something like this: 'When a circumcised man moves in and out of a woman without "the gliding movement" caused by the foreskin, it can have a painful effect on the woman's mucous membrane. This could explain the pain and the tendency towards dryness that some women with circumcised men experience', says the Danish epidemiologist Morten Frisch in an interview (ScienceNordic 2011). Further, according to Frisch, the circumcised man has to work harder to reach an orgasm, due to the desensitised glans of the penis, and that can lead to a painful experience for the woman.
7. For an ongoing debate on the pros and cons of male circumcision, including the issue of sexual pleasure, see Svoboda and Van Howe (2013); Frisch et al. (2013); and the AAP Task Force on Circumcision (2013, American Academy of Pediatrics).
8. E.g. Obermeyer (2005); Berg et al. (2010).
9. E.g. Gruenbaum (2006).
10. E.g. Foldès et al. (2012).
11. E.g. Krieger et al. (2008).
12. E.g. Kim and Pang (2007).
13. E.g. Evans (2011).
14. Conferring with studies by Kinsey, showing the enormous variation in the US in the 1940s (among uncut women, if not men). A prominent in-group variation like this – among cut and uncut women alike – was also what was found in these studies (Berg et al. 2010).
15. Obviously, another central organ is the brain. The prevalence of sleep orgasms (or nocturnal orgasms) in men and women – in absence of tactile genital stimulation – demonstrates that sexual pleasure is not exclusively a matter of genital tissue.

References

AAP Task Force on Circumcision. 2013. "Cultural Bias and Circumcision: The AAP Task Force on Circumcision Responds." *Pediatrics* 131: 801–804.

Alsibiani, S. A., and A. Rouzi. 2010. "Sexual Function in Women with Female Genital Mutilation." *Fertility and Sterility* 93 (3): 722–724.

Ansell, J. S., and J. Rajfer. 1981. "A New and Simplified Method for Concealing the Hypertrophied Clitoris." *Journal of Pediatric Surgery* 16 (5): 681–684.

Bell, K. 2005. "Genital Cutting and Western Discourses on Sexuality." *Medical Anthropology Quarterly* 19 (2): 125–148.

Berg, R., E. Denison and A. Fretheim. 2010. *Psychological, Social and Sexual Consequences of Female Genital Mutilation/Cutting (FGM/C): A Systematic Review of Quantitative Studies.* Oslo: Norwegian Knowledge Centre for the Health Services.

Berg, R. C., and E. Denison. 2012. "Does Female Genital Mutilation/Cutting (FGM/C) Affect Women's Sexual Functioning? A Systematic Review of the Sexual Consequences of FGM/C." *Sexuality Research and Social Policy* 9 (1): 4–56.

Braun, V. 2005. "In Search of (Better) Sexual Pleasure: Female Genital 'Cosmetic' Surgery." *Sexualities* 8 (4): 407–424.

Bronselaer, G. A, J. M. Schober, H. F. L. Meyer-Bahlburg, G. T'sjoen, R. Vlietinck, and P. B. Hoebeke. 2013. "Male Circumcision Decreases Penile Sensitivity as Measured in a Large Cohort." *BJU International* 111 (5): 820–827.

Cameron, D., and D. Kulick. 2003. *Language and Sexuality*. Cambridge: Cambridge University Press.

Darby, R., and J. S. Svoboda. 2007. "A Rose by Another Name? Rethinking the Similarities and Differences between Male and Female Genital Cutting." *Medical Anthropology Quarterly* 21 (3): 301–323.

DeLaet, D. L. 2009. "Framing Male Circumcision as a Human Rights Issue? Contributions to the Debate over the Universality of Human Rights." *Journal of Human Rights* 8: 405–426.

Dustin, M. 2010. "Female Genital Mutilation/Cutting in the UK: Challenging the Inconsistencies." *European Journal of Women's Studies* 17 (1): 7–23.

Ehrenreich, N., and M. Barr. 2005. "Intersex Surgery, Female Genital Cutting, and the Selective Condemnation of 'Cultural Practices'." *Harvard Civil Rights – Civil Liberties Law Review* 40 (1): 71–140.

Elchalal, U., B. Ben-Ami, R. Gillis, and A. Brzezinski. 1997. "Ritualistic Female Genital Mutilation: Current Status and Future Outlook." *Obstetrical and Gynecological Survey* 52 (10): 643–651.

Elnashar, A. M., K. E. Ibrahim, M. M. El-Desoky, O. M. Ali, and M. E. M. Hassan. 2007. "Female Sexual Dysfunction in Lower Egypt." *British Journal of Obstetrics and Gynaecology* 14 (2): 201–206.

Esho, T., P. Enzlin, S. Van Wolputte, and M. Temmerman. 2010. "Female Genital Cutting and Sexual Function: In Search of an Alternate Theoretical Model." *African Identities* 8 (3): 221–235.

Evans, M. 2011. "Circumcision in Boys and Girls: Why the Double Standard?" *British Medical Journal* 342: 442.

Foldès, P., B. Cuzin, and A. Andro. 2012. "Reconstructive Surgery After Female Genital Mutilation: A Prospective Cohort Study." *The Lancet* 380 (9837): 134–141.

Fox, M., and M. Thomson. 2009. "Foreskin is a Feminist Issue." *Australian Feminist Studies* 24 (60): 195–210.

Frisch, M. 2012. "Author's Response to: Does Sexual Function Survey in Denmark Offer Any Support for Male Circumcision Having an Adverse Effect?" *International Journal of Epidemiology* 41 (1): 312–314.

Frisch, M., Y. Aigrain, V. Barauskas, R. Bjarnason, S.-A. Boddy, P. Czauderna, R. P. E. de Gier, et al. 2013. "Cultural Bias in the AAP's 2012 Technical Report and Policy Statement on Male Circumcision." *Pediatrics* 131: 796–800.

Frisch, M., M. Lindolm, and M. Grønbæk. 2011. "Male Circumcision and Sexual Function in Men and Women: A Survey-based, Cross-Sectional Study in Denmark." *International Journal of Epidemiology* 40: 1367–1381.

Gagnon, J., and W. Simon. 1973. *Sexual Conduct: The Social Sources of Human Sexuality*. Chicago: Aldine.

Gruenbaum, E. 2006. "Sexuality Issues in the Movement to Abolish Female Genital Cutting in Sudan." *Medical Anthropology Quarterly* 20 (1): 121–138.

Hinton, D. E., D. Howes, and L. J. Kirmayer. 2008. "Toward a Medical Anthropology of Sensations: Definitions and Research Agenda." *Transcultural Psychiatry* 45 (2): 142–162.

Hughes, I. A, C. Houk, S. F. Ahmed, P. A. Lee, Lawson Wilkins Pediatric Endocrine Society (LWPES)/ European Society for Paediatric Endocrinology (ESPE) Consensus Group. 2006. "Consensus Statement on Management of Intersex Disorders." *Journal of Pediatric Urology* 2: 148–162.

Johnsdotter, S., and B. Essén. 2010. "Genitals and Ethnicity: The Politics of Genital Modifications." *Reproductive Health Matters* 18 (35): 29–37.

Johnson, M. 2010. "Male Genital Mutilation: Beyond the Tolerable?" *Ethnicities* 10 (2): 181–207.

Karkazis, K. 2008. *Fixing Sex: Intersex, Medical Authority, and Lived Experience*. Durham: Duke University Press.

Kelly, B., and C. Foster. 2012. "Should Female Genital Cosmetic Surgery and Genital Piercing be Regarded Ethically and Legally as Female Genital Mutilation?" *British Journal of Obstetrics and Gynaecology* 119: 389–392.

Kim, D., and M.-G. Pang. 2007. "The Effect of Male Circumcision on Sexuality." *BJU International* 99 (3): 619–622.

Krieger, J. N, S. D. Mehta, R. C. Bailey, K. Agot, J. O. Ndinya-Achola, and C. Parker. 2008. "Adult Male Circumcision: Effects on Sexual Function and Sexual Satisfaction in Kisumu, Kenya." *The Journal of Sexual Medicine* 5 (11): 2610–2622.

Lean, W. L., J. M. Hutson, and A.V. Deshpande. 2007. "Clitoryplasty: Past, Present and Future." *Pediatric Surgery International* 23: 289–293.

Lightfoot-Klein, H. 1989. *Prisoners of Ritual: An Odyssey into Female Genital Circumcision in Africa*. New York: The Haworth Press.

Maharaj, N. R., A. Dhai, R. Wiersma, and J. Moodley. 2005. "Intersex Conditions in Children and Adolescents: Surgical, Ethical, and Legal Considerations." *Journal of Pediatric and Adolescent Gynecology* 18 (6): 399–402.

Malmström, M. 2009. "Just Like Couscous: Gender, Agency and the Politics of Female Circumcision in Cairo." Doctoral dissertation, School of Global Studies, Göteborg University.

Morris, B. J., J. H. Waskett, and R. H. Gray. 2012. "Does Sexual Function Survey in Denmark Offer Any Support for Male Circumcision Having an Adverse Effect?" *International Journal of Epidemiology* 41 (1): 310–312.

Njambi, W. N. 2004. "Dualisms and Female Bodies in Representations of African Female Circumcision: A Feminist Critique." *Feminist Theory* 5 (3): 281–303.

Nour, N. M. 2012. "Using Facts to Moderate the Message." *The Hastings Center Report* 42 (6): 30–31.

Obermeyer, C. M. 2005. "The Consequences of Female Circumcision for Health and Sexuality: An Update on the Evidence." *Culture, Health & Sexuality* 7 (5): 443–461.

O'Connell H. E., K.V. Sanjeevan, and J. M. Hutson. 2005. "Anatomy of the Clitoris." *The Journal of Urology* 174: 1189–1195.

Osinowo, H. O., and A. O. Taiwo. 2003. "Impact of Female Genital Mutilation on Sexual Functioning, Self-esteem and Marital Instability of Women in Ajegunle." *Ife Psychologia* 11 (1): 123–130.

Renganathan, A., R. Cartwright, and L. Cardozo. 2009. "Gynecological Cosmetic Surgery." *Expert Review of Obstetrics & Gynecology* 4 (2): 101–04.

Richters, J. 2009. "Bodies, Pleasure and Displeasure." *Culture, Health & Sexuality* 11 (3): 225–236.

ScienceNordic. 2011. "Male Circumcision Leads to a Bad Sex Life." Accessed May 2, 2013. http://sciencenordic.com/male-circumcision-leads-bad-sex-life

Shweder, R. A. 2002. "'What about Female Genital Mutilation?' And Why Understanding Culture Matters in the First Place." In *Engaging Cultural Differences: The Multicultural Challenge in Liberal Democracies*, edited by R. Shweder, M. Minow, and H. R. Markus. New York: Russell Sage Foundation.

Shweder, R. A. 2013. "The Goose and the Gander: The Genital Wars," manuscript available from Richard A. Shweder at this e-mail address: rshd@uchicago.edu

Solomon, L. M., and R. C. Noll. 2007. "Male Versus Female Genital Alteration: Differences in Legal, Medical, and Socioethical Responses." *Gender Medicine* 4 (2): 89–96.

Svoboda, J. S., and R. S. Van Howe. 2013. "Out of Step: Fatal Flaws in the Latest AAP Policy Report on Neonatal Circumcision." *Journal of Medical Ethics,* published online March 18, 2013 [Epub ahead of print].

The Public Policy Advisory Network on Female Genital Surgeries in Africa. 2012. "Seven Things to Know About Female Genital Surgeries in Africa." *The Hastings Center Report* 42 (6): 19–27.

Tiefer, L. 2004. *Sex Is Not a Natural Act and Other Essays*. Oxford: Westview Press.

Toubia, N. 1994. "Female Circumcision as a Public Health Issue." *New England Journal of Medicine* 331: 712–716.

Veale, D., and J. Daniels. 2012. "Cosmetic Clitoridectomy in a 33-year-old Woman." *Archives of Sexual Behavior* 41: 725–730.

Wade, L. 2012. "The Function of Balance in US News Coverage of Uncontested Issues: The Case of Female Genital Cutting." *Journalism* 13 (7): 869–885.

WHO. 2012. "Female Genital Mutilation." Accessed April 30, 2013. http://apps.who.int/iris/bitstream/10665/77428/1/WHO_RHR_12.41_eng.pdf

WHO, UNAIDS, and JHPIEGO. 2009. "Manual for Male Circumcision under Local Anaesthesia." Accessed April 30, 2013. http://www.who.int/hiv/pub/malecircumcision/who_mc_local_anaesthesia.pdf

Woodhouse, C. R. J. 2004. "Intersex Surgery in the Adult." *BJU International* 93 (suppl. 3): 57–65.

Critiquing circumcision: in search of a new paradigm for conceptualizing genital modification

Zachary T. Androus

Independent Scholar

In this article, I advance two separate but related critiques of current approaches to classifying and analyzing culturally, socially, and medically motivated genital modifications: first that the widely employed categories of female circumcision and male circumcision separate these practices in gendered terms that are inconsistent with both the reality of these practices and fundamental social scientific principles, and second that the practice of neonatal male circumcision that emerged from Anglophone medical practice to become an entrenched social norm in the United States merits a critical evaluation beyond that which it has heretofore been subjected. These critiques lead me to propose an alternative approach to the conceptual classification of genital modification practices, one in which the extent of the modification, the meanings of the practice to those involved, whether it is motivated by a group or individual desire, and the developmental stage of the individual form a framework for analysis, rather than the geographically and gender-based approaches that have resulted in the profoundly ethnocentric exceptionalism that characterizes most current research, writing, and activism on the matter. The differential attention paid to male and female circumcision fails to reflect the cultural sensibilities of those whose practices are in question and creates a de facto exceptionalism by which US practices are exempted from the same scrutiny afforded by others. I address specifically the gendered approach to African circumcision practices, including the recent attention that male circumcision has received as a potential anti-HIV intervention, and I argue the need for a much more vigorously critical scholarly attention to US circumcision practices. My approach is influenced by critical medical anthropology, which frames its inquiries around a focus on the human body and which does not accept biomedical knowledge as factual a priori, but rather seeks to contextualize it within the socially and culturally relevant system of knowledge that has produced it. I draw also on the history of circumcision, campaigns for both its promulgation and elimination, and my own ethnographic work with US parents on how they make the decision whether to circumcise their newborn sons.

In this article, I identify a set of problems with the gender-specific approach to genital modification practices taken by many scholars, activists, and institutions that address the genital modification of females while excluding that of males. Such a gender-restricted focus is usually predicated on a set of assumptions including the intrinsic harm of female genital modifications, their automatic violation of the rights of women and girls, and the impossibility of their having medical value, while male circumcision instead is assumed to be categorically not harmful, which is why it has the possibility of being medically beneficial and, according to Rahman and Toubia (2000, 21), why it is not considered an equivalent violation of rights compared to acts of female genital mutilation (FGM). This widely held idea is problematic because so many different groups of people in so many different parts of the world practice such a variety of genital modifications that a categorical division on the basis of gender immediately fails to adequately describe or account for the ways in which many of those people experience the practices in which they participate. Removing gender as an a priori distinction is not an attempt to remove gender as a factor of classification, but to move toward a framework that actually reflects the variety of ways that gender is understood in the world in relation to the modification of people's genitals. In respect to the questions of harm, risk, and human rights, these are most effectively addressed in terms of their actual association with specific practices because some practices will carry more risk or be more harmful than others. The extent of risk or harm is determined by the character of the practice more so than the sex of the genitals on which it is being performed: a simple operation performed on an adolescent in a hospital will carry less risk than a complex operation performed on an adolescent in a rural camp, irrespective of the sex of the individual. In respect to human rights, no basis exists to restrict males from enjoying the same rights to self-determination and freedom from harm frequently invoked in the case of female genital modifications.

Solving these problems will require a different way of thinking about genital modification practices, which in turn will require a different way of talking about them. In this article, I strive to develop a more accurate descriptive terminology for making reference to genital modification practices to make more meaningful classificatory distinctions than those between sexes. This reflects my firm conviction that scholarly attention to cultural and social practices ought to be critical, which is to say not based simply on the universalization of one particular culture-bound perspective as a design for classificatory and analytical frameworks, examples of which are all too frequent.

The widespread tendency in scholarship, law, and medicine to classify genital modification on the basis of gender and geography is often related to a particular cultural perspective typically described as 'Western' (Bell 2005; Sardi 2011). Scheper-Hughes and Lock are comfortable referring to a 'Western epistemology' as part of their description of the 'radically materialist thinking characteristic of clinical biomedicine' rooted in Aristotle and Hippocrates and fully developed by Descartes (1987, 8, 9). Despite its repeated deployment in debates over these practices, I find the term Western to be unsatisfactory and inadequate. Instead, I prefer designating it as a biomedical perspective, following Kleinman's preference for 'biomedicine' over 'Western medicine' (1995, 25). This perspective and the practices it supports are not static or homogenous; they are reflective of the historical particularities of their development and deployment in the world (Kleinman 1995, 23). Despite its inherent 'heterogeneity', defining characteristics of this perspective can be located in the persistently fundamental 'scientific paradigm' around which it is organized (1995, 25, 26). This leads to a series of defining characteristics that underlie the perspective on genital modifications typified by the position of Rahman and Toubia cited above: an 'extreme insistence on materialism as the grounds of knowledge' and a 'corresponding requirement that single causal chains must be used to specify pathogenesis in a language of structural flaws' (Kleinman 1995, 29). Two other features of biomedicine as described by Kleinman help to explain some of the contradictions inherent in the gender-based double standard for the acceptability of genital modifications: first, the 'set of deep dualisms between male and female, mind and body, strength and weakness, [and] wealth and poverty' (1995, 30) manifests in the tendency to determine the fundamental consequence of genital modification on the basis of gender insofar as it is conceptually impossible to harm strong male bodies by modifying their genitals, while it is impossible to modify female genitals without doing harm to their weak bodies. Second, the premise that '*nature* is physical… [and] knowable independent of perspective or representation', because 'the psychological, social, and moral are only so many superficial layers of epiphenomenal cover that disguise the bedrock of truth… the real stuff: biology as an architectural structure and its chemical associates' (Kleinman 1995, 30), allows for the absolute association of harm with any modification of the weak female body. My intention is not to pass judgment on this perspective itself; my goal is to explore alternatives to the problems created by using it as a basis for cross-cultural analyses. This is important in the case of genital modifications because the tremendous range of such practices in the world means that using one set of normative values as the basis for developing the categories to describe genital modifications globally guarantees a framework that distorts rather than clearly represents.

The biomedical perspective on genital modification practices has facilitated the dissemination of two interrelated values relating to gender and geography: that modifications performed on males are fundamentally different from those performed on females and that the practices performed in Africa are fundamentally different from those performed in other parts of the world. This paradigmatic framework shapes research agendas and guides the approaches of national and international governmental and non-governmental organizations to the creation of their political and legal instruments and information campaigns. While some scholars and activists have adopted this framework as an operational perspective on the matter, others have criticized it on various grounds, but there are few proposals for thinking about the practices collectively in a fundamentally different way. In the rest of this article, I explore some possibilities for the cross-cultural classification of genital modifications based on other attributes including local meaning, the developmental stage at the time of modification, whether the modification is motivated by an individual or group value, and the extent of the modification. Kuhn (1996) explains that new paradigms develop from the use of current ones to explore anomalies, and I am hoping to contribute to just such a process in respect to the conceptualization of genital modification practices on a global scale, but at this stage, the terms are still set by a biomedical paradigm. The different ways to describe genital modifications that I propose below are not a scientific revolution that will replace the biomedical perspective, but they are part of 'a more or less extended exploration of the area of anomaly' (Kuhn 1996, 53) between the premise that female genital modifications are categorically problematic while male ones are not and the ethnographic and epidemiological data to the contrary.

Before moving on, some discussion of terminology is necessary. In English language scholarship, the unqualified term circumcision generally refers to a procedure performed on young males. Adding qualifiers, such as female or adult, distinguishes other cases. I prefer alternative terms to avoid confusion with popular usages, and so I forego variations on the term circumcision in favor of the phrase genital modification. This term is qualified to varying degrees to allow the specific degree of reference necessary for the analytical or classificatory purposes at hand, with the unqualified phrase genital modification serving as a globally collective reference. (Whether a global category is a meaningful or legitimate level of classification is obviously a debatable point in its own right, but it must be named before its legitimacy can be debated.) Additional degrees of specification are added flexibly to facilitate the purposes of a given discussion, from very broad classifications like Maasai genital modification or initiatory genital modification to quite specific classifications like Egyptian minors genitally modified in hospitals for religious motives. I support an adjustable terminology that allows for specific or comparative reference when necessary. Both of my first examples, Maasai and initiatory, are categories that include a range of practices that differ in many important ways, but they are also each meaningful ways to group practices for the purposes of better understanding the associations between risk, harm, rights, and motivation for genital modifications of different types. When I make reference to other authors, I follow their usage, so common terms like male circumcision and coinages like FGM appear in those cases.

Although I have my own opinions on global genital modification practices, I am attempting not to advocate for a position in this article, beyond the claim that approaches to genital modification should be critically informed and culturally relative rather than ethnocentric. Of course, I will explain my own position, so that the reader may reach his or her own conclusion as to how successful I am in this attempt. My research until now has been informed largely by critical medical anthropology and has focused on male genital modification in the forms promulgated by the professionalized biomedical enterprise over the course of the nineteenth and twentieth centuries. I have carried out specific projects with US parents on their decisions about whether to circumcise their newborn sons and with men who elected circumcision as adults. My broader participant-observation includes time spent with the intactivists and their public at demonstrations and as a part of the interdisciplinary mix of attendees and presenters at two of the National Organization of Circumcision Information Resource Centers International Symposia. Since moving to Europe from the United States, I have also been party to a series of events organized by immigrant groups representing various points of view on the importation of their genital modification practices into host societies with no corollary practice of their own. My own experience as a US-born male raised there by parents from a European society where circumcision as it is known in the United States is generally considered undesirable certainly contributes to my personal opinion that everyone in European and descendant societies, including males born in the United States, should have a right to make their own decisions about genital modification. I see this position as wholly consistent with the strong tradition of individual rights these societies have developed since the nineteenth century. I am deeply skeptical of medical justifications for male circumcision, mostly because of circumcision's historical promotion as a treatment or prophylaxis for a series of conditions such as masturbation, paralysis, epilepsy, syphilis, cancer, urinary tract infections, and most recently, HIV, all of which are now understood to be primarily influenced by other factors (for the history of medical promotion of circumcision, see Darby (2005), Glick (2005) and Gollaher (2000)).

In social and cultural contexts other than my own, I do not see an ethical bright line in terms of age, gender, religion, culture, or geography. I struggle with the contradictions that I imagine must confront anyone who surveys the range of voices to be heard on genital modification: almost immediately upon beginning my research, I encountered people who felt harmed and others who felt helped for having been genitally modified in the same manner as members of their same ethnic group, gender, or nationality, and the same range of feelings among those who had not been. I quickly learned that gender, geographic origin, and genital status are not reliable indicators of what a given person's opinion or experience of their own cultural tradition might be. My anthropological training developed in me a very strong non-interventionist attitude towards non-European and descendant practices, as well as a vigorous skepticism of overly deterministic notions of culture as an index of people's feelings on any given matter. Despite my disciplinary allegiance to the familiar ethos of anthropological cultural relativism, I see the debates over the appropriateness of intervention in non-Western practices as intellectual exercises more akin to philosophy than policy at this point. For centuries, the concerted intervention in societies around the world by European and European descendant colonial and development enterprises have meant that it is no longer possible to disentangle native and interventionist ideas and approaches. In respect to biomedicine, Kleinman describes the spread of biomedicine as a process by which the biomedical perspective itself is affected by the indigenous perspectives it comes into contact with over the course of its globalization (1995, 24). This makes it impossible to predict the framework of meanings through which any given individual will understand and experience his or her body and its culturally or socially motivated modification.

One further reflection on cultural relativism and my motivation to address some of the problems I see with the current approach to understanding genital modification before I discuss them: Early anthropologists modeled their nascent discipline on the natural sciences while simultaneously struggling to distinguish their enterprise from them. I understand the natural and social sciences to share the basic goal of generating reliable descriptions of the world around us, but the social sciences struggle with the dilemma of objectivity more than do the natural sciences. Cultural relativism is one of the necessarily imperfect strategies we developed to help deal with the problem of making reliable descriptions of other peoples' worlds from our subjective positions. I say necessarily imperfect because I cannot imagine a totally effective resolution of this dilemma. What I can imagine is a descriptive framework based on observable facts about genital modification practices. I understand that any such claim to observable facts is highly susceptible to certain critiques addressing the ultimately contextual nature of all knowledge, but the point of my effort here is to explore alternate ways of thinking within our inescapable subjectivities rather than to succumb to the paralyzing philosophical dilemma over whether anything can be known at all that occasionally threatens to emerge from a strong appeal to cultural relativism.

Gender exclusivity in expert discourse on global genital modification

Prior to the 1970s, anthropologists treated male and female circumcision together in places where they occurred together. Neither they nor the sociologists were paying much attention to the medicalized male circumcision craze that swept English speaking societies around the world over the course of the twentieth century, but when they looked to the famous 'other', they described in gender-inclusive terms the genital modifications that were practiced. For example, John G. Kennedy (1970) treated what he called male circumcision and female excision together in his survey of Nubian practices and attendant discussion of the applicability of popular explanatory theories for genital modifications as rites of passage. Horace Miner (1942, 622, 635) saw fit to include clitoridectomy in his discussion of initiatory male circumcision among the Songhoi, even though they did not practice it, because it was present among other groups in the vicinity. The tone of anthropological writing on African genital modification practices changed after the 1980s, undoubtedly reflecting the postmodern crisis of representation and the rise of the international anti-FGM movement, both of which had by then gained strength.

A gender-based distinction between male circumcision and what widely became known as 'female genital mutilation' (FGM) had become paradigmatic by the end of the 1990s. FGM is named as an international public health issue by the World Health Organization (2000), and various NGOs are committed exclusively or in part to its eradication, while male circumcision is being promoted as an anti-HIV intervention by many of the very same agencies. Material appearing since the first publication of *The Hosken Report: Genital and Sexual Mutilation of Females* in 1982 (Hosken 1995) reflects the pervasive influence of Hosken's insistence on addressing female modifications to the exclusion of male ones, especially in African contexts. The international anti-FGM campaign has many critics, with anthropologists at the forefront. Criticism of the international anti-FGM movement has generally focused on refuting popular claims about meaning, motivation, and harm. For example, while acknowledging that it cannot be 'objectively' tested, Ahmadu reports that her 'research [among Kono and Mandinka women] and experience contradict received knowledge regarding the supposedly negative effects of removing the clitoris on women's sexuality' (2000, 304). Gruenbaum demonstrates that 'by no means is female circumcision a single phenomenon with a single purpose such as "controlling women" or "suppressing female sexuality"' (2001, 47). Hale takes on the politics of knowledge related to female circumcision by asking 'whether and how' women from developed regions of the world can selectively and voluntarily take up the issues of 'so-called Third World women' (2005, 209). Shell-Duncan and Hernlund agree with those who 'have argued that the discussion of female "circumcision" by Westerners has been excessive, essentializing, and paternalistic' (2000, 2). By answering the claims of the international anti-FGM campaign, however, these scholars implicitly reproduce the a priori gender-based distinction that characterizes them. This has led some to omit male genital modifications from their analysis, even while acknowledging its local relevance.

For example, Shell-Duncan and Hernlund (2000) describe the interrelationship of meaning between male and female genital modifications in several societies during their discussion of marriageability as a rationale for female 'circumcision' (2000, 21). They present a cogent critique of the unfounded assumptions inherent in the anti-FGM discourse, but they never address its gender exclusivity in such terms. Shell-Duncan, Obiero, and Muruli (2000) also describe the occurrence of male and female genital modification practices together before addressing only female 'circumcision' among the Rendille of northern Kenya. Their investigation of the ways in which 'female "circumcision" and surrounding attitudes change as a society experiences the transformation brought about by settlement [which replaced nomadism] and development' (2000, 112) raises the question of the degree to which attitudes around male circumcision do or do not change as well. The authors' explanation that a single word in the Rendille language refers to both female and male circumcision (2000, 114) suggests that Rendille speakers understand the practices to be related in some way. The authors offer no justification or explanation for not addressing the operations performed on males; they simply move directly into a gender-specific discussion of female 'circumcision'. In a subsequent discussion of the tension surrounding the medicalization of female 'circumcision', they make passing reference to the use of anesthesia by a local nurse who circumcised a number of 'warriors' during their initiation, sparking a discussion of anesthesia for women (2000, 117). As part of the explanation of how persistently traditional the practice is, they report that only 0.2% of Rendille women were circumcised by a trained nurse (2000, 120). The persistence of tradition for the women while biomedical elements slip into the initiation of warriors is enough to warrant attention from the authors, but the fact that the community itself is incorporating both male and female practices into their discussions makes the authors' decision to not do so all the more difficult to understand.

Christine J. Walley encountered female genital operations in a village that included two ethnic groups: one whose genital modification practices affected only boys, and the other both boys and girls (1997, 409). When Walley describes her own 'inner distress' about clitoridectomy, she mentions nothing about her feelings towards the circumcision of the male initiates (1997, 410). In fact, in her capacity as an English teacher, she gave the students the option of writing essays about female circumcision, and though she reflects on the possible influences of the anti-FGM campaigns on their responses, she never comments on the kind of message that might be sent implicitly by an absence of discussion about male circumcision for these teenagers, male and female, who were all initiated together (1997, 411). Walley repeatedly makes reference to male circumcision in various contexts, but never includes it in any of the questions that she directs toward female circumcision in these contexts (1997, 414–417). Throughout, she references the initiation of boys into manhood, but restricts her search for voices and penetrating questions about meaning and experience to female initiation without offering a justification for this focus in her otherwise engaging, personal, and reflective essay. A suggestive possibility is raised by Walley's cogent explanation of the way that women often become symbolic bearers of 'hardened notions' of culture and tradition (1997, 425–427). Walley appears to me as to be complicit in this sort of discursive construction of women's bodies as sites for the deployment of essentialist notions of culture by using female circumcision and the anti-FGM campaigns to represent tradition and modernity, respectively.

This kind of implicit acceptance of a gendered framework for approaching genital modifications is not restricted to anthropologists. Historian Lynn Thomas (2000) provides an illuminating discussion of the local responses to efforts by British colonial administrators to end female circumcision in the Meru district of Kenya during the early and middle twentieth centuries, but by focusing on female circumcision, she ends up telling only part of the story. Thomas includes one tantalizing reference to something much larger when she reports that at a meeting of the local colonial administrative unit in 1956, 'the medical officer proposed that boys should be circumcised between the ages of six months to one year instead of at adolescence, and female "circumcision" should be abandoned entirely' (2000, 134). At the mid-twentieth century, early circumcision of males was being widely promoted in British medicine at the same time that medicalized genital surgery for females was falling out of favor (Darby 2005; Glick 2005); it appears that the medical officer was proposing that Meru initiation practices be adjusted to reflect contemporaneous British circumcision patterns. An exclusive focus on women's genitals characterizes the rest of Thomas' chapter, so much so that in the ensuing analysis regarding responses to the female side of the medical officer's proposal, there is not a single further mention of anything to do with male initiation among the Meru, then or now (2000, 134–138). This is despite her introductory explanation that both male and female initiations were influential aspects of Meru social organization at the time (2000, 131).

These authors exhibit one of the fundamental problems with the gender exclusive approach: the artificial separation of related practices under a rubric of gender ends up reflecting the cultural sensibilities of the observer or historian more than that of the people whose practices and experiences are being described. This gender exclusivity contributes to a sense of geographic exclusivity insofar as the African practices overlooked by these scholars are normalized by the biomedical perspective insofar as they are male genital modifications. Physicians in Britain, and its postcolonial descendants in Anglophone North America and the Pacific, vigorously promoted medicalized male genital modification through the nineteenth and twentieth centuries. Certain female genital surgeries were promoted as well during this time (Green 2005; Kandela 1999), but they declined in popularity while male circumcision became so widespread as to be considered routine. This broad trend created the conditions by which a generic male circumcision can presently be promoted as an intervention against HIV in sub-Saharan Africa by the same international governmental organizations that are campaigning against FGM. The process by which male circumcision emerged as a normative category in the twentieth century among English speaking societies of the world is directly related to the institutionalization of biomedicine as a profession. I see this as the foundation for the current campaign to promote the procedure as an anti-HIV intervention in sub-Saharan Africa because there have been English speaking doctors advocating for circumcision as a public health measure against some disease for over a hundred years (Darby 2005). Understanding the significance of the African male circumcision campaigns requires understanding of the practice of neonatal circumcision in the United States for two reasons: first, US researchers and institutions play a central role in the development of what they call male circumcision as an anti-HIV intervention and second, because their approach is determined in large part by the perceived characteristics of genital modification widespread in the United States and also known as male circumcision.

American (male) circumcision

Trends

Call for the universal circumcision of boys as a public health measure appears in the US medical literature as early as the mid-nineteenth century (e.g., Delaney 1849), but circumcision was more likely to be prescribed as a treatment at that time, often for masturbation or the nervous diseases which were then believed to result from it, such as epilepsy and paralysis (Gollaher 2000, 75–78). Over the course of the twentieth century, circumcision developed into a prophylactic measure carried out at a younger age, until the circumcision of male neonates was a routine aspect of hospital birth by the 1950s (Glick 2005, 180–181). While circumcision is widespread in the United States today, it is not absolute. The National Health and Nutrition Examination Survey from 1999 to 2004 found that a total of 79% of US males were circumcised, with 88% of whites, 73% of blacks, 42% of Mexican Americans, and 50% of 'others' reporting that they were circumcised (Xu et al. 2007, 479). The rate of circumcision appears to be declining: the most recent data estimates that between 50% and 60% of newborn males are being circumcised in the United States (NHDS 2009).

Despite this trend, it is important to note that circumcision remains a strongly normative category in the shared cultural imagination of the United States. Almost every one of the many non-specialists with whom I have had occasion to discuss the matter in the course of my research typically assumes that any given man is circumcised, irrespective of their own circumcision status or that of the men they know. For example, a volunteer in my study of parental decision making repeatedly stated that, like himself, every one of his male friends was circumcised. Yet I also interviewed one of those friends who, it transpired, was not circumcised. On another occasion, a nurse with whom I was discussing my research informally explained to me that her husband was not circumcised. I was struck at the time by the shift in her nonverbal communication style at that point: the volume and pitch of her voice both lowered, and she leaned towards me before using the word 'actually' to preface her explanation of her husband's status as if revealing a sort of secret. Her language throughout the rest of our conversation clearly indicated that she saw US men as categorically circumcised despite her husband's status.

Changing medical motives

The rise of scientific medicine over the course of the twentieth century saw the decline of theories that justified circumcision as a treatment for nervous disorders and masturbation.

Increased understanding of the mechanisms of sexually transmitted diseases and cancer led the American Academy of Pediatrics to include a comment in their 1971 edition of *Standards and Recommendation for Hospital Care of Newborn Infants* that 'there are no valid medical indications for circumcision in the neonatal period' (American Academy of Pediatrics Committee on Fetus and Newborn 1971, 110). The next official word, issued by a committee in 1975, introduced what was to become the defining feature of all subsequent AAP policy statements on neonatal male circumcision: the claim that parents have an absolute right to elect circumcision despite the absence of any medical indication for the procedure (Thompson et al. 1975, 610). The latest policy statement dates from 2012 and was accompanied by a separate Technical Report (Blank et al. 2012). The prior statement, issued in 1999 (Lannon et al.) and reaffirmed in 2005 (American Academy of Pediatrics), found the benefits of circumcision insufficient to recommend the procedure. However, the 1999 Task Force did reiterate the usual exceptions about circumcision being potentially desirable for social or cultural reasons, granting parents the freedom to elect it for their infant sons as they see fit (Lannon et al. 1999, 686). The recommendation that health care providers cover the cost of circumcision (Blank et al. 2012, 585) is the only additional feature of the 2012 Policy Statement not present previously.

Circumcision is obviously exceptional, insofar as no other neonatal surgical procedure can be elected by parents independent of medical necessity, which itself is typically determined by physicians rather than parents. The concept of 'potential benefits' (Lannon et al. 1999, 686, 691) is used to describe the phenomenon by which some men still contract diseases that show reduced rates among circumcised populations, or confounding factors, like behavior, that can mitigate the protective effects of circumcision. Both neonatal circumcision in the United States and phrophylactic male circumcision in Africa are based on the premise that a *potential* benefit justifies male circumcision, but the possibility of such benefit can be easily negated by confounding factors. As with the debates in the medical literature over the putative benefits of neonatal circumcision, there is no consensus in the medical literature on the usefulness of circumcision as an HIV intervention, despite frequent claims to the contrary. The observed correlations between lower rates of HIV and circumcising groups that motivated the trials were themselves balanced by the observations of de Vincenzi and Mertens (1994) and Ntozi (1995), who found no such lower rate of HIV among certain circumcising groups before the trials took place. After the publication of the trials, Garenne (2008) reported higher rates of HIV among circumcised groups in Cameroon, Lesotho, and Malawi. The trials themselves have been roundly criticized both for their design and the extrapolation of their results to general claims about the relationship between circumcision and HIV (Boyle and Hill 2011; Lie and Miller 2011; Rogowska-Szadkowska 2010). Individually maintained internet sites such as www.circumcisionandhiv.com and www.circumstitions.com/hiv have done a fine job of collecting resources that challenge circumcision's usefulness as an anti-HIV intervention. Perhaps it should be instructive that the very same pattern of initial observational correlations between a circumcising population and lower rates of disease played out a century earlier in the cities of the United States with Jewish populations (Glick 2005, 150–209). In the case of both US circumcision and the African anti-HIV circumcision campaign, the best possible outcome that can be claimed for circumcision is only one of reduced risk whose benefit can be erased by behavioral factors. This has been insufficient to recommend the procedure in the United States (Lannon et al. 1999) and well below the expected efficacy of a typical vaccine in Africa (Garenne 2006), not to mention incompatible with the concept of vaccination itself.

The biomedical perspective on circumcision bears responsibility for facilitating both the international anti-FGM movement and the current campaigns to promote male circumcision as an anti-HIV intervention in sub-Saharan Africa. I have touched on some of the problems created by using one particular cultural perspective, the biomedical, as a basis for responding to genital modification practices globally. In the following sections, I explore some possibilities for thinking about genital modifications in novel ways by talking about them in novel ways.

An alternative conceptual framework for genital modification

I propose that all possible modifications of the human external genital structures can be classified according to four sets of characteristics. The first set of characteristics includes the ways in which the practitioners themselves understand the meaning, motivation, consequence, and significance of the practice. To populate this category with specific types of meaning, motivation, consequence, and significance as understood by practitioners requires listening to the voices of the people themselves who are carrying out the modification in question. The second characteristic is the developmental stage of the individual in terms of the local meaning that constitutes the first category. This is not only an age-related value like child or adolescent (each of which is locally defined in a number of ways), but can include any stage of status or condition during an individual's life, including initiate, patient, or spouse. The third characteristic refers to whether the modification is an expression of a widely shared group expectation or is an individually elected procedure. To be clear, this is not about who decides, but rather whether the decision reflects a broadly shared expectation of modification or if modifications occur idiosyncratically. Finally, the fourth characteristic is based on the extent of the modification. This is in some ways the most challenging category in which to achieve specificity, but with that aim in mind, I feel safe distinguishing between the implantation of single or multiple objects, manipulation sufficient to reshape, cutting without removing tissue, and cutting that removes tissue. These four categories are designed to support an adaptable terminology by which labels can be as general or specific as necessary. I am not attempting to exhaustively catalog global genital modifications by way of the few examples I offer for each category. The point is to develop a framework sturdy enough to describe any given genital modification in the world on its own terms without resorting to the biomedical paradigm. I return to the relationship between terminology and the framework after explaining each of the four categories in more depth.

First category: local meaning

A comprehensive framework must be able to account for the meaning and significance of any given genital modification to the people by whom it is enacted. In this first category should appear the meanings, motivations, or local understandings of why genital modifications are performed. Are they part of an initiation, some other kind of rite of passage, a generalized social norm, an expression of a specific aesthetic value, a medical practice, or some combination thereof? Giving biomedical genital modifications equal consideration is crucial to any alternative framework, because many of the troubling inconsistencies in the current model result from their exemption from ethical standards applied to other types of modification (Somerville 2000, 212, 213). To be clear, this is not intended to identify the practitioner or the context, as when physicians happen to perform ritually or religiously motivated modifications; it is the *motive* driving the practice that constitutes the classification. A lot of careful work would need to be done to actually classify the range of explanations that people have offered the ethnographic record, but that would provide an effective means of making cross-cultural comparisons without having to rely on one particular culture-bound perspective from which to view global genital modifications.

Second category: developmental stage

Every genital modification happens to an individual who is at a particular stage in the course of their life. While there are no culturally universal stages, every human society makes some distinction between different stages of life. The determination of what particular stage an individual is occupying at the time of their genital modification relies on understanding the local knowledge of what stages there are in a human life and how individuals pass through them. These can include age-related stages like infant, child, adolescent, or adult or other socially and culturally demarcated classifications like initiate, patient, spouse, or parent. Flexibility and permeability are necessary for this framework to function, so there must be the possibility of overlap and multiplicity between the categories, so that, for example, socially normative initiatory genital modification of Kono adolescents can be distinguished from socially normative non-initiatory childhood genital modification of males in Turkey. This allows for a much more nuanced and accurate discussion of practices that may bear no social or geographic relationship to one another, but are related in other ways, as in the two above examples.

Third category: individual or group value

The distinction between individual and group modification is designed to account for the fact that certain modifications are elected by individuals, while other modifications are elected more or less on behalf of individuals by virtue of widespread group expectations that lead individuals themselves or their relatives to have certain modifications carried out. Within this category can always go an ethnic or social label like Jewish or Yoruba, the heterogeneity of belief within any given ethnic group and ethnic composition within any given social group notwithstanding. It is very important to understand that my intention is not to describe group behaviors, but rather to create the possibility of classifying any given genital modification that is carried out on the basis of values associated with a shared identity. Not every Jewish or Yoruba person is genitally modified, and among those who are not, everyone was necessarily modified for the reasons typically associated with the shared values expressed by the genital modifications commonly practiced within those groups. A new paradigm for classifying genital modification will necessarily be incompatible with heretofore conventional groupings, and so will cut across what otherwise appear to be natural divisions among practices.

Fourth category: extent

This fourth category lacks the depth of the others, but its classificatory possibilities possess tremendous breadth insofar as they address the mechanics of the modifications. While the human capacity for inventing meaning is essentially unlimited, the genital structures themselves present a finite range of modifiability. Within this range can be distinguished manual manipulation that results in visible change, as described, for example, by Villa and Grassivaro Gallo (2006); manipulation using external devices, as described to Vale and Juno by Fakir Musafar (Vale and Juno 1989) and by Schultheiss et al. (1998); cutting without removing tissue, cutting with the manipulation of tissue, as described by Glick (2009); cutting with the removal of tissue; and the implantation of single or multiple objects. Using anatomical conceptualizations of the genital structures derived from the biomedical tradition is necessary, but this should not be taken as an endorsement or deployment of the philosophical premises that characterize the biomedical perspective as a belief system.

A sort of dilemma is created by trying to make specific descriptions of extent that can be used to make comparisons of practices performed in unrelated contexts: on the one hand, objective descriptions would be the most useful for this purpose, but on the other hand, the structure of the genitals themselves is always a cultural understanding. In principle, the scientific anatomical model is on equal ground with other classifications, such as the physiological expression of an inherent bisexual nature that requires transformation into absolutely male or female parts through complex rituals that include the removal of certain elements from the structure of the genitals. This view is described by Ahmadu (2000, 284–289) as being widespread among her Kono informants. Care must be taken to distinguish references to the extent of a modification that rely on sets of shared cultural meanings by way referencing locally understood features. Such classifications, like the male parts of a woman that Ahmadu's informants might recognize, or the foreskin that a US American might recognize, fit more comfortably in the first category along with esthetic descriptives like smoothing the vagina or exposing the glans, insofar as they are culturally subjective understandings, but they play an important role in contextual discussions of modifications in practice.

Using the alternative framework to describe known practices

With the generic scheme of the alternative framework laid out, we can now experiment with using it to describe some of the better known practices described in the scholarly literature. I want to stress that I am aiming towards a re-classification of these practices, a complete conceptual reordering, and not simply the replacement of one set of labels with another. With this in mind, let us consider some well-described practices from the literature and how they may be described and conceptualized alternatively using the framework proposed above.

Data from the social demographic surveys completed by a few thousand of the 20 million Yoruba people of southwestern Nigeria and reported on by Orubuyole, Caldwell, and Caldwell (2000) provide the basis for my first example. While the authors choose to focus on female genital modifications, the social demographic surveys whose results they are reporting include information about genitally modified males as well. Let us imagine a hypothetical pair of Yoruba brothers who are among the small percentage of these Yoruba respondents not genitally modified during the first week of their life. Upon reaching adulthood, they each elect a procedure that they call circumcision. When asked by researchers why, one explains that he was persuaded by the public health campaigns in Africa that promote circumcision as an anti-HIV measure, while the other explains that he felt somehow less Yoruba for being unmodified genitally, since every other Yoruba person with whom he has had occasion to discuss the matter have been so modified themselves and bewildered that he was not. The first of these would have to be described as a medical, adult, individually motivated modification that removed tissue by cutting, while the second would be an ethnic-identified, socially normative, adult, group motivated modification that removed tissue by cutting. Although the full complexity of their motives may not be captured by labeling in the fashion I have suggested, I hope my example demonstrates how conventional classifications that would not distinguish between two adult male Yoruba circumcisions risk obscuring the complexity inherent in these practices.

An example that diverges more radically from currently paradigmatic understandings of genital modification can be made of practices in the Nubian region of Sudan described by Janice Boddy (1989) in her in-depth ethnographic analysis of a gendered possession cult from that region. That Boddy requires chapters of a book to even begin explaining what these practices mean to the women of a village in northern Sudan speaks to the limits of any collective typology. Nevertheless, these practices can be briefly described for classificatory and comparative purposes using the categories I have explained: in terms of local meaning, these are fertility related and gender constituting, they take place during a locally recognized stage of childhood self-awareness, they are motivated by local, widely shared values that maintain that male genitals must be 'exposed' by cutting that removes tissue while female genitals must be 'concealed' by a combination of cutting that removes tissue and specific techniques of scar formation. In both of these examples, gender is a component of the descriptive classification because it is meaningful locally, not because it is an intrinsically meaningful distinction to make.

The normalization of male circumcision in Anglophone society was a necessary condition for the emergence of the paradigmatic gender distinction that characterizes European and descendant cultural, social, and political responses to African genital modification practices. I feel it fair to say that circumcision is afforded exceptional status in scientific medicine, especially in the United States. This feature has been described (Bell 2005; Sardi 2011) and criticized (Somerville 2000; Darby and Svoboda 2007), but conceptual alternatives are limited. My goal in proposing an alternative framework is to introduce the possibility for more radical rethinking of genital modification itself as a remarkable category of the human experience, rather than ordinary and extraordinary practices being defined by the sex of the body that bears them.

References

Ahmadu, F. 2000. "Rites and Wrongs: A Insider/Outsider Reflects on Power and Excision." In *Female "Circumcision" in Africa: Culture, Controversy, and Change*, edited by B. Shell-Duncan and Y. Hernlund. Boulder, CO: Lynne Reinner.

American Academy of Pediatrics. 2005. "AAP Publications Retired and Reaffirmed." *Pediatrics* 116 (3): 796.

American Academy of Pediatrics Committee on Fetus and Newborn. 1971. *Standards and Recommendation for Hospital Care of Newborn Infants*. 5th ed. Evanston, IL: American Academy of Pediatrics.

Bell, K. 2005. "Genital Cutting and Western Discourses on Sexuality." *Medical Anthropology Quarterly* 19 (2): 125–148.

Blank, S., M. Brady, E. Buerk, C. Waldemar, D. Diekema, A. Freedman, L. Maxwell, and S. Wegner. 2012. "Task Force on Circumcision: Circumcision Policy Statement." *Pediatrics* 130 (3): 585–586.

Boddy, J. 1989. *Wombs and Alien Spirits: Women, Men, and the Zār Cult in Northern Sudan*. Madison: University of Wisconsin Press.

Boyle, G. J., and G. Hill. 2011. "Sub-Saharan Randomised Clinical Trials into Male Circumcision and HIV Transmission: Methodological, Ethical, and Legal Concerns." *Journal of Law and Medicine* 19: 316–334.

Darby, R., and J. S. Svoboda. 2007. "A Rose by Any Other Name? Rethinking the Similarities and Differences Between Male and Female Genital Cutting." *Medical Anthropology Quarterly* 21 (3): 301–323.

Darby, R. J. 2005. *A Surgical Temptation: The Demonization of the Foreskin and the Rise of Male Circumcision in Britain*. Chicago, IL: University of Chicago Press.

de Vincenzi, I., and T. Mertens. 1994. "Male Circumcision: A Role in HIV Prevention?" *AIDS* 8 (2): 153–160.

Delaney, M. G. 1849. "Congenital Phimosis." *American Journal of the Medical Sciences* 18: 35–38.

Garenne, M. 2006. "Male Circumcision and HIV Control in Africa." *PLoS Med* 3 (1): e78.

Garenne, M. 2008. "Long-Term Population Effect of Male Circumcision in Generalized HIV Epidemics in Sub-Saharan Africa." *African Journal of AIDS Research* 7 (1): 1–8.

Glick, L. B. 2005. *Marked in Your Flesh: Circumcision from Ancient Judea to Modern America*. Oxford: Oxford University Press.

Glick, L. B. 2009. "Real Men: Foreskin Cutting and Male Identity in the Philippines." In *Circumcision and Human Rights*, edited by G. C. Denniston, F. M. Hodges, and M. F. Milos. Berlin: Springer.

Gollaher, D. L. 2000. *Circumcision: A History of the World's Most Controversial Surgery*. New York: Basic Books.

Green, F. J. 2005. "From Clitoridectomies to 'Designer Vaginas': The Medical Construction of Heteronormative Female Bodies and Sexuality Through Female Genital Cutting." *Sexualities, Evolution & Gender* 7 (2): 153–187.

Gruenbaum, E. 2001. *The Female Circumcision Controversy: An Anthropological Perspective*. Philadelphia: University of Pennsylvania Press.

Hale, S. 2005. "Colonial Discourse and Ethngoraphic Residuals: The 'Female Circumcision' Debate and the Politics of Knowledge." In *Female Circumcision and the Politics of Knowledge: African Women in Imperialist Discourse*, edited by O. Nnaemeka. Westport, CT: Praeger.

Hosken, F. P. 1995. *The Hosken Report: Genital and Sexual Mutilation of Females*. 4th revised ed. Lexington, MA: Women's International Network News.

Kandela, P. 1999. "Sketches From The Lancet: Clitoridectomy." *The Lancet* 353: 1453.

Kennedy, J. G. 1970. "Circumcision and Excision in Egyptian Nubia." *Man* 5 (2): 175–191.

Kleinman, A. 1995. *Writing at the Margin: Discourse Between Anthropology and Medicine*. Berkeley: University of California Press.

Kuhn, T. S. 1996. *The Structure of Scientific Revolutions*. 3rd ed. Chicago, IL: University of Chicago Press.

Lannon, C. M., A. G. D. Bailey, A. R. Fleischman, G. W. Kaplan, C. T. Shoemaker, J. T. Swanson, and D. Coustan. 1999. "American Academy of Pediatrics: Circumcision Policy Statement." *Pediatrics* 103 (1): 686–693.

Lie, R. K., and F. G. Miller. 2011. "What Counts as Reliable Evidence for Public Health Policy: The Case of Circumcision for Preventing HIV Infection." *BMC Medical Research Methodology* 11: 34.

Miner, H. 1942. "Songhoi Circumcision." *American Anthropologist* 44 (4): 621–637.

National Hospital Discharge Survey, National Center for Health Statistics, and Centers for Disease Control and Prevention. 2009. "Estimated Number of Male Newborn Infants, and Percent Circumcised During Birth Hospitalization, by Geographic Region and Race: United States, 1979–2008."

Ntozi, J. P. M. 1995. "The East Africa AIDS Epidemic and the Absence of Male Circumcision: What is the Link? Forum." *Health Transition Review* 5: 97–117.

Orubuloye, I. O., P. Caldwell, and J. Caldwell. 2000. "Female 'Circumcision' Among the Yoruba of Southwestern Nigeria: The Beginning of Change." In *Female "Circumcision" in Africa: Culture, Controversy, and Change*, edited by B. Shell-Duncan and Y. Hernlund. Boulder, CO: Lynne Rienner.

Rahman, A., and N. Toubia. 2000. *Female Genital Mutilation: A Guide to Laws and Policies Worldwide*. London: Zed.

Rogowska-Szadkowska, D. 2010. "Letter to the Editor: Is Adult Male Circumcision a Viable Public Health Strategy for HIV Prevention Outside Sub-Saharan Africa?." *AIDS Patient Care and STDs* 24 (12): 751–752.

Sardi, L. M. 2011. "The Male Neonatal Circumcision Debate: Social Movements, Sexual Citizenship, and Human Rights." *Societies Without Borders* 6 (3): 304–329.

Scheper-Hughes, N., and M. M. Lock. 1987. "The Mindful Body: A Prolegomenon to Future Work in Medical Anthropology." *Medical Anthropology Quarterly* 1 (1): 6–41.

Schultheiss, D., M. C. Truss, C. G. Stief, and U. Jonas. 1998. "Uncircumcision: A Historical Review of Preputial Restoration." *Plastic and Reconstructive Surgery* 101 (7): 1990–1998.

Shell-Duncan, B., and Y. Hernlund, eds. 2000. "Female 'Circumcision' in Africa: Dimensions of the Practice and Debates." In *Female "Circumcision" in Africa: Culture, Controversy, Change*. Boulder, CO: Lynne Reiner.

Shell-Duncan, B., W. O. Obiero, and L. A. Muruli. 2000. "Women Without Choices: The Debate Over Medicalization of Female Genital Cutting and Its Impact on a Northern Kenyan Community." In *Female "Circumcision" in Africa: Culture, Controversy, Change*, edited by B. Shell-Duncan and Y. Hernlund. Boulder, CO: Lynne Reinner.

Somerville, M. 2000. *The Ethical Canary: Science, Society and the Human Spirit*. Toronto: Viking.

Thomas, L. 2000. "'Ngaitana (I Will Circumcise Myself)': Lessons From the Colonial Campaigns to Ban Circumcision in Meru, Kenya." In *Female "Circumcision" in Africa: Culture, Controversy, Change*, edited by B. Shell-Duncan and Y. Hernlund. Boulder, CO: Lynne Reinner.

Thompson, H. C., L. R. King, E. Knox, and S. B. Korones. 1975. "Committee on Fetus and Newborn: Report of the Ad Hoc Task Force on Circumcision." *Pediatrics* 56 (4): 610–611.

Vale, V., and A. Juno. 1989. "Fakir Musafir." In *Modern Primitives: An Investigation of Contemporary Adornment and Ritual*, edited by V. Vale and A. Juno. San Francisco, CA: RE/Search.

Villa, E., and P. Grassivaro Gallo. 2006. "Psycholinguistic Approaches to Ritual Labia Minora Elongation Among the Baganda Women of Uganda." In *Bodliy Integrity and the Politics of Circumcision: Culture, Controversy, and Change*, edited by G. C. Denniston, P. Grassivaro Gallo, F. M. Hodges, M. F. Milos, and F. Viviani. Berlin: Springer.

Walley, C. J. 1997. "Searching for 'Voices': Feminism, Anthropology, and the Global Debate Over Female Genital Operations." *Cultural Anthropology* 12 (3): 405–438.

World Health Organization. 2000. "Fact Sheet No. 241 Female Genital Mutilation." Electronic document. Accessed May 3, 2004. http://www.who.int/mediacentre/factsheets/fs241/en/

Xu, F., L. E. Markowitz, M. R. Sternberg, and S. O. Aral. 2007. "Prevalence of Circumcision and Herpes Simplex Virus Type 2 Infection in Men in the United States: The National Health and Nutrition Examination Survey (NHANES), 1999–2004." *Sexually Transmitted Diseases* 34 (7): 479–484.

A reply to "Critiquing circumcision: in search of a new paradigm for conceptualizing genital modification"

Jennifer Coffman

James Madison University, Harrisonburg, VA, USA

This is a reply to:

Androus, Zachary T. 2013. "Critiquing circumcision: in search of a new paradigm for conceptualizing genital modification." *Global Discourse.* 3 (2): 266–280. http://dx.doi.org/10.1080/23269995.2013.813282

Genitals can indeed be fascinating, at least occasionally, as many of us know. Zachary Androus (2013) argues that some people's genitals (e.g., African girls/women) may be disproportionately fascinating to certain individuals or groups, while others' genitals (those of boys/men) undergo various modifications without much critical concern. He wants us to think about why that might be. Toward this end, he proposes a framework that, he says, will conceptualize and classify genital modifications globally while 'fore [going] both geography and gender in its descriptive analytics'. Despite the difficulty in achieving such a framework, which does not entirely succeed, I applaud the attempt to contribute to a more comprehensive record of current practices, as well as encouraging a more holistic approach to how and why individuals undertake genital modifications.

Androus summarizes his own critical position regarding genital modifications as being heavily influenced by his European parents who themselves came from a background in which circumcision was not practiced. Still, he describes popular 'Western' (which he locates culturally and geographically in 'European and descendant societies') sentiment as claiming that female genital modifications are without medical value and thus violate the rights of women and girls, whereas male circumcision is considered medically beneficial and therefore not a violation of rights. His concern is less that genital modifications occur, but rather why certain forms are prohibited by late twentieth/early twenty-first century versions of the repugnancy rule, while others are actively promoted by international health campaigns. Gender is an inevitable part of this answer, but Androus' suggested framework subsumes gender into the matrix of components that may help move some people away from the 'female genital mutilation' and 'circumcision for healthy males' dichotomy. He does this by proposing four major characteristics to map genital modifications: (1) the qualitative, self-reflective input of practitioners, or, as he says, 'the ways in which the practitioners themselves understand the meaning, motivation, consequence, and significance of the practice'; (2) the person's societal role and status or 'the developmental stage of the individual in terms of the local meaning that constitutes the first category'; (3) sociocentric and/or egocentric origins of the choice to modify or 'whether the modification is an expression of a widely shared group expectation or is an individually elected procedure'; and (4) the physical manifestation or extent of the modification. Providing details for each of these characteristics should enable readers to make sense of drivers such as 'esthetic values' and 'rites of passage', even though these are also classifications themselves that may bear the bias of the recorder of events. Still, it is unclear how these characteristics will then be sorted into a classification system, *per se*, instead of simply comprising a detailed – and no doubt very interesting – list of different individuals' experiences with genital modifications. If Androus can populate the system with examples and then rethink the utility of this system's approach, it may indeed prove to serve as a tool to summarize complex events, beliefs, values, and importantly, variety. His framework may also help make the various procedures lumped together as 'female genital mutilation' less stark and also highlight the questions about male circumcision that he and others (e.g., Sardi 2011) raise.

A bit of history provides some context about the inescapability of gender and geography. While female genital cutting became increasingly relevant in various parts of Europe because of colonial endeavors that began well over a century ago, the rise of the term 'female genital mutilation' coincided with the United Nations Decade for Women (1975–1985). Despite many practitioners' claims that genital modifications beautified and protected girls and women, making them socially safe and valuable, the United Nations adopted the term 'female genital mutilation' and crafted it as a human rights violation. Attendant global activist campaigns, oriented toward eradication and largely focused on Africans, maligned a variety of procedures as disfiguring and potentially life-threatening, even suggesting that such modifications were pursued with the *intention* to harm (Coffman 2007; Shell-Duncan and Hernlund 2000).

There has never been an equivalent campaign of moral outrage against 'male genital mutilation' – hence Androus' proposed classification system. Androus does not take a stand on whether genital modifications are inherently good or bad, but rather suggests that if someone wants to be critical about them, he or she must first be informed and, second, be careful about condemning or praising practices that occur among females, while ignoring practices that occur among males. After all, men are gendered, too. And, if gender can generally be perceived as a significant aspect of a person's role in a particular society where local constructions of gendered identities are culturally important, especially in societies in which popular culture indicates that gender may be achieved or enhanced via genital modification, then the proposed framework cannot escape gender. This by no means suggests there is only one way to be a Kono woman or Yoruba man, for example. Obviously, things change, procedures happen or do not happen at particular times in individuals' lives, and people move. And that moving part links us back to another significant factor: place.

The places where genital modifications are praised or condemned and how these practices are pursued or prohibited, and all in between, indicate that geographic contexts remain key to this new framework, too. Even if condemnation happens in the nebulous space of UN-based activism, the people who undergo or refuse genital modifications exist somewhere more locatable. Thus, the action of genital modification may bear different kinds of consequences based on state and/or local policies governing those inhabiting the geographic location in which the operation occurs. This, too, can be subsumed in the matrix Androus proposes, and thus can be accorded a less salient role than in the kinds of campaigns he critiques. This gets us closer to what Lyons (2007) suggests is a polythetic approach – one that complicates debates about why individuals pursue genital modifications and what sorts of implications such modifications may have. But, we must first see how this classification system gets implemented with real examples and to know when we as readers – and he as the designer – are satisfied that the system is comprehensive enough, at least for the moment.

To borrow from Clifford Geertz (1973, 30), when we look at the symbolic dimensions of social actions such as genital modifications, we do not 'turn away from the existential dilemmas of life for some empyrean realm of de-emotionalized forms; [we] plunge into the midst of them'. As Geertz goes on to note, our recording of procedures and narratives linked to them is an interpretive endeavor, but may not lead to satisfying answers to our deepest questions. Rather, we will 'make available to us answers that others… have given, and thus… include them in the consultable record of what [humans have] said' and done (Geertz, with some liberties, 1973, 30). From there, we may choose.

References

Androus, Zachary T. 2013. "Critiquing Circumcision: In Search of a New Paradigm for Conceptualizing Genital Modification." *Global Discourse* 3 (2): 266–280.

Coffman, Jennifer E. 2007. "Producing FGM in US Courts: Political Asylum in the Post-Kasinga Era." *Africa Today* 53 (4): 59–84.

Geertz, Clifford. 1973. *The Interpretation of Cultures: Selected Essays*. New York: Basic Books.

Lyons, Harriet. 2007. "Genital Cutting: The Past and Present of a Polythetic Category." *Africa Today* 53 (4): 3–17.

Sardi, Lauren M. 2011. "The Male Neonatal Circumcision Debate: Social Movements, Sexual Citizenship, and Human Rights." *Societies Without Borders* 6 (3): 304–329.

Shell-Duncan, Bettina, and Ylva Hernlund. 2000. "Female 'Circumcision' in Africa: Dimensions of the Practice and Debates." In *Female "Circumcision" in Africa: Culture, Controversy, and Change*, edited by Bettina Shell-Duncan and Ylva Hernlund, 1–40. London: Lynne Rienner.

New lives for old: modernity, biomedicine, traditional culture and HIV prevention in Lesotho

Nicola L. Bulled

Department of Anthropology, University of Connecticut, 354 Mansfield Road, U-1176, Storrs, CT 06269, USA

Traditional male circumcision practices have been strongly discouraged by HIV prevention campaigns in Lesotho. Traditional circumcision rituals are perceived as a possible transmission route for HIV because of the reuse of unsterilized cutting instruments. While individuals living in urban areas and the lowlands have increasingly considered traditional circumcision a practice of the past, foregoing the procedure all together, those dwelling in rural areas continue to consider the practice vital in the construction of male national identity. Initially, the national government voiced strong concern over the publicizing of medical male circumcision (MMC) – conducted by surgeons in sterile clinics. There have been claims that male circumcision (either traditional or MMC) does not have the same level of protective benefit against HIV in Lesotho that research suggests it has in other countries in the region. This article critically examines the development of government responses to international expectations on MMC scale-up. It also explores the impact of government responses on the attitudes of youth who serve to benefit most from such biomedical HIV prevention measures. Given the existing distinction between traditional practices and MMC, recent international calls for male circumcision in the region are positioned at the divides of modern/traditional, urban/rural, educated/ignorant, uninfected/infected.

Introduction

In 2006, the World Health Organization (WHO) released a statement acknowledging the demonstrated effects of MMC in reducing the risk of HIV infection in men in response to three randomized control trials conducted in the AIDS belt of Africa (Auvert et al. 2005; WHO 2006; Bailey et al. 2007; Gray et al. 2007). MMC as an HIV prevention strategy involves complete clinical removal of the foreskin from the head of the penis. It is believed that by removing the foreskin, HIV and other sexually transmitted pathogens are less likely to survive as there is no longer the warm, moist subpreputial space. Further, lesions and microtears in the mucosal surface of the inner foreskin, which allow pathogens through the physical skin barrier, no longer occur. Most importantly, the HIV target cells on the inner surface of the foreskin, which are highly susceptible to HIV infection, are removed (Patterson et al. 2002; McCoombe and Short 2006).

However, the WHO and UNAIDS warned that circumcision does not provide complete protection against HIV infection. Consequently, they called for the inclusion of MMC as part of a comprehensive prevention package to include behaviour change strategies of delayed onset of sexual relations, reduction in the number of sexual partners, correct and consistent use of male and female condoms, routine HIV screening and HIV treatment. At the time, the WHO and its international partners did not offer specific policy recommendations for governments and non-governmental institutions interested in expanding or promoting MMC. Rather they noted barriers to offering MMC more widely, including limitations in infrastructure, the need for well-trained practitioners and sanitary settings and the importance of developing procedures for informed consent and confidentiality. They emphasized the need for correct and continuing information dissemination to ensure individuals do not develop a false sense of security and consequently engage in high-risk behaviours, which negate the protective effects of male circumcision. They also stressed cultural sensitivity.

By 2007, the WHO had officially endorsed MMC as a strategy for HIV prevention. Together with UNAIDS and Jhpiego,[1] the WHO generated a procedural guide for performing MMC under local anaesthesia to ensure that resource-limited settings could continue to meet increases in local demand (WHO/UNAIDS/JHPIEGO 2007). Recent publications show that several countries in southern Africa, including Tanzania, Kenya, Zambia, Swaziland, Namibia, Botswana and Rwanda, are planning to or have introduced or expanded MMC programs. These expansions are heavily backed by international funding agencies including the US President's Emergency Plan for AIDS Relief (PEPFAR), the Agence Nationale de Recherche su la SIDA, the Bill and Melinda Gates Foundation, the US National Institutes of Health and the Global Fund.

According to the international HIV community, concerns about the cultural acceptability of MMC in Africa are unwarranted (Weiss et al. 2008). Thirteen acceptability studies from nine countries in sub-Saharan Africa have shown that approximately 62% (29–81%) of uncircumcised men wish to become circumcised, 50–79% of women favour circumcision for their partners and 50–90% of women would circumcise their sons (Westercamp and Bailey 2007). This data, however, does not indicate whether the desired circumcisions are MMC conducted in sterile clinics or traditional circumcisions conducted during initiation ceremonies, which have routinely been conducted by certain groups throughout Africa for centuries.

This article draws on ethnographic research conducted in the small southern African Kingdom of Lesotho to argue that current discourse on MMC highlights defined and established inequities in global power dynamics. In Lesotho, traditional male circumcision has and continues to be an important yet repeatedly challenged element in initiation rites (*lebollo*). Since the arrival of Christian missionaries in Lesotho in the 1800s, *lebollo* practices involving the circumcision of boys between the ages of 15 and 25 years have been discouraged. The advent of the AIDS era offered further cause to abandon the practice, given concerns that the reuse of unsterilized cutting instruments for initiation associated rituals, particularly male circumcision, contributes to HIV transmission. In recent years, increasing reports from neighbouring South Africa have made apparent the significant dangers associated with traditional circumcision practices. During the 2006–2007 initiation season, 27 initiates reportedly died in the Eastern Cape province (on the southern border of Lesotho), 63 underwent penile amputations and 562 were hospitalized (reported in Vincent 2008a). Certainly, individuals in Lesotho are not naïve to the risks associated with initiation-associated circumcisions, with individuals citing these risks as reasons for electing not to engage in *lebollo* practices. More recently, expectations of modernity have impacted the people of Lesotho, becoming a cultural factor in popular attitudes about *lebollo*-associated circumcision. As stated by a young fashionably dressed Masotho woman while we talked together with her German boyfriend in a chic café in the bordering South African town of Ladybrand, 'You can't put "From the Mountain" on your resume'.

Although the importance placed on *lebollo* practices, and the practice itself, have changed over time, *lebollo* is still considered by some to be vital in the construction of male national identity. Recent data suggest that over half of Basotho men self-identify as circumcised, with the vast majority of these circumcisions occurring during the traditional initiation process of *lebollo* (MoHSW 2009). The situation in Lesotho, therefore, presents a compelling and emblematic case study of the friction involved in incorporating global HIV directives such as MMC into local cultural contexts. In addition, unlike neighbouring South Africa, with its extensive and often conflicting racial/ethnic diversity and from where much of the circumcision literature has emerged, people in Lesotho share a single national identity, the Basotho. Consequently, conflicts between global and local discourse on male circumcision become more evident.

In this article, I trace the development of Lesotho government responses to international expectations on MMC. I explore the impact of these international expectations and local government responses on the attitudes of youth in Lesotho who serve to benefit most from HIV prevention measures such as MMC and conclude by offering possible combination approaches for making the best of the old in a world of the new. By examining current discourse surrounding male circumcision in Lesotho as it relates to international directives, this article looks beyond the content of informational health education messages to examine the ideological constructions of how biomedical knowledge is produced, circulated and received. In so doing, I draw on the theoretical perspective of biocommunicability (Briggs 2003; Briggs and Mantini-Briggs 2003; Briggs 2005; Briggs and Hallin 2007; Briggs and Nichter 2009; Briggs and Hallin 2010), which evolved from Foucauldian notions of governmentality and biopower. Anthropologist Charles Briggs (2005) notes that by examining how biomedical information flows from creators to consumers, the relationship between political economy and governmentality is exposed or the effects of global and local power dynamics are revealed.

Research site and methods

Formerly Basutoland, a protectorate of Britain, Lesotho gained independence in 1966 and is governed now by a constitutional monarch. Lesotho is small in size, about 30,000 square kilometres, 11,178 square miles, roughly the size of Belgium and completely surrounded by South Africa. It is a very mountainous country, with 77% of inhabitants living in rural areas, most of them concentrated in the 'lowlands', a narrow crescent of land lying along the western perimeter of the country. Adjacent to the lowlands to the east is the much larger yet sparsely populated 'mountain' zone.

Lesotho is one of the poorest nations in the world and, in 2011, ranked 160 out of 187 countries on the United Nations Development Program's Human Development Index (2011). More than 50% of Lesotho's rural inhabitants live in poverty (Rural Poverty Portal 2013). However, a growing middle class has been established following recent developments, which include increasing foreign investment in Lesotho's urban textile industries, rural dam projects and diamond mines (Foulo and Moleko 1995; DFID 2008). These developments have allowed a certain sector of the population, particularly those in urban areas, to engage with global media, purchase global commodities and identify with global cultural trends and understandings. According to the World Bank (2010), mobile cellular subscriptions in Lesotho have increased from 1.1 per 100 people in 2000 to 32.0 in 2009. Ownership of personal computers has increased from 0.1 to 0.3 per 100 people in the same time period, and the per cent of households with television sets increased from 12% to 13%. This industrial growth and development and increasing incorporation in the global market have made Lesotho one of the most unequal nations in the world with a Gini index of 63.2 (CIA 2010).

Economic inequality significantly contributes to the local HIV epidemic. Currently, Lesotho has the third highest prevalence of adult HIV/AIDS in the world (23.3% of people aged 15–49 years) behind Botswana (24.1%) and Swaziland (33.4%) (UNAIDS 2010). While the population annual growth rate averaged 2.2% from 1970 to 1990, it has dropped to 0.08% since that time (WHO 2009a). Life expectancy has fallen to 45 years, 21 years less than what it would have been without AIDS (Hassan and Ojo 2002), and 58% of the population is under the age of 19. Immediate factors contributing to infection include unsafe heterosexual intercourse and mother-to-child transmission (NAC 2009). Underlying structural causes include both economic and gender inequality and migratory labour practices, which have contributed to social dislocation (World Bank 2000; WHO 2005).

To explore the impact of global HIV directives on local knowledge, explanatory accounts and practices of youth in Lesotho, I conducted a 15-month multi-sited, multi-method ethnographic study of students attending classes at the Lesotho College of Education between the years 2010 and 2012. The Lesotho College of Education (LCE) is the only tertiary level education facility in Lesotho offering a diploma in education. Approximately 5000 students from the 10 national districts of Lesotho come to LCE for a 3-year teacher certification programme, receiving a government bursary to cover tuition and living expenses. The majority of students self-identify as originating from a rural area; many have never ventured to the country's capital city Maseru before registration and orientation. Females comprise the majority of the student population. The median age of students is 23 years.

Research methods included ethnographic observations and interviews with students at both the urban Maseru campus and a satellite campus in the mountain town of Thaba-Tseka. Ethnographic examination of students (aged 18–26 years) focused on factors impacting HIV risk, including exposure to different sources of information that offer norms of sexual behaviour impacting HIV risk (i.e., religious leaders, teachers, health personal, peers, sexual partners, media), engagement with industries of modernity (i.e., television, magazines, music, the Internet, fashion), social environments (i.e., curfews, restrictions on who might visit your room, access to sexual partners), and socioeconomic status (i.e., family assets and household cooking, water and ablution facilities). Students were asked about their own HIV risk by soliciting certain details of current and past romantic and sexual relationships, sexual behaviours and risk reduction strategies.

Ethnographic material was augmented by examination of HIV policy documents and discussions with local HIV stakeholders, health care providers and traditional healers. In addition, newsprint text of the two largest local newspapers from the past decade offered insight on local HIV discourse. Analysis included any news article, feature, editorial, column or opinion piece with the words HIV or AIDS in the headline or with a central focus on HIV/AIDS, published between January 2000 and May 2011. The total number of articles included in the analysis amounted to 320 of various lengths. The articles were reviewed, and those specifically addressing 'culture', population segments at risk of HIV infection, knowledge or education were coded using the same codebook established for analysis of student interviews.

Government negotiations with traditional and modern circumcision practices

To date, national guidelines on male circumcision (MMC or *lebollo*-based) in Lesotho have not been finalized or released. Neighbouring South Africa released the Application of Health Standards in Traditional Circumcision Act No. 6 of 2001 in an effort to monitor traditional circumcision ceremonies. However, *lebollo*-based practices in Lesotho have not been regulated. International directives on MMC have only been released in recent years, requiring the national government to consider modern biomedical strategies for male circumcision.

The national government references a number of concerns as reasons for their delay in developing a national male circumcision policy. These include practical concerns over the implementation of new modern biomedical strategies such as funding limitations and infrastructural weakness, as well as potential conflicts arising from an increase in the monitoring of traditional strategies to ensure they comply with modern standards (see Vincent 2008b for a discussion of the outcry about regulation). In addition, they have argued that there is no evidence to suggest that male circumcision (either MMC or traditional) is an effective HIV prevention strategy in Lesotho. MMC and traditional circumcision are viewed by the lay-public as synonymous practices further complicating policy development efforts. Ministry of Health and Social Welfare (MoHSW) officials have noted that a semantic distinction needs to be made between '*lebollo*-based circumcision' and 'clinic-based foreskin removal', yet currently no such distinction has been made publicly.

In what follows, I examine the Lesotho government's concerns regarding the development of official male circumcision policy. I also examine why the government may be unwilling to put forward a sharp distinction between MMC (as an HIV risk reduction surgery, foreskin removal or 'new circumcision') and initiation-embedded circumcision to endorse male circumcision as a health promotion without either criticizing or embracing lay practices.

The current public confusion around MMC and *lebollo*-based circumcision is evident in a newspaper article published in a popular national newspaper in 2009. In the article, a speech by Chief Advocate Borenahaborkhete Sekonyela given in 2007 is cited to offer clarification between *lebollo*-based circumcision and MMC practices. Sekonyela is quoted as saying:

> We have initiation schools which have existed from time immemorial. They are meant to socialize the young men and women who are about to graduate from teenage years into facets of adulthood or adult life. It is a process which builds a complete human being with values and deep morals. But unfortunately the term *lebollo* has been misused and misunderstood to refer to the surgical part done in hospitals. That is not *lebollo*. (Nyaka 2009, 3)

Advocate Sekonyela argues that there has been a misapplication of the rich cultural term, *lebollo*, which is inappropriately used to imply 'circumcision', rather than an initiation rite. However, the article's author further states, 'under Sesotho customs and traditions there was no circumcision' (Nyaka 2009, 3) as part of *lebollo* practices. This claim is inaccurate. Both self-reported and visual medical examination data, as well as ethnographic documentation of initiation rites in the region, suggest that circumcision, partial or complete removal of the foreskin, has been a principal component of *lebollo* practices in Lesotho.

The primary reason for delaying official national policy is the government claim that there is no evidence to suggest that male circumcision is protective against HIV infection in Lesotho. The Lesotho Demographic and Health survey (DHS) notes that the relationship between *self-reported* male circumcision and HIV 'does not conform to the expected pattern of higher prevalence among uncircumcised men' (2009, 212). HIV prevalence is in fact higher in circumcised men than in uncircumcised men (21% compared to 16%). However, the DHS data do not account for distinctions in type of circumcision performed (traditional *lebollo* or MMC), and visual confirmation of circumcision status is not obtained.

One possible explanation for the contradictory pattern between male circumcision and HIV in Lesotho is the age at which circumcision is performed in Lesotho. Traditional circumcision occurs after sexual debut (average in Lesotho is 15 years). Young men may have been exposed to HIV before circumcision. Should some initiation candidates be infected with HIV before circumcision, they risk transmitting infection to their fellow initiates should traditional healers not use sterile instruments or procedures to perform the surgery (see Brewer et al. 2007). This was noted by Mathoriso Monaheng (Staff reporter 2003, 10), former Director of Administration at the Lesotho AIDS Program Coordinating Agency, who argued that 'the problem [of initiation rites] is that they are using one knife to circumcise boys, that knife is used by everybody'. However, warnings of the dangers of sharing cutting instruments have compelled people to supply their own sterile razor blades when seeking health care from traditional healers. It is likely that initiation candidates currently do the same.

The Lesotho government further argues that cost and limitations in infrastructure have further halted a full scale-up of MMC initiatives. The MoHSW is only considering clinic-based circumcision surgeries performed by trained surgeons. The national guidelines (not yet finalized or released) stipulate that the 'sleeve/dorsal slit method' is the standard method for MMC in Lesotho. Of the three methods, forceps guided, dorsal slit and sleeve, sleeve is considered the most difficult followed by dorsal slit. Forceps guided is considered the easiest method, which can be performed by trained health professionals (nurses or even traditional healers) and need not be performed by surgeons.

In addition, with 50% of men already circumcised (mostly through traditional methods), mathematical models that suggest increasing the proportion of men circumcised to the level of 80% may only reduce the population prevalence of HIV slightly and only if male circumcision remains consistently high (Gray et al. 2003; Williams et al. 2006; Nagelkerke et al. 2007). The estimated cost of scaling-up MMC to achieve a level that would effectively reduce HIV prevalence is 125 million LSL (15 million USD), an annual cost of 10 million LSL (1.22 million USD) (MoHSW 2008). Scale-up of such a magnitude would, it is estimated, prevent one HIV infection for every 6.1 individuals circumcised. It would also save 2136 LSL ($262 USD) per individual infection averted in life-long antiretroviral treatments and other prevention measures (USAID 2007). Lesotho currently does not have a sufficient number of surgeons to perform MMC and have few health care facilities in rural areas with the capacity for performing sterile surgical procedures.

The MoHSW has argued that in addition to barriers offered by limited funding and infrastructure, culture has been an obstacle to developing a national male circumcision policy that would involve the support and implementation of MMC services. In 2009, the Director General of Health, Dr. Mpolai Moteetee, was quoted in a newspaper article titled *Health Ministry has no intention of campaigning for circumcision* arguing that 'circumcising young children [neonatal circumcision] is against the Basotho culture' (Linake 2009, 8). Her statement suggests that circumcision still serves as a marker of manhood to be performed during adolescence, thus an important part of cultural and individual identity.

According to the MoHSW, disagreements with traditional healers have further limited progress. While the MoHSW neither regulates nor supports the circumcision procedures performed during initiation, they have suggested the implementation of standardized certification requirements for all traditional healers perhaps in an effort to more closely monitor *lebollo* circumcision practices (Linake 2010). Traditional healers argue that they have been appointed by the forefathers and consequently require no certification from the government. By supporting the most difficult method of MMC, the MoHSW will remove any possibility that traditional healers could perform government-supported safe and effective circumcision surgeries as part of initiation rites even with government sponsored training. This may result in a significant reduction in clientele for traditional healers who perform circumcisions as a livelihood.

Despite these limitations and objections towards male circumcision (traditional and MMC), private, non-governmental and even government efforts are being made to appeal to international directives on HIV prevention measures. In 2007, a male clinic was established in Lesotho's capital city, Maseru, run by the Lesotho Planned Parenthood Association. According to Programme Officer Tefo Lephowa, 240 men, aged 17 and above, undergo MMC at the clinic every month (Matope 2010). Demand has continued to increase to the point where men are placed on an ever expanding waiting list (personal communication). Beginning in 2012, international organizations (funded by PEPFAR, with the operational assistance of Jhpiego) will provide six international medical doctors whose sole duties will be to perform MMC (personal communication with John Nkonyana [MoHSW] and Todd Koppenhaver [PEPFAR]). The non-governmental organization Population Services International (PSI) is also launching an MMC effort in collaboration with the Lesotho Defence Force (personal communications with PSI/Lesotho Director Dennis Walto and Technical Services Advisor Brian Pedersen). These efforts are not attempts to scale-up services to the level of 50% or 80% population coverage necessary to reduce the population prevalence of HIV. Rather they are efforts to reduce the backlog of increasing demand. This strategy will be in place for 2 years at which time a new plan will be developed.

The concerns raised by the Lesotho government over developing national policies for male circumcision position the issue of male circumcision at the divide between modern and traditional. The international community supports new sanitary methods for male circumcision that are 'safe and proper' and to take place in *modern* hospitals. This, by implication, is in opposition to the unsafe and improper circumcisions that take place at *traditional* initiation schools (Vincent 2008a, 81). By supporting MMC, the government might be seen as undermining long practiced traditions. Since the influx of Christian missionaries in the 1800s, followed later by colonists, and now development workers, public health strategists and global media, the tradition has increasingly been linked with savagery, irrationality, superstition and outdated dangerous beliefs. Traditional practices are positioned in stark contrast to the progressive, civilized and sanitary practice of the modern.

An old cultural practice in decline

Historical ethnographic analyses conducted in sub-Saharan Africa suggest that male circumcision is an ancient practice among Bantu speakers. Theorists posit that male circumcision is performed in celebration of cultural particularity, group membership and ethical duties. Given that the practice is performed anywhere from infancy to adulthood, Paige and Paige (1981) have argued that male circumcision is a way for fathers to demonstrate their allegiance to a family, clan or village – the fraternal interest group theory. Circumcision ceremonies occur at a time when the father's political and military potential becomes a source of concern to his lineage. A father demonstrates his group loyalty by submitting his son to initiation, knowing the brutality of the acts his son will have to undergo, including circumcision, which can result in infection, castration and even death (Paige and Paige 1981). Turner argued that rituals such as initiation rites act as a 'social glue', 'compensat[ing] to some extent for the limited range of effective political control and for the instability of kinship and affinal ties to which political value is attached' (1957, 291).

Particularly, important elements of traditional circumcision include the pain, suffering and danger involved in performing surgery in non-sterile conditions without anaesthetic. Enduring the perils of the ritual in addition to the other demanding aspects of initiation demonstrates manhood, fitness and respect for communal ties. Ethnographies conducted in southern Africa during the first half of the twentieth century, before the global spread of HIV, reveal that initiations generally involve three phases (see Wagner 1949; Junod 1962; Estermann 1979). Using the terms offered by van Gennep (1909), these can be divided into separation rites, marginal rites and aggregation rites. The first phase involves physical withdrawal from society. The initiation candidates are taken away from their homes and villages to a secluded location, symbolically leaving behind their former social status. The end of this phase is marked with the act of circumcision. Former South African President Nelson Mandela recalls in his autobiography, *Long Walk to Freedom*, his circumcision experience at the age of 16 years, lined up with other boys:

> Before I knew it, the old man was kneeling in front of me [...] his hands moved so fast they seemed to be controlled by an otherworldly force. Without a word, he took my foreskin, pulled it forward, and then, in a single motion, brought down his assegai [spear]. I felt as if fire were shooting through my veins; the pain was so intense that I buried my chin in my chest. Many seconds seemed to pass before I remembered the cry, and then I recovered and called out, '*Ndiyindoda!*' (I am a man!). (Mandela 1994, 32)

The second phase involves a period of seclusion and 'marginality' in the sense that initiates are removed from society and stoically endure the pain associated with circumcision. During this time, they are also instructed in both practical and theoretical knowledge. They undergo physical hardship including nakedness in the cold winter months, beatings, starvation, torture and harassment and surviving the pain and possible complications of the healing circumcision. The initiates are forbidden to escape under penalty of death or social ostracism. They prove their emotional strength through tests of memorization and sleep deprivation. The final phase is associated with the candidates returning to society in their new status. This may involve great festivities and celebration. In some cases, the lodge where the initiation rites took place is burnt, along with all the old possession of the initiates. The duration of these initiation rites can vary from a few weeks to many months. In essence, traditional circumcision is not simply about the removal of a piece of skin and, therefore, cannot easily be replaced by MMC.

While ethnographic accounts suggest that initiation rites involve generally the same elements, circumcision practices vary considerably in the region. In some groups, circumcision as a part of initiation rites has even been abandoned and replaced by ritualistic cuts. Other groups, communities, families or individuals have completely abandoned the practice of traditional initiation. The Zulus of South Africa abandoned the practice during the reign of King Shaka as all boys of initiation age were needed for military service. It was believed that 10 years of military service was sufficient to prove loyalty to their chief. Other groups likely abandoned the practice of circumcision or initiation as a consequence of modernizing Western influences (Wagner 1949; Marck 1997) including the rise in cultural value placed on individual agency.

Recent data from Lesotho indicates that circumcision as an element of initiation rites may have been modified to accommodate new situations and circumstances including reduced demand or interest in initiation practices. A study conducted among a sample of young adult men undergoing physical examinations during the Lesotho Defence Force recruitment process found that of the individuals self-reporting circumcision by initiation, only 28% had complete foreskin removal (Thomas et al. 2011). Almost half (42%) had no foreskin removed. In comparison, of those recruits circumcised by medical personnel, 73% had complete circumcisions.[2]

The mystery that still enshrouds initiation rites in Lesotho contributes to often contradictory local opinions of the practice. Although some cheer for the boys arriving back from initiation school, smeared with dirt and wrapped in blankets as they are driven in trucks through the capital city, others cluck their tongues, jeer and shake their heads. Few men will admit to attending initiation school and none will reveal the details of what occurs during their time in seclusion. Men who elect not to attend initiation school often cite fear of the unknown as their rationale. Others explain that in contemporary society, one cannot afford to spend 6 months (the standard time of contemporary ceremonies) away from formal education or employment. Some explain that their family could not afford to pay the initiator's fees or associated expenses such as a blanket, food and new clothing for when one emerges.[3] Still others argue that initiation rites are contrary to their religious doctrine or that initiation rites are the practices of people who are neither educated nor modern. Before Christian missionary introductions of schools, education took place during initiation, which served as an important marker in the passage to adulthood. Missionaries objected to initiation rites, citing it as a backwards and ungodly practice, so it, and consequently circumcision, became rare during colonial years except among a certain clan, the *Tlokoa*, in the mountains (Magubane 1998).

Currently in Lesotho, 52% of Basotho men self-identify as circumcised, with 90% of these occurring during the traditional initiation process of *lebollo* (MoHSW 2009). According to the recent Demographic and Health survey (MoHSW 2009), self-reported circumcisions, and thus attendance at initiation schools, vary with regards to dwelling area, education level and socioeconomic status. Men living in rural areas (59% rural versus 34% in urban), those with less education (79% of those who had never been to school versus 24% and 26% of those who had completed primary or secondary school, respectively) and lower economic status (74% lowest wealth quintile versus 29% highest) were more likely to report circumcision. These statistics indicate that while traditional circumcision remains an important marker of male individual or collective identity in certain sectors of the population, its significance as a cultural practice is declining in others.

Recent literature from the region suggests that male circumcision conducted as part of traditional initiation rites is a way for youth to claim an identity to transition from boy to man. Stevens and Lockhat argue that the democratic era in southern Africa has forced black youth to shift their identities to accommodate to rapidly globalizing economic markets, noting that 'new role models, economic structures and dominance of western ideologies [...] have now encouraged an ideological shift from collectivism to individualism' (1997, 253). The transition has been easier for some than others. For those marginalized by rapid social change, the stability offered by centuries of tradition may provide protection from uncertainty and loss of status. As noted by Vincent among the Xhosa in South Africa, 'Far from being regarded as an outdated relic, it is often youth – frequently marginalized urban youth, in search of stable identities in troubled times – who insist on ritual circumcision in the face of opposition from parents, elders and guardians' (2008, 90).

While urban youth in neighbouring South Africa may continue to feel politically and economically marginalized even in the post-apartheid era, turning to traditional circumcision as a way of gaining status (Vincent 2008b), this is not clearly the case in Lesotho.

Youth in urban areas with higher levels of education and employment potentials hold superior social positions as manhood is increasingly demonstrated through advancement in education, career success and even by having many sexual partners as proof of virility. In addition, increases in urbanization and modernization in Lesotho have weakened clan ties and consequently the need for fathers to demonstrate clan affiliation by sending their sons to *lebollo* ceremonies. Many youth in Lesotho justify their lack of circumcision in terms of their father's lack of circumcision.

The rise of a new modern approach

Urban men and boys may elect instead to be circumcised in modern biomedical clinics. Modern biomedical MMC is performed in government health facilities, hospitals, filter clinics or private surgeries at a cost that varies from 50 to 600 LSL (6–74 USD). Only medical doctors are authorized to perform MMC in Lesotho. According to a recent assessment of male circumcision, approximately 4000–6000 MMC are performed each year (MoHSW 2008). Rural health facilities have neither the facilities nor the personnel to perform circumcision surgeries even if there was demand. Further, the costs of MMC remain prohibitive for many individuals, especially those in rural areas who are not engaged in the formal economy and have the additional expense of travelling to a service facility.

The majority of clients seeking services are adult men (60%) in urban areas. Men seeking MMC do so for varied reasons. Some cite the perceived health benefits of reduced sexually transmitted infections and HIV prevention. Others, generally the younger men aged 17–20 years, have been forced to undergo MMC by their parents. Given the age of the boys, one can assume that MMC may have replaced *lebollo* practices as a marker of manhood for modern urban dwelling individuals.

Unclear government directives regarding MMC as an HIV prevention strategy have resulted in growing speculation and considerable confusion among youth. I asked 556 students whether 'A circumcised man's chances of getting HIV from occasional exposure through unprotected sex are lower than a man who has never been circumcised'.[4] One third disagreed. Many students are not aware that circumcision can be performed in a clinic-based setting as they are only familiar with *lebollo*-based circumcision. As noted previously, 'circumcision' and 'initiation' are synonymous terms among lay-people in Lesotho. Some students did clarify that if a man were circumcised in a clinic, his chances of HIV infection declined, while if circumcised during initiation, his risk of HIV increased. However, still others noted that only if the clinic used a new sterile blade to perform the surgery would risk of HIV infection not increase during circumcision. Few students, even those who had undergone MMC, clearly understood that by removing the foreskin, risk of HIV infection is reduced.

Take, for example, the following student responses to my question regarding male circumcision and HIV risk:

> Student 1: No, I do not believe. Because if you are circumcised or if someone is not circumcised and you have sex with someone who is HIV positive both of them not using condoms, both of them are going to contract HIV. It does not matter whether you are circumcised or not (female, Maseru campus, urban, 21 years).
>
> Student 2: I don't think it is 100% safe. I think that whether or not he is circumcised he will still get HIV. I saw them at my place, died because of HIV, even if they come from circumcision. I mean traditional, I don't know those from hospitals (female, Maseru campus, rural, 26 years).

> Student 3: I am not sure. Is it true that when a male is circumcised he has a less chance of being infected? That I am not quite sure of (male, Maseru campus, urban, 24 years).

Male circumcision performed as part of *lebollo* practices is considered by many as a risky behaviour. Though few students knew the particulars of *lebollo* or the associated circumcision ceremony having not attended themselves, most were aware of the educational messages warning of the sharing of cutting instruments. This is clear in the statements of two female students: 'We don't know what is happening there. We don't know if they are using different blades (at the initiation schools)'; 'In the Basotho culture, where people go for initiation and they are circumcised. I don't really know what happens in the process of circumcision, if they use one blade or they use different blades. If they use only one blade that means there is transmission of AIDS there'.

Being students at a tertiary level education institution, they perceive themselves as engaged in a rapidly modernizing world. Their education status separates them from the individuals who engage in initiation rites or those who practice 'Basotho culture'. This distinction is clearly evident in a situation that caused much concern among a collection of traditional healers serving as cultural representatives. A school principal refused to allow entry to young boys returning from their initiation ceremonies. The initiates had missed months of schooling while away in 'the mountains'. The principal claimed that the boys had missed too much schooling and were too far behind the other students to be readmitted. Although not specifically stated by the school principal, the traditional healers in meetings with the concerned parents and in speaking with the school board on the parents' behalf suggested that the principal believed formal education in schools and traditional education during initiation were at odds. In returning from 'the mountains', the boys were anticipated to be violent, aggressive and no longer possessing the restraint necessary for formal schooling.

The continued practice of Basotho customs and traditions including belief in the virgin cure, witchcraft, lack of condom use, consultations with traditional healers and finally engagement in initiation rites is linked to individuals residing in rural areas. Rural dwelling individuals are also perceived to have lower levels of education, including awareness and basic knowledge of HIV, given their limited access to media (television, newspapers, radio and Internet) and health facilities. Notes a male student, 'Rural dwelling people are uneducated because most still hold cultural beliefs. They are sent to circumcision schools in the mountains. When they come back they should marry each other and work in the fields'. The students attending LCE are living in a world that no longer practices traditional cultural rites, particularly those that the international community has identified as increasing risk of HIV transmission.

National data support youth perceptions that individuals who are less educated are less aware of HIV and HIV transmission routes and that these individuals live in the rural mountainous areas (MoHSW 2009). Men and women with no education are least likely to have comprehensive knowledge of HIV (13% and 25%, respectively) as compared to individuals with education beyond primary school (49%).[5] Further, the proportion of men who recognized that HIV could be prevented by using a condom when having sexual intercourse was lowest among men from mountain regions (68%) as compared to men in the lowlands where most urban centres are located (86%). Despite data indicating that individuals in rural areas have reduced knowledge of HIV and continue to engage in cultural practices that are considered locally to place them at risk for HIV (i.e., circumcision by traditional healers), cases of HIV infection are proportionally lower among individuals in rural areas (21% compared to 27%).

Higher rates of HIV in urban areas suggest that conditions in the urban space drive greater involvement in HIV risk behaviours (i.e., multiple sex partners, transactional sex, inter-generational sex). In addition, it may indicate that traditionally performed circumcisions are actually protective against HIV for men in rural areas, though data collected to date is too limited to tease out any rural/urban distinction. Nevertheless, the fundamental failure of Lesotho government agents and the local HIV community to conduct the cultural work necessary to introduce a new public health intervention has made youth unaware of the function of male circumcision as an HIV prevention strategy. Vincent (2008a, 433) notes that, 'campaigns for circumcision aimed at curbing HIV can be very confusing because they are layered onto other messages – of abstinence, sexual restraint and sexual responsibility on one hand, and the rights and privileges that go along with [...] manhood on the other'. Consequently, international debates about MMC versus traditional circumcision are positioned at the divides of modern/traditional, educated/ignorant, urban/rural and uninfected/infected. For urban youth in Lesotho, MMC circumcision has little if any significance; it is regarded merely as a modernization and sterilization of traditional Basotho culture.

A view to combining traditional and modern strategies

Lebollo practices continue to serve an important role in the maintenance of social structures and national identities among a significant portion of Basotho society. As circumcision is an integral part of local initiation rites, alternative local strategies could be considered and implemented that combine the strengths of biomedicine (objectivity) with the continued relevance of *lebollo* (subjectivity).

In meetings with traditional healers, initiation instructors and others involved in the preservation and revitalization of Basotho culture, two possible compromise solutions were offered. First, though perhaps the less popular option, initiation candidates could schedule their MMC before attending initiation schools. This medicalized approach has been adopted in some communities in Zimbabwe (Harmon 2011), South Africa (Vincent 2008b) and Kenya (WHO 2009b). Alternatively, male medical doctors and nurses could attend the initiation ceremonies to conduct the circumcision. In this way, the initiates receive safe, sterile and complete surgeries that are integrated into the *lebollo* practice.

Second, traditional healers could receive training on how to perform appropriate and effective circumcision surgeries that would offer protection against HIV. This approach has been implemented in the Eastern Cape Province of South Africa (Kanta 2004), following the Application of Health Standards in Traditional Circumcision Act No. 6 of 2001. The law stipulates that circumcision instruments must be approved, sterilized, and used only one time. Permission must be obtained from a health officer to hold an initiation/circumcision school, and health officers have the right to inspect any initiation ritual. Evaluation of the trainings found significant improvements in knowledge related to sexually transmitted infections and HIV, circumcision practice and abnormal anatomy, and attitudes towards collaborations with biomedical health care providers (Peltzer et al. 2008). Traditional healers in Lesotho view this approach as more empowering as it ensures that (1) an important cultural practice is maintained; (2) practices of traditional healers do not contribute to the transmission of HIV and (3) traditional healers will perform a service that offers some protection to the people of Lesotho.

Traditional healers believe that the MoHSW inappropriately claim that 'culture' is a barrier to the scale-up of MMC services. They view such individuals as vilifying *lebollo* practices and denying their nation's culture. Vincent argues that traditional healers, or other community leaders involved in the preservation of traditional culture, resist 'the intrusion of state influence into a domain where some of the poorest and most marginalized in the society seek to maintain a limited hold on power' (2008, 87). She suggests that such individuals have limited marketable skills and opportunities for the assertion of power or status. As the region becomes more integrated into global markets, these individuals do not have ready access to any other currency or currency which they can readily covert into the coinage of the modern liberal capitalist order (2008, 89). Consequently, 'tradition' is viewed as a limited currency with which to trade for power and one that state regulations risk further devaluing.

Conclusion

In Lesotho, two circumcision practices exist side-by-side. Though waning as a practice, rural men continue to undergo circumcision through traditional *lebollo* ceremonies. Men in urban areas have either elected not to be circumcised or are circumcised in modern MMC facilities. The Lesotho government has remained essentially silent on the issue of male circumcision as an HIV prevention strategy. Though government sponsored educational campaigns have communicated the risk of traditional circumcision in transmitting HIV, *lebollo* ceremonies and the traditional healers or initiators involved in such ceremonies are not regulated. Furthermore, other than defining which type of MMC surgery can be performed in Lesotho, the government has resisted international directives calling for the scale-up of MMC services, offering neither support nor hindrance to non-government and private attempts to offer such services.

The government may not have wanted to support either traditional or modern circumcision practices for two primary reasons. First, collaborations with *lebollo* instructors and traditional healers could suggest the government of Lesotho supports traditional cultural practice. For years, government officials in Lesotho and elsewhere in Africa have distanced themselves from such traditions in an attempt to identifying themselves and their countries as modern, democratic and capitalist. Second, given the considerable objection raised in South Africa to government regulation of traditional circumcision practices, the Lesotho government's unwillingness to publicly announce their decisions about circumcision may have been a political step given that national elections were held in early 2012.

As indicated by data gathered from youth, the silence has resulted in considerable local confusion. Traditional and clinic-based circumcisions are viewed as one and the same, having no association with HIV other than increasing the risk of infection if unsterilized cutting instruments are used. Consequently, what could potentially be an effective public health intervention is mired in discourse pitting global-modern against local-traditional.

In Lesotho, the cultural practice of *lebollo*-based circumcision is in decline largely as a consequence of modern influences. The link between HIV and male circumcision has further stimulated interest in replacing traditional practices with modern methods. By presenting the debate as a modern value system clashing with a traditional is at risk of suggesting that cultural practices are pristine and static, contaminated by outside interference. With biomedical HIV directives largely produced by international agencies that have the financial capacity to ensure their directives are implemented, HIV prevention strategies such as MMC can be viewed as the 'contaminating outside interference'.

Calls for MMC place male circumcision, a practice routinely conducted during traditional ceremonies in the bush or mountains, within the restricted purview of the modern biomedical community. Biomedicine has justified its need to oversee and control life events, such as male circumcision, by grounding itself in science wherein knowledge about the body and disease is systematized and objective. As Foucault (1973, 54) argued, medicine 'assumes a normative posture, which authorizes it not only to distribute advice as to a healthy life, but also to dictate the standards for physical and moral relations of the individual and of the society in which he lives'. Observations and causative experimentation based on germ theory and employing gold standard randomized control trials provide the evidence needed to rationalize surgical removal of foreskin from every boy and man in the AIDS belt. By employing statistical surveys, biomedicine has defined 'healthy' and 'pathology' relative to an act that continues to hold significant meaning. Notes Vincent (2008a, 81), 'doctors and hospitals are one of the primary mechanisms through which certain practices are authorized and rendered legitimate while others are marginalized and rendered illegitimate'. Poor and marginalized individuals, particularly those who are not integrated into the global system from which directives come, may turn to traditions as a way of gaining or maintaining social standing in the local community.

However, with appropriate communication strategies, cultural work and collaborations within specific cultural contexts, HIV prevention strategies such as MMC do not need to be positioned at a divide between the modern and traditional, global and local. The strengths of one can be used to enhance the other by incorporating rather than isolating strategies. By so doing, cultural identities and traditions become dynamic as the 'old' can be deconstructed and reconstructed in 'new' forms.

Notes

1. Founded as The Johns Hopkins Programme for International Education in Gynaecology and Obstetrics in 1974, Jhpiego is an independent organization affiliated with Johns Hopkins University providing technical support, training and policy guidance on matters related to reproductive health.
2. This is a troubling statistic as it suggests that even clinic-based circumcision surgeries often are not done in a manner that will afford protection from HIV. Note, however, that the question did not ask if the circumcision was performed in a clinic, but rather phrased in terms of who performed the circumcision. Misunderstanding or differences in definitions whereby a traditional healer may be considered medical personnel may account for some, though likely not all, of the incomplete circumcisions.
3. A local traditional healer, Liao, contradicts this point, saying that no set fees are established, rather individuals and families donate to a central fund (personal communication).
4. This question did not specify between MMC and *lebollo*-associated circumcision as if the foreskin is completely removed using sterile instruments, either practice should theoretically afford the individual protection from HIV.
5. Comprehensive knowledge means knowing that consistent use of condoms during sexual intercourse and having just one uninfected faithful partner can reduce risk of HIV infection, knowing that a healthy-looking person can have HIV and rejecting the two most common local misconceptions about HIV transmission – that HIV can be transmitted by mosquito bites and a person can become infected by sharing food with an HIV positive individual.

References

Auvert, B., D. Taljaard, E. Lagarde, J. Sobngwi-Tambekou, R. Sitta, and A. Puren. 2005. "Randomized, Controlled Intervention Trial of Male Circumcision for Reduction of HIV Infection Risk: The ANRS 1265 Trial." *PLoS Medicine* 2 (11): e298.

Bailey, R. C., S. Moses, C. B. Parker, K. Agot, I. Maclean, J. N. Krieger, C. F. Williams, R. T. Campbell, and J. O. Ndinya-Achola. 2007. "Male Circumcision for HIV Prevention in Young Men in Kisumu, Kenya: A Randomised Controlled Trial." *Lancet* 369 (9562): 643–656.

Briggs, C. L. 2003. "Why Nation-States and Journalists can't Teach People to be Healthy: Power and Pragmatic Miscalculation in Public Discourses on Health." *Medical Anthropology Quarterly* 17 (3): 287–321.

Briggs, C. L. 2005. "Communicability, Racial Discourse, and Disease." *Annual Review of Anthropology* 34: 269–291.

Briggs, C. L., and D. C. Hallin. 2007. "Biocommunicability: The Neoliberal Subject and its Contradictions in New Coverage of Health Issues." *Social Text* 25 (4): 43–66.

Briggs, C. L., and D. C. Hallin. 2010. "Health Reporting as Political Reporting: Biocommunicability and The Public Sphere." *Journalism* 11 (2): 149–165.

Briggs, C. L., and C. Mantini-Briggs. 2003. *Stories in the Time of Cholera: Racial Profiling in a Medical Nightmare*. Berkeley: University of California Press.

Briggs, C.L., and M. Nichter. 2009. "Biocommunicability and the Biopolitics of Pandemic Threats." *Medical Anthropology* 28 (3): 189–198.

CIA. 2010. *The World Factbook: Africa, Lesotho*. Central Intelligence Agency. Accessed March 27, 2011. https://www.cia.gov/library/publications/the-world-factbook/geos/lt.html

DFID. 2008. *Helping Lesotho's Factory Workers to Stitch up HIV and AIDS*. Accessed May 11, 2011. http://www.dfid.gov.uk/casestudies/files/africa/lesotho-factory.asp

Estermann, C. 1979. *The Ethnography of Southwestern Angola II. The Nyaneka-Nkumbi Ethnic Group*. London: Africana Publishing Company.

Foucault, M. 1973. *The Birth of the Clinic: An Archeaology of Medical Perception*. New York: Vintage.

Foulo, T., and M. Moleko. 1995. *Survey of Basotho Migrant Mineworkers*. Maseru: Central Bank and Bureau of Statistics.

Gray, R. H., G. Kigozi, D. Serwadda, F. Makumbi, S. Watya, F. Nalugoda, N. Kiwanuka, et al. 2007. "Male Circumcision for HIV Prevention in Men in Rakai, Uganda: A Randomised Trial." *Lancet* 369 (9562): 657–666.

Gray, R. H., X. Li, M. J. Wawer, S. J. Gange, D. Serwadda, N. K. Sewankambo, R. Moore, F. Wabwire-Mangen, T. Lutalo, and T. C. Quinn; The Rakai Project Group. 2003. "Stochastic Simulation of the Impact of Antiretroviral Therapy and HIV Vaccines on HIV Transmission: Rakai, Uganda." *AIDS* 17 (13): 1941–1951.

Hassan, F., and O. Ojo. 2002. *Lesotho: Development in a Challenging Environment. A Joint World Bank-African Development Bank Evaluation*. Geneva: World Bank Publications.

Junod, H. A. 1962. *The Life of a South African Tribe*. New York: University Books.

Linake, M. 2009. "Health Ministry has No Intentions of Campaigning for Circumcision." *Informative* 8, July 13.

Linake, M. 2010. "Male Circumcision Crucial in Reducing Chances of HIV Infection." *Informative*, October 26. Accessed May 11, 2011. http://www.informativenews.co.ls/index.php/archives/2420-male-circumcision-crucial-in-reducing-chances-of-hiv-infections-

Magubane, P. 1998. *Vanishing Cultures of South Africa: Changing Customs in a Changing World*. New York: Rizzoli International Publications.

Marck, J. 1997. "Aspects of Male Circumcision in Sub-Equatorial African Cultural History." *Health Transition Review* 7 (Suppl): 337–359.

Matope, T. 2010. "Men Throng Clinic for Circumcision." *Public Eye*, October 18. Accessed March 27, 2011. http://www.publiceyenews.com/2010/10/18/men-throng-clinic-for-circumcision/

McCoombe, S., and R. Short. 2006. "Potential HIV-1 Target Cells in the Human Penis." *AIDS* 20: 1491–1495.

MoHSW. 2008. *Situation Analysis Report: Male Circumcision in Lesotho*. Maseru: Lesotho Ministry of Health and Social Welfare.

MoHSW. 2009. *Lesotho Demographic and Health Survey 2009*. Maseru: Lesotho Ministry of Health and Social Welfare, Bureau of Statistics, ORC Macro.

NAC. 2009. *Quarterly Report on the National Response to HIV/AIDS: Reporting period July through September 2009*. Maseru: Lesotho National AIDS Commission.

Nagelkerke, N. J., S. Moses, S. J. de Vlas, and R. C. Bailey. 2007. "Modelling the Public Health Impact of Male Circumcision for HIV Prevention in High Prevalence Areas in Africa." *BMC Infectious Diseases* 7 (16). doi: 10.1186/1471-2334-7-16.

Nyaka, L. 2009. "Male Circumcision Can Reduce HIV [...] but No Panacea, can't Replace Condoms." *Public Eye* 3, June 12.

Paige, K. E., and J. M. Paige. 1981. *The Politics of Reproductive Ritual*. Berkeley: University of California Press.

Patterson, B., A. Landay, J. Siegel, Z. Flener, D. Pessis, A. Chaviano, A. Chaviano, and R. C. Bailey. 2002. "Susceptibility to Human Immunodeficiency Virus-1 Infection of Human Foreskin and Cervical Tissue in Explant Culture." *American Journal of Pathology* 16: 867–873.

Rural Poverty Portal. 2013. "Rural Poverty in Lesotho." Accessed May 31, 2013. http://www.ruralpovertyportal.org/country/home/tags/lesotho

Staff reporter. 2003. "Culture Undermines Prevention Efforts in Lesotho." *Public Eye* 10, September 26.

Stevens, G., and R. Lockhat. 1997. "Coca Cola Kids: Reflections on Black Adolescent Identity Development in Post-Apartheid South Africa." *South African Journal of Psychology* 27 (4): 250–255.

Thomas, A. G., B. R. Tran, M. Cranston, M. C. Brown, R. Kumar, and M. Tlelai. 2011. "Voluntary Medical Male Circumcision: A Cross-Sectional Study Comparing Circumcision Self-Report and Physical Examination Findings in Lesotho." *PLoS One* 6 (11): e27561.

UNAIDS. 2010. "Joint United Nations Programme on HIV/AIDS."Accessed March 12, 2010. http://www.unaids.org/en/KnowledgeCentre/HIVData/default.asp

UNDP. 2011. *Human Development Report 2011, Sustainability and Equity: A Better Future for All*. Geneva: United Nations Development Program.

USAID. 2007. *Costing Male Circumcision in Lesotho and Implications for the Cost-Effectiveness of Circumcision as an HIV Intervention*. Washington, DC: United States Agency for International Development.

van Gennep, A. 1909. *The Rites of Passage*. London: Routledge.

Vincent, L. 2008a. "'Boys will be boys': Traditional Xhosa Male Circumcision, HIV and Sexual Socialisation in Contemporary South Africa." *Culture, Health & Sexuality* 10 (5): 431–446.

Vincent, L. 2008b. "Cutting Tradition: The Political Regulation of Traditional Circumcision Rites in South Africa's Liberal Democratic Order." *Journal of Southern African Studies* 34 (1): 77–91.

Wagner, G. 1949. *The Bantu of North Kavirondo*. London: International African Institute.

Weiss, H. A., D. Halperin, R. C. Bailey, R. J. Hayes, G. Schmid, and C. A. Hankins. 2008. "Male Circumcision for HIV Prevention: From Evidence to Action?" *AIDS* 22 (5): 567–574.

Westercamp, N., and R. C. Bailey. 2007. "Acceptability of Male Circumcision for Prevention of HIV/AIDS in Sub-Saharan Africa: A Review." *AIDS and Behavior* 11 (3): 341–355.

WHO. 2005. *Summary Country Profile for HIV Treatment Scale-up: Lesotho*. Accessed November 11, 2009. http://www.who.int/hiv/HIVCP_LSO.pdf

WHO. 2006. *Statement on Kenyan and Ugandan Trial Findings Regarding Male Circumcision and HIV.* Geneva: World Health Organization. UNFPA, UNICEF, World Bank and UNAIDS Secretariat.

WHO. 2009a. *Country Cooperative Strategy at a Glance: Lesotho*. Geneva: World Health Organization.

WHO. 2009b. *Traditional Male Circumcision Among Young People: A Public Health Perspective in the Context of HIV Prevention*. Geneva: World Health Organization.

WHO/UNAIDS/JHPIEGO. 2007. *Manual for Male Circumcision Under Local Anaesthesia*. Geneva: World Health Organization.

Williams, B. G., J. O. Lloyd-Smith, E. Gouws, C. A. Hankins, W. M. Getz, J. Hargrove, I. de Zoysa, C. Dye, and B. Auvert. 2006. "The Potential Impact of Male Circumcision on HIV in Sub-Saharan Africa." *PLoS Medicine* 3 (7): e262.

World Bank. 2000. *Lesotho-the Development Impact of HIV/AIDS-Selected Issues and Options*. World Bank Macroeconomic Technical Group. Unpublished report.

World Bank. 2010. *Information and Communication Techonology (ICT) at a Glance Table: Lesotho*. Geneva: World Bank.

New lives for old: modernity, biomedicine, traditional culture and HIV prevention in Lesotho (a response to Nicola L. Bulled)

Louise Vincent

Department of Political and International Studies, Rhodes University, South Africa

This is a reply to:

Bulled, Nicola L. 2013. "New lives for old: modernity, biomedicine, traditional culture and HIV prevention in Lesotho." *Global Discourse.* 3 (2): 284–299. http://dx.doi.org/10.1080/23269995.2013.804700.

Nicola Bulled makes the important point that there is a distinction between what the Lesotho Ministry of Health and Social Welfare refer to as 'lebollo-based circumcision' and 'clinic based foreskin removal'. There is much more than semantics at stake here. Throughout Africa, 'circumcision' is properly understood as one small part of a much wider process of male initiation. On this basis, many object to the term 'circumcision' which focuses in a misleading way on a single surgical event, whereas initiation is one of the most significant events in the entire life of a person.

The clamour for circumcision to be employed as a protector against HIV infection misses this nuance. In support of state regulation of ritual circumcision, South African doctors have called for 'safe and proper circumcisions' to take place in hospitals. For many, this would appear as the ideal solution to the problematic rate of death and injury associated with traditional male circumcision. Bulled herself favours a fusion of some sort between traditional and medical circumcision which she feels could be achieved through 'appropriate communication strategies, cultural work, and collaborations within specific cultural contexts'.

But there are many cultural constraints on the medicalisation of any aspect of male initiation from the point of view of the precepts of tradition. To suggest incorporation in this way, moreover, risks underestimating what is at stake. It is to deploy a rationalist logic of progress in favour of sanitising the least appealing elements of 'tradition' seen from a westernised point of view. It is a position that purports to value diversity and advocates tolerance but within strict limits imposed by a western liberal imaginary within which western medical practices are not just different but better. A radical departure from this point of view would entail accepting practices alien to western world views, discomforting, repugnant even, as part of a genuine politics of tolerance.

This would require taking seriously the many ways in which medical circumcision offends the assumptions that are central to male initiation practices in many different settings. First, the use of anaesthetic disregards the important part that pain and suffering play in the ritual as part of the process of demonstrating manhood and fitness for the respect and communal privileges that go along with that approbation. The endurance of physical brutality, seclusion, dietary taboos and testing are a typical and central part of the practice in many different cultural settings (see for example, Beidelman 1965; Hambly

1935; Heald 1986; Holdredge and Young 1927) and initiates are commonly 'expected to endure circumcision stoically' (Silverman 2004, 421). As Wilson et al. (1952, 202) note, 'it is the undergoing of hardships and bearing of pain (*ukunyamzela)* that are necessary to becoming a man. If a boy undergoes those, then his manhood is not disparaged'.

Hospital circumcision removes the heart of the practice which has always been about hardship, suffering and the sacrificing of comforts. Initiates acknowledge this and expect little mercy at the hands of traditional surgeons and nurses as is suggested in the naming of these schools after war-torn cities and countries: Afghanistan, Kuwait, Beirut, Bosnia, Rwanda and Panama City.[1] The initiation into manhood at the hands of a spear or knife-wielding traditional surgeon is meant to be agonising while traditionally, the mutilations and deaths that followed inevitable slips of the hand were dismissed as 'a sign that the victim had not been destined to reach manhood' (Russell 1997, 27). The initiation ritual is not merely a psychological journey into manhood but is centrally a bodily one with healing part of the transformation process.

Likewise, it is one of the most basic tenets of traditional circumcision that it is a ritual reserved for males. Married women should be excluded from all contact with the initiate during the entire period of the ritual. This presents a serious problem for those who are forced to be hospitalised as a result of complications following traditional circumcision. It also means that proposals for incorporation of circumcision within western medical practice are problematic, since once hospitalised it is very difficult to prevent contact with married females, be they nurses, doctors or visitors to the institution.

Moreover, the private and individualised nature of hospital circumcision removes from the practice its necessarily public dimension in which the community bears witness to the individual's changed social and legal standing. John Mbiti, in his *Introduction to African Religion* (1999, 93), argues that initiation has a religious significance which is dependent upon the (public) shedding of blood. The blood shed binds the person to the land and hence to the ancestors (Momoti 2002, 58). Mbiti argues that once the individual sheds his blood, he 'joins the stream of his people and truly becomes one with them' (1997, 93). In this sense, the scars of initiation are also the scars of identity (Momoti 2002, 60). The public ceremonies, feasting and celebration associated with initiation serve to strengthen communal bonds and renew the vitality of a community.

Advocates of hospital circumcision overlook the reality of the poor access that people in rural societies in Africa have to effective medical care in the formal health sector and the enormous contribution that the traditional healing sector makes to public health in the context of this overall lack. South Africa, for instance, has one doctor for every 1500 people but in rural areas, where ritual circumcision is most commonly practiced, this figure falls to one in 26,000. There are an estimated 200,000 traditional healers in the country in contrast to some 31,000 'western trained' medical practitioners (ibid.). According to the Medical Research Council, between 75 and 80 per cent of South Africans regularly consult traditional healers. A medical doctor told the Pretoria High Court that hospitals in the Northern Province 'were so badly run that patients had to be sent home for lack of running water; they had to lie in their own urine for days; equipment was regularly stolen; and essential medication was either out of stock or not provided' (Schlemmer and Wilson 2001, 54).

It is then somewhat disingenuous to hold up public health facilities in this context – in many instances already groaning under the weight of the HIV crisis – as the answer to the medical problems that surround traditional circumcision.

Many young males find themselves under pressure from their families to be circumcised in a hospital; but the negative social consequences that would follow if it were to become known that they had not 'gone to the mountain' are so severe that they often go against the wishes of their families to be circumcised in the bush. Thembu chief and grandson of former President Nelson Mandela describes how he chose to go against the wishes of both his grandfather and father when the responsibility fell on him to arrange for the circumcision of his younger brother:

> Ten years into my manhood, the time had come for my brother to undergo the journey. He had listened to the stories told by his brother and … he aspired to take the same journey I had travelled. In December 2002 he mentioned his intentions to the elders and he was told to go to hospital. He found it hopeless to take them to task …. A year later he approached me to take up the challenge with him. We approached our grandfather and father about the matter. Once again, they stood firm on their position. He would have to go to hospital. [They] were motivated not only by the increased rate of death at circumcision schools that was being reported in the local press but also by the risk of HIV/AIDS infection. Even though I assured them that I would attend to the matter myself, they remained firm on the surgery being performed in a hospital. But this is unacceptable in our culture and you would never be recognised as a man if it was found that you had been circumcised in a hospital. (Interview, Chief Mandla Mandela)

The suggestion of hospital circumcision for Chief Mandla Mandela's brother echoed the family's approach to his own circumcision:

> I approached my elders in the summer of 1993 for guidance as I felt my time had come to undergo this journey into manhood. From the get go my grandfather as well as my father were uncertain about the safety of this ritual. Their concern was the increase of deaths in these circumcision schools during recent years. They suggested that I go to a hospital for the surgery and then go to a school for the remainder of the initiation process.

What Chief Mandla Mandela's story reflects is the fact that contrary to what one might intuit, it is not the case that the younger generation favours the modernisation of tradition and the ease and simplicity offered by hospital circumcision. In contrast, contemporary youth often blame their elders for the erosion of culture that occurred during the years of the anti-apartheid struggle and, in a time when the certainties of struggle identities have given way, are turning to tradition for the ingredients of their own contemporary identity construction. Nor is the defence of tradition a phenomenon of illiterate people in rural backwaters. Chief Mandla Mandela, who grew up in urban Soweto, is a university graduate and successful businessman as well as being a Thembu chief. The intergenerational family conflicts that occur around hospital circumcision are thus a window into a much wider social process that is underway.

Chief Mandla Mandela reflects on his feelings about being urged to go to hospital to become a man:

> Many thoughts rushed into my head. I wondered if our move to Johannesburg had conquered our traditions. Have we become prejudiced towards our own identity, or traditions, our culture and values. Within three generations apartheid had conquered and eradicated all the traditional values we had in my family…. I rejected their proposal [to go to hospital] because I was never going to become the weak link in my family. Every man that had come before me had travelled this journey so why did it have to be different in my time? Defiance had come alive again but this time not directed at the state or its agents.

As a result of this decision, Chief Mandela's circumcision had to take place in the absence of his closest male relatives.

> I found myself lost and lonely as these were the men whose support I needed to gain.... It was in December 1993 that I parted with my boyish ways in the hills surrounding Tsolo. During the seven weeks I spent there I learnt more than what I had been taught about my own identity in school. My ceremony as a young man was held at the Great Place in Bumbane and my host was the Thembu King Zwelibanzi. It was him and Mqoma that came up with my manhood name in the absence of both my father and my grandfather. The greatest thing about being one of the sons of the Great Place is that the occasion was blessed with the presence of Thembu chiefs.

Another rare first-hand account comes to us in the groundbreaking novel, *A Man who is Not a Man* (2009), in which Thando Mgqolozana controversially breaks with tradition, ignoring strong social prohibitions against speaking about male initiation and circumcision. He does so very knowingly. As he has his narrator, Lumkile's Oom Dan say, 'what happens on the mountain, stays on the mountain'. 'Transgression of this taboo was not a decision to be taken lightly. I was aware that to do so would have heavy consequences'.

Why take this step then? While the narrator's suppurating septic penis is the unavoidably powerful focal point for the opening chapter, the novel is about much more than merely revealing the secrets of initiation. The action quickly turns to zol, 'Operation Redistribution' in the Southern Suburbs of Cape Town, girls, carjacking, football and jail. In short, it is a chronicle of young black South African masculinity, of dysfunctional families and schools, of a world in which boys seek to become men as a frantic escape route from being regarded as no more than a dog.

The imperative of tradition in this context is brought home by the stark choice that the narrator faces – between a life of criminality punctuated by the drunken rages of a frequently absent father in an urban shack and life in a rural dust bowl. The narrator finds redemption in the hierarchies and certainties of rural life – 'the greenness of sowing fields, the thorniness of bush, the shape of mountains' – which offer an escape from what he refers to as the 'revolving-door-syndrome' that is 'the crux of the young black story in South Africa.... You either ended up doing time in prison, or they buried you, or both'.

There is also a love story here which evokes a further central element of the male circumcision saga in contemporary Africa. To be an uncircumcised male in some cultural settings is to be denied access to the respect and rights afforded to men including the right to be legitimately married, to legitimately father children and to inherit. When Lumkile falls for the beautiful Yanda, his manhood is literally on the table: 'She widened her eyes at its bulkiness, and I felt a spurt of manly pride'. Youthful sexuality is negotiated in a context suffused with talk of STDs, HIV, serial abortion, substance abuse and domestic violence.

Lumkile is disarmingly candid about 'the cut' being what he fears most of all. What do they use? How long does it take? Do they chop fast or peel it away little by little? Are you supposed to watch while it is happening or close your eyes? The journey into manhood is meant to be painful – to teach endurance and to impart the resources that will be needed to deal with life's difficulties. Similarly to 'fail' in this journey, far from being interpreted merely as bodily incapacity, is an indication of permanent failure to become a full adult human being.

Botched circumcision is regarded as a blight on the good name of the culture and the initiate himself is to blame (for drinking water, sleeping, having sex on the eve of circumcision, taking drugs or any of a number of possible transgressions of protocol). Reports of unskilled, fly-by-night traditional surgeons using the same instrument to circumcise again and again while under the influence of alcohol and the fact that circumcision takes place in the heat of December in huts crafted with tin and plastic do nothing to dent the certainty that an initiation gone wrong is a sure sign of a man who was never meant to be.

Mgqolozana documents the routine cruelties, the jibes and physical brutality that go to a particular construction of masculinity associated with violence, imperviousness to pain and suppression of feeling. The ritualised exclusion of women from the process is also a symbolic eschewing of the feminine denoted by the derided tears and secret letters to mother associated with city boys who lack endurance on the mountain. This is a construction of masculinity as being in undiluted contradistinction to femininity. To seek medical intervention, as Lumkile inevitably must when his penis begins to rot, is to be indelibly marked as weak, womanly and therefore shameful.

When what should have been the triumphant moment of entry into manhood marked by the burning of the circumcision hut and the welcoming of the initiate into the community as a man, turns instead into Lumkile being set upon by an angry crowd of villagers and their dogs, he reflects that this is not simply about the mob expressing its scorn for him, but is also about a culture turning on itself. 'My failure was not only mine, but the culture's.... Nothing was as it should be'. In the end, he rejects that culture's demarcation of 'the men' from the 'not men' as spurious and chooses instead to define manhood for himself.

But if Mgqolozana wants us to learn something from what he calls his 'sermon on the mount', it is that traditions, including those concerning ideal masculinity, are to be understood as dynamic rather than calcified. He has Oom Dan, the person who is the embodiment of pure manhood in the narrative, telling Lumkile that 'the times are changing and we have no choice but to adapt to them'.

Note

1. Available at: http://www.iol.co.za/news/south-africa/circumcisions-now-at-kuwait-beirut-bosnia-1.218276#.UXqI5yspb20

References

Beidelman, T. 1965. "Notes on the Boys Initiation Among the Ngulu of East Africa." *Man* 65 (4): 123.

Hambly, W. 1935. "Tribal Initiation of Boys in Angola." *American Anthropology* 37: 36–40.

Heald, S. 1986. "The Ritual Use of Violence: Circumcision among the Gisu of Uganda." In *The Anthropology of Violence*, edited by D. Riches, 70–85. London: Blackwell.

Holdredge, C., and K. Young. 1927. "Circumcision Rites among the Bajok." *American Anthropology* 29: 661–69.

Mbiti, J. 1997. *Introduction to African Religion*, 93 p. London: Heineman.

Mgqolozana, T. 2009. *A Man Who is not a Man*. Durban: University of KwaZulu-Natal Press.

Momoti, N. 2002. "Law and Culture in the New Constitution with Specific Reference to the Custom of Circumcision as Practiced in the Eastern Cape." Unpublished Master of Laws Thesis, Rhodes University, South Africa.

Russell, A. 1997. "Ancient Practice of Tribal Circumcision Divides South Africa." *Daily Telegraph*, January 23, p. 27.

Schlemmer, L., and J. Wilson. 2001. *'Social Development', in South Africa Survey 2001/2002*, 54. Johannesburg: South African Institute of Race Relations.
Silverman, E. 2004. "Anthropology and Circumcision." *Annual Review of Anthropology* 33: 419–445.
Wilson, M. 1952. *Social Structure: Keiskammahoek Rural Survey Vol. II*, 202. Pietermaritzburg: Shuter and Shooter.

The production of sexual mutilation among Muslim women in Cairo

Maria Frederika Malmström[a,b,c,d]

[a]*Nordic Africa Institute, Uppsala, Sweden;* [b]*Department of School of Global Studies, University of Gothenburg, Sweden;* [c]*Center for the Study of Gender and Sexuality, New York University, New York, USA;* [d]*Performance Studies, Tisch School of Arts, New York University, New York, USA*

Female circumcision has become a global political minefield, with 'Western' interventions affecting Egyptian politics and social development, not least in the area of democracy and human rights. As younger generation of women in Egypt informed by international human rights discourse begins to question norms still upheld by the previous generation, new dilemmas and tensions emerge. In this article, I discuss the risk that international interventions designed to modify local practices may fail when the local moral worlds in which such practices are embedded are inadequately understood. Rather than increasing women's agency, such interventions may reduce it and instead produce a sense of sexual mutilation among women.

Introduction

The issue of female circumcision has become a global political minefield, with 'Western' interventions affecting many 'third-world' countries' political and social development, not least in the area of gender equality, democracy and human rights. The politics of female circumcision should not be analysed as controversy between 'African women' and 'Westerners', since these simplified binaries reduce a wide range of different categories and positions (Moore 2007). However, the presentation of female circumcision as female genital mutilation (FGM) in interventionist discourse contradicts, and is negligent of, the perception of the practice in many countries where it is prevalent. This article examines, through participant observation, the consequences of this discourse on the self-perception of women who have undergone female circumcision in one such country: Egypt.

In FGM discourse, female circumcision is presented as mutilation of healthy body parts to inflict patriarchal control over women's bodies and sexuality. This stance is linked to a specific cultural context and to international women's political movements. Much contemporary academic literature and activist understanding of female sexuality is informed by post-Freudian Western conceptions of sexuality, according to which the clitoris is seen as essential for pleasure. There is clear neglect of cultural diversity in the interpretation of female circumcision in the social science literature (Dopico 2007), with little interest in the various local meanings or lived experiences of the practice. Anthropological studies, such as those of Ahmadu (2007), Johansen (2007) and Malmström (2004), are exceptions. Dellenborg (2004) notes that because the Western world makes such a strong link between sexuality, identity and individual development, excision of the clitoris has come to be understood as having consequences for women's emancipation (cf. Basson 2000). Masters and Johnson's (1966) research about female sexuality from the 1960s claimed that all female orgasms are caused by stimulation of clitoris and this claim often became a focal point for the women's liberation movement in the 1970s in the struggle for women's sexual autonomy. Clitoral orgasm became a prerequisite for good sex, and this was associated with female identity and emancipation in general. It is, therefore, unsurprising that clitoral excision is a charged topic in the West, where it has been equated with deprivation of femininity and natural sexual well-being.

This view has assumed hegemonic status in political, policy and activist discussions, subsuming other voices in the global FGM discourses. This article tries to make room also for less dominant voices: those of different generations of Muslim women from two lower income neighbourhoods of Cairo. The first area, located in the centre of the city, consists of classical Islamic districts. The second is in the suburbs of Cairo, where there are newer buildings. For ethical reasons, I have chosen not to identify the neighbourhoods by name. The women I spent time with lived in low-income areas of Cairo but their lifestyles were not strictly associated with economic class or consumption (cf. Early 1993 for a further discussion about class categories in Egypt). The group included women from various socio-economic and educational backgrounds and women of different generations, marital status and sexual preferences. The political controversy about FGM in Egypt reveals that the practice represents very different things to different kinds of actors, nationally and internationally. The practice has gained particular symbolic force in a global political context of modernisation, gender and human rights, but also Islamisation and security concerns about the region. However, this article will focus on global politics, sexuality and women in lower-income areas of Cairo and will not discuss any class-based or other distinctions in relation to the multifaceted meanings of the practice (Malmström 2009a, 2009b).

The aim of this article was to discuss the risk that international interventions designed to modify local practices may fail when the local moral worlds in which such practices are embedded are inadequately understood. As the younger generation of women in Egypt, whom I met, prompted by international human rights discourse, begins to question the norms still upheld by the previous generation, new dilemmas and tensions emerge. Drawing on fieldwork in Cairo, carried out from August 2002 until July 2003, I will show that rather than increasing women's agency, such interventions may reduce it. These interventions have tended to undermine pre-existing forms of female agency in Cairo and have called into question the norms regarding female sexuality upon which agency was formerly based. This article is part of an extensive study about constructions of gender through the prism of female circumcision and the interplay with the wider social dynamics in Egypt in the early 2000s.

Theoretical framework: social constructivism, agency and embodiment

My goal in this article is not just to provide an ethnographic account of the global politics of female circumcision and my interlocutors' strategies developed to meet these challenges in Egypt. It is also a theoretical attempt to broaden key analytical concepts in social scientific theory and detach agency from the goals of progressive politics. I will discuss constructions of cultural norms related to sexuality, where I base my framing of the conceptualisation of subjectivity as a process of becoming – through relations of difference and power – in line with Butler's (1990) notion of reiteration as a means of constructing identity. My theoretical framework, in this article, is to combine more generative theories of agency with those of embodiment to tease out the broader implications of my ethnographic study and discuss the relevance of a constructivist theoretical framework.

Agency and embodiment

Agency is both a universal human capacity for action and a socio-culturally mediated capacity (Ahearn 2001) defined locally in particular social worlds (Mahmood 2005). Agency does not have to act against dominant norms in society but 'individuals may respond in unanticipated and innovative ways which may hinder, reinforce or catalyse social change' (McNay 2000, 5). Abu-Lughod's (1990) understanding of resistance as diagnostic of power relations marks a vital analytical step within anthropology: to move beyond the coupling of resistance and subordination and the teleology of freedom and emancipation. By submitting to norms, which women deem to be positive, women may manifest their agency in practice (cf. Mahmood 2005). Hence, resistance is only one act among many other modes of action.

Mahmood's practice-oriented embodied approach develops the poststructuralist and feminist liberal notions of subjectivity formation by bringing embodiment into the analysis. Embodied agency may express struggles for other desires than emancipatory politics. I have earlier (2009, 2011) suggested alternative thinking about agency, including embodied capacities and means of subject formation. My former findings (2009) showed how the body was taught and expected to bear hardship, showing endurance without complaining. It also revealed agency of the body, with the body[1] not always capable of fulfilling one's or others' demands. Following Mahmood (2005), I understand embodied agency as a means of developing the self's potentiality – in its Aristotelian meaning – the abilities one obtains through particular kinds of embodied training and knowledge.

Exploring the body as a medium for the self (Mahmood 2005) has political consequences. The body has the ability to act, to tell a larger story, to be evidence and to be de/reformed (Scheper-Huges 2004). The body may also signify contradictions, since it is able to both reaffirm and transform forms of domination (cf. Peteet 1994). Bodies are, in different contexts, also sacrificed, which may be understood, not as acts of self-destruction, but as social acts of construction with political significance (Linos 2010). The embodied experience of female circumcision is an important field to examine, since political actions are expressed and acted out through the body. The global politics of FGM may in fact change experiences and notions of the individual body. McNay's (2004) theory of agency assists in helping us to understand how the subject is made through the interplay of the global hegemonic structures of power and the subjects' lived experiences (cf. Malmström 2009a, 2009b).

Essentialism and social constructivism: sexuality and female circumcision

Sexual desire and pleasure are complex. While sexuality is highly individual, it is also socially and politically moulded. Forms of expression and meaning are historically and culturally construed and linked to power structures and to gender ideologies in any particular society (cf. De Beauvoir 1953; Foucault 2002 [1976]). It is, therefore, important to examine the individual's perspective to understand such a complex phenomenon as sexuality. As late as 1950s, female circumcision was performed in both the United States and the United Kingdom to treat hysteria and mental illness (Barker-Benfield 1976), though it was uncommon to use the procedure for cosmetic reasons, as in the case of 'designer vaginas' among some Western women today (cf. Malmström 2009a).

Up to the 1970s, the majority of social scientists, including Sigmund Freud and Alfred Kinsey, analysed sexuality as an immanent force. Here, the general view was that, even if the expression could vary, sexual desire was seen as a result of a universal, biological sexual drive. More recently, scholars have postulated the notion of sexual scripts, questioning the concept of universal sexuality without cultural and historical differences. The theory of sexual scripts suggests that sexuality is always socially constructed and locally anchored, holding that biology can never cause or explain sexual practices, but merely provide sexuality with its prerequisites and parameters (Johnsdotter 2012a). As Bryant and Schofield phrase it:

> A discursively constructed self is understood as being constituted by a series of shifting, insecure and incommensurable subject positions. These are constituted by normative discourse, and while the process involved is dynamic and unstable, it renders largely impossible a unified subject capable of resisting normative inscriptions and inculcations. (Bryant and Schofield 2007, 322)

Johnsdotter (2012a, 2012b) discusses the tensions between essentialism and constructivism and the boundaries between body and mind in relation to sexuality in general and in relation to sexuality and female circumcision (see Fredriksen 2008) in particular (see Switankowsky 2000). She highlights the differences between the physical body and the social body and shows how these bodies are woven together on the same surface (with or without cutting), as well as how the surface of bodies constitute the interface between people and the society. She argues that it is not enough for the body to recognise sensations to perceive sexual lust and pleasure. The body also has to interpret the bodily sensations in relation to cultural and social meanings of the sensations in the specific context, as 'a shared sense of erotic meaning' (Cameron and Kulick 2003, 15). Also, as Tiefer points out: 'A psychocultural history kicks in, experiences get hooked to meanings and pleasures and can move far beyond the sensory or sensorimotor' (Tiefer 1995, 210). Thus, as Johnsdotter (2012a) claims, in line with many other scholars, sexual lust is embedded in individual, meaningful symbolically charged experiences, which can only be reached if the socio-cultural significance to it is ascribed. Hence, the significance of sexuality needs to be understood through the singularity of experience, not only as a form of social interaction (and not as objective physiology), but as linked to social structures and discourses, as we will see with the example of Cairo later in this article.

Nevertheless, in earlier studies of female circumcision, such as El-Deefrawi et al. (2001) and Koso-Thomas (1987), there is an assumption that female circumcision severely reduces libido, with claims that more than 90% of infibulated women have no sexual pleasure evident (cf. Johansen 2007). However, the literature is mixed. One recent study suggests that cut women have more sexual problems than uncut women (Berg and Denison 2010), although other studies demonstrate that differences among cut and uncut women are exceptionally limited (Elnashar et al. 2007). Moreover, Lightfoot-Klein's (2009) study of infibulated Sudanese women, 90% had the ability to reach orgasm, although there were variations among the women in terms of intensity and length of their orgasms. However, similar variations (including the 5–10%, which never achieved orgasm) can also be found among uncut women (Crooks and Bauer 2005). Catania et al.'s (2007) study of women subject to different types of the practice shows similar results, but with an unexpected finding in which 91% of the infibulated women reached orgasm, while 86% of women reached orgasm with other forms of less invasive cutting. Cut women with sexual dysfunctions can and, as they underscore, must be cured, since these women have the right to an appropriate sexual therapy. Johansen (2007) found in her study that Somali women, who were infibulated in Somalia and now living in Norway, did not talk about time-limited repeated sensations. They talked instead about desire, pleasure and orgasm as taking a long time and also as uninterrupted processes. However, all the Diaspora women she spoke to claimed that infibulation had affected their sexual lives – the sexual pleasure was perceived as either reduced or different. The women in the study who spoke about reduced sexual emotions talked about a sense of loss, in relation to both the actual body parts and the sexual feelings (Johansen 2007, 268). The other group of women stated that the clitoris was the most sexually sensitive part in uncut women, but underscored that the whole body in fact is sexual. One of these women described it as: 'If you are in love and young, just the touch of the fingertips can make you shake all over' (Johansen 2007, 269). Body parts that were considered more sensitive than other ones among these women were their breasts, abdomens, thighs and buttocks. Gruenbaum, in turn, discusses the issue of re-inbulation and its complexity in relation to sexuality in Sudan. One example she describes is the case of a married woman with more than 10 children, who had been tightly re-inbulated after each childbirth: 'It was obvious to me in Sadiya's description that although there may be pain, frustration and discomfort involved with sex, there is also a great deal of excitement, a common goal, and pleasure that she and her husband share' (Gruenbaum 2001, 140). This literature suggests that cultural influence can change the perception of pleasure and that cut women have the possibility of reaching orgasm.

Another vital aspect of understanding sexual pleasure in relation to female circumcision is the ill-defined nature of physiological prerequisites. The fact that the inner part of clitoris is approximately 10 centimeters may be of sexual significance among cut women (O'Connell 2005). Einstein (2008) points out that a neurobiological analysis will deepen the understanding of 'how cultural practices inscribe meaning on central nervous system structures, affecting mind as well as body' (Einstein 2008, 84). This, according to Einstein, affects neural signaling to target structures and transforms sensory perception (cf. Heiman 2007). She argues that the brain and spinal cord will respond to female circumcision precisely as any other loss of neural targets, which means a rearranging of neural networks. The neural rewiring may result in (clitoral) phantom sensations and neuropathic pain (such as vulvodynia, which is sometimes induced by surgical treatment for cancer of the vulva). Einstein also discusses the possibility of a shift in sites of pleasure, which means an altered sensation instead of an absence of sensation, something which Johansen's (2007) study also indicates (cf. Okonofua et al. 2002). Paradoxically, she claims that, among some cut women, an increase in sexual desire may occur, 'because to the extent that these neurons degenerate, inhibition from the brain to the spinal cord will be affected' (Einstein 2008, 93). Nevertheless, among some cut women, circumcision induced chronic pain. Einstein concludes with an exhortation of listening to the voices of the cut women (which means diverse and unexpected accounts of the outcomes of circumcision on body and mind) with regard to what they actually feel to understand the impact of circumcision on the body (cf. Johnsdotter 2012a).

What is frequently ignored, as Ahmadu (2007) points out, is that many uncut women also report never reaching orgasm. Historically, though, this may not have been problematic: sexuality is experienced in the context of history and it is discursively constructed according to regimes of power (Foucault 2002): 'the meaning of sexual satisfaction is not constant, but dynamic. Each generation reinterprets it according to their culture and history. What once was considered satisfaction may no longer be valid' (Dopico 2007,

246f). Images and discourses of female sexuality may, therefore, always be at odds with what many women actually experience (Malmström 2009a).

Politically sensitive vocabularies and modernisation

In the context of historical, cultural construction of sexuality, it is difficult to find an appropriate term for such a politicised practice as female circumcision, the meaning of which is in such a state of flux. The Egyptian concept for the practice is ṭahâra (purity), which is the term I used when speaking about the practice in the field. The culturally sensitive choice in Egypt is otherwise ẖitân el-banât (girl's circumcision) in contrast to the politicised et-taświh el-ginsi (sexual mutilation). In classical Arabic, it is called ẖafaḍ (to lower, depress, abase, make gentle).

The radical feminist Fran Hosken coined the term FGM during the seventies. Today, this term is the most frequently used within the dominant discourse (see the discussion about various voices with different power in the introduction) among international organisations and African feminists/activists, who consistently identify FGM as a 'harmful practice'. This suggests how politically charged the practice has become. The issue, as mentioned earlier, does not involve a binary between 'the West' and 'non-West'. Instead, there are divisions and disagreements within 'Western' as well as 'non-Western' countries. In the dominant discourse and academic literature, the practice has been reformulated, as Hernlund points out, 'from "circumcision" to "genital mutilation", from a "traditional practice" to "a human rights violation", and (by some) from "culture" to "torture"'(Hernlund 2000, 5). My choice of term is female circumcision, since it has less stigmatising connotations than FGM and is closer to local understandings. Female circumcision is also broader and encompasses different forms and degrees of cutting (cf. Omoigui 2000). Like other writers on this issue, I am well aware of the problem of the term female circumcision having euphemistic connotations (e.g. Boddy 2007).

The term FGM is used when referring to juridical or activist understandings or when referring to 'Western' FGM discourse. This term has been at the heart of a powerful human rights discourse of opposition to the practice in Africa for the last two decades (cf Kassamali 1998), putting pressure on the states in which the practice is widespread to exhibit their devotion to international ideals (Boyle 2002). Within this discourse, FGM is seen to violate seven human rights conventions: The Universal Declaration of Human Rights (1948); The United Nations Convention on the Rights of the Child (1959); The African Charter on the Rights and Welfare of the Child (1990); The United Nations Convention on the Elimination of All Forms of Discrimination Against Women (1992); The United Nations Declaration on Violence Against Women (1993); The World Conference on Human Rights Declaration and Programme of Action, Vienna (1993) and the United Nations High Commission on Refugees Statement Against Gender-Based Violence (1996). From a human and women's rights perspective, FGM is identified as discriminatory because the practice is understood as rooted in gendered power imbalances and inequalities (UNFPA/UNICEF 2011). From a children's rights perspective, FGM is perceived as a violation of the rights of the child to development, protection and participation (United Nations Children's Fund 2005). From a sexual and reproductive health human rights approach, rape and other forms of sexual violence, which encompass FGM, represent serious breaches of sexual and reproductive freedoms and are inconsistent with the right to health (United Nations Economic and Social Council 2004), bodily integrity and freedom from torture (United Nations 1993, Article 2). However, from a cultural rights perspective, every human being has also the right to culture, including the right to enjoy and cultivate cultural identity. Cultural rights, however, are not unlimited. The right to culture is limited at the point at which it infringes on another human right (United Nations Background Note 1995).

Eradication of FGM is seen to be an integral part of modernisation (Beijing Declaration 1995). Modernisation is, of course, never a linear or predictable process, as numerous critics have shown. Latour (1993) argues that notions of modernity are based on untenable intellectual divisions such as those between modern and traditional and between objective facts of nature and subjective knowledge of culture. Modernity may instead be understood as a set of discourses that appeared in European classical social theory in the second half of the nineteenth century. These discourses, processes and practices have been widely circulated by different social groups in various parts of the world (cf. Spencer 1996). The concept of modernisation, on the other hand, may be interpreted as a way to adopt discourses, practices, ideologies, views and techniques of modernity. Modernisation processes have often been seen as Westernisation. However, as Ghannam argues,

> Modernity can no longer be viewed as a totality or a master narrative that entails similar changes in different societies, as modernization theory has argued. Nor can it be seen as a whole that is either taken or rejected. As active agents, people are able to selectively appropriate certain aspects of what they see as modern. (Ghannam 2002, 137)

The Arabic words that refer to notions of modernity are taġarrub (Westernisation), taṭawwur (development) or tamaddun (becoming modern or sophisticated) (cf. Ghannam 2002). Additionally, when people in Egypt spoke about 'modern' practices, such as the medicalisation of female circumcision, they used terms such as môḍa (fashion). In early 2000s, modernisation processes took two directions. The first one was the course of the Western-oriented government of Mubarak that drew on a more liberal, secular discourse. The other direction was the religious and 'moral' modernisation of political Islamists. For people among the lower economic strata, modernity has comprised both, but in varying degrees. The majority of my interlocutors strived for welfare and 'a better life', particularly with regard to economic security, higher education for girls and boys, increased consumption, medicalisation, new values regarding appearance (thin body and tight clothes) and nuclear families. Secularisation was not valued, with people longing for a modern way of life with Islamic principles and morals.

In this light, although human rights are regarded as universally applicable, the values on which they are based can be traced to a specifically European history and tradition of thought (though this is contended by Sen 2004). In countries where female circumcision is performed, states have adopted policies that prohibit the practice even when the laws do not reflect what the majority of the population want (Boyle 2002). To improve human rights, there is a need to understand and engage local contexts (Obiora 1997). Abu-Lughod's (2010) recent post-colonial study on 'Muslim women's rights' is, in this respect, valuable, illustrating in various settings in the Middle East and in North Africa the numerous meanings and shapes of human rights (which may also accumulate meanings from different sources). Scholars such as An-Na'im (1992) have used such cases to argue that human rights constantly develop in relation to socio-cultural, economic and political changes, where Western influence is only one out of many.

This has, perhaps, been lost in current understandings of the debate on female circumcision and human rights. International organisations have not always seen female circumcision as a significant global political issue worthy of intervention in the affairs of states in which female circumcision was practiced. The United Nations first requested that the World Health Organization (WHO) examine the practice in 1958. The WHO argued that it was outside their area of competence; that it was a cultural and social phenomenon rather than a medical one and that WHO policy was to avoid interfering in the domestic politics of sovereign states. Today, however, the international community and non-governmental organisations are deeply involved in globally eradicating FGM and seem to have no qualms in shaping the domestic politics of concerned states. This may appear particularly troubling since there is disparity in treatment of female circumcision/genital mutilation, which is seen as non-Western, and male circumcision/genital mutilation, which is practised widely in the West (cf Dellenborg 2009). The discursive representations of female circumcision as devastating and male circumcision as relatively innocuous, as Johnsdotter (2012b) points out, elucidates the extent to which discourses are influenced by political currents at a specific time in history. International organisations, such as the International Monetary Fund and the World Bank, have linked economic aid to reforms concerning FGM, and the International Inter-governmental Organisation (IGO) and the WHO have stated that they condemn the practice as a violation of women's rights (Boyle 2002). The tendencies of these interventions to dis-embed female circumcision from its complex social and cultural context has meant that they are often perceived locally as an attack on the cultural integrity of the group.

Female circumcision in Egypt: doxa and modernisation

Contrary to the interventionist discourse, female circumcision is not an isolable phenomenon. In Egypt, female circumcision is deeply interwoven into all aspects of social, cultural and political life. It is this embeddedness that has given female circumcision its cultural necessity and moral force. Older Cairo women, particularly among the lower income strata, view the excised female body as complete, beautiful and normal and as essential to the making of moral Muslim womanhood and motherhood. From an emic (local) perspective, circumcision protects the young woman from sexual relations before marriage and puts the married woman into balance with her spouse. The meaning of female circumcision in Egypt has been challenged by several global political processes, such as military interventions in the Arab region and neo-liberal economic politics coupled with secular modernisation processes, as well as by global interventions into the most intimate part of Egyptian women's lives, as will be elaborated later. The politicisation of female circumcision in Egypt may be interpreted as the beginning of a crisis in the universe of what Bourdieu refers to as doxa, 'the pre-verbal taking-for-granted of the world that flows from practical sense' (Bourdieu 1990, 68). From this perspective, the politics of female circumcision make a rift in the doxa, since, among my interlocutors, female circumcision before the politicisation of the issue in Cairo had been embedded in the private world of the family, in the life-long creation of femininity and in lived Islam.

The process of modernisation that has contributed to this rift in Egypt is twofold. First, there was the long-term modernisation process initiated by Nasser, which resulted in new patterns of family and consumption and new employment opportunities for both women and men. Second, there are the neo-liberal economic policies of a more recent date, which have had negative consequences for both sexes, bringing rising unemployment, higher food prices and expensive public services.

Egypt has, in recent decades, undergone substantial social, political and economic changes that have affected men's and women's lives in different ways. All of the older women I met during my year in Cairo had experienced great hardships, and they shared many experiences, such as poverty, early marriages, miscarriages, deaths of spouses and children, poor health and lack of formal education. They were all illiterate and were working either as housewives or in low-paid employment as cleaners, laundresses, petty sellers and so on. The women's daughters had a different outlook on life from their mothers. They had not experienced absolute poverty, lack of education or child marriage. Their goals, expectations and visions of a good life contrasted sharply with those of their mothers. The majority of the young women were living at home with their parents, many were university educated and unmarried. They were influenced by different aspects of the on-going social transformation around them. There were similarities in their notions of a good life, including individual freedom, consumption and increased space for action. Many of them dreamed of having an apartment of their own in a middle class neighbourhood and a profession (even after marriage, which would ideally be with an intellectual husband). They also cherished new bodily ideals; the young women wanted to be slim and have trendy, tight clothes. However, the younger generation was not homogenous. While the majority of the young women did not consider the role of housewife to be desirable, some wanted to devote themselves to their family after marriage. These women wanted to take care of the household and bring up their children well. All the young women I interviewed agreed about the importance of education. A modern woman had to be educated. Those young women who wanted to become housewives were, however, often the ones who had found political Islam to offer the code for the right way of living – acode that contrasted with their families' interpretation of Islam. These young women faced problems, sometimes within their families but also in relation to the state. Their choice of clothing was problematic. They publicly demonstrated their submission to God through Islamic dresses such as niqâb. Because of their clothing, these women often encountered problems on the state labour market and in contact with state authorities in general. Some young women used a veil, they said, not only to show their faith but also to follow fashion or as a strategy to enhance their individual freedom. The young women who never used a veil also faced problems, though not with the state but in relation to local society, where they were humiliated and gossiped about.

My findings show common patterns of intergenerational tension where young people's desire for freedom conflicts with their parents' and families' norms. Here, the issue revolves around marriage and many young women's desire to decide for themselves, but for married women, there are also tensions surrounding polygyny, divorce and loss of spouses. It is clear that the majority of young women challenge 'conventional' models of womanhood and the need to endure hardships as a route to becoming 'proper' women, but they do so in different ways.[2] The new generation of urban Egyptian women is at the crossroads between the old and the new. However, all these women, regardless of age, valued university education.

The hopes of both young and older women to achieve a 'good life' have come to nothing largely because of the effects of structural adjustment policies of the 1990s and of neo-liberal economics in general (El-Kholy 2002). The poor of all generations find themselves excluded from many of the benefits supposedly offered by modernisation and are instead forced to forgo the desires prompted by modern flows of information, even though they have to conform to modern norms. Consumer goods such as VCRs, colour TVs, mobile phones, flushing toilets, ceramic wash basins and new water heaters were all objects of desire. Villas, fancy cars, summer cottages, weddings celebrated at luxury hotels, the private American University of Cairo, summer vacations, journeys abroad and more were, however, beyond the reach of most of the women I spoke to (Amin 2000). Many of the older women felt that doomsday was approaching, and this view was shared by younger women who adhered to the political Islamist movement.

Many of the young women I met were dissatisfied with their lives and were despondent about their futures. The economic problems relating to housing, marriage and parenthood meant adolescence became extended, and it was difficult to become a fully-fledged adult. Housing was crucial to the presentation of self in everyday life. As Ghannam notes:

> The apartment, its physical features and furniture, embodies messages that manifest the family's financial abilities. If one knows how to read spatial signs, it is possible to learn many things about the unit's residents, such as their religious identity and socio-economic status. Blankets and clothes that women hang outside the apartment's balcony, for instance, are read by other women as indicators of the family's ability to invest in accumulating household goods [...] The apartment is not only important to a woman's own identity but also central to how a woman views other families. (Ghannam 2002, 53f)

Being a 'generous housewife' still gave a woman moral status. Marriage, housing and motherhood were essential ingredients of an adult woman's identity but, for many young women, this identity had remained unattainable, and the girls I met had to remain living with their parents well beyond the age of 20. The young women realised that their goals were impossible to fulfil. Their dreams were also kept secret from their families.

The Politicisation of female circumcision in Egypt

Gender constructions and women's agency have been greatly affected by the politicisation of female circumcision. The first external intervention in Egypt began in Cairo in 1994 with the United Nations International Conference on Population and Development (ICPD). The conference encompassed a wide range of positions, national as well as international, represented by the Egyptian state, feminists, human rights activists, academics and medical, legal and religious professionals. The ICPD conference broke the national taboo of speaking publicly about female circumcision and sparked off highly politicised both in Egypt and the West.

The increased politicisation of female circumcision in Egypt after the ICPD conference intensified another internal struggle over what kind of modernisation Egypt should seek: whether to follow the course of Mubarak's Western-oriented government or that of the political Islamists. The effects of privatisation and structural adjustment policies in Egypt are perceived by the people whom I met to constitute unwanted Western political interference. The women I spoke with reacted with anger and dissatisfaction about the Egyptian state's economic mismanagement and weakness towards the Western world. The Islamist movement, in turn, strives for a religious and 'moral' modernisation, supporting female circumcision as an Islamic virtue.

The fact that female circumcision is performed in an Arab Muslim country provides further global political ramifications. The events of 9/11 and the fear of Arab terrorism and anti-Muslim intolerance this generated fuelled global interventions into Egyptian national affairs. The interventions in turn generated fear, paranoia and a sense of hopelessness among the Egyptian population. With the Iraq war and the deteriorating situation in Palestine, many felt threatened and believed that a complete colonisation of Arab countries was approaching. Many did not understand what they felt were unfair Western perceptions of Muslims and Arabs. The deteriorating conditions of life and the instability in the region contributed to a loss of control and undermined individual and collective security. Thus, social and political dynamics, such as modernisation, the after effects of 9/11 and more recent events concerning female circumcision, have together begun to dis-embed female circumcision from the socio-cultural context in which it was previously taken for granted (Malmström 2009a).

More recent changes, such as the after-effects of the Arab uprising, on the issue of circumcision remain to be seen. The people elected both Muslim Brotherhood and the Salafi politicians in the parliamentary elections of 2011/2012 and a Muslim Brotherhood President in 2012. The question is whether circumcision's strong position as a national political tool between the state and political Islam will be affected by changes (whether long-term or temporary) in domestic power relations.

Sexual desire and creative agency

As elsewhere, Egyptian women's desire and pleasure are shaped by cultural norms, though they may consciously challenge or reformulate some of these. There is always an interaction between subjects' experiences of phenomenal immediacy and normative models and power structures (McNay 2000, 2004; Malmström 2011). After many months of intensive fieldwork in Cairo, I understood that moral virtues among the women in the lower income neighbourhoods were acquired through bodily practices that actually shape one's character. These women cultivated a proper, sexual, feminine self, and their feelings were shaped by the interplay of mind, body, agency, social structures and cultural repertoire. The repetition of terms for female libido as well as the idea of disreputable female sexuality – the ambiguous 'sexual dream woman and prostitute' – teach women how to feel and behave. The tropes of cold, hot and sharp-edged are repeated, instructing women about the emic ideal gender balance according to which men and women should be different yet complementary. The norms of balance occur not only in discourses of sexuality but also in notions of the stable, 'perfect' Arab society. Local notions of open and closed female bodies teach women when the body must be closed and when it should be open. These are inculcated from early childhood through concern with protection of the 'hymen' (since social virginity is essential) and through female circumcision.

A woman is taught to be shy in her sexual relation with her husband and to make her husband feel that he has to initiate their lovemaking. Many women agreed that: 'If she wants more, she cannot express it since she should not have knowledge about it. Men are often afraid if their women show that they like sex, since they may be not able to satisfy them'. Women internalise the ideals of el-ḥayâ (modesty) for instance through the taboo upon discussing sexuality with mothers or husbands and the prescriptions for manners of speech and movement. In these ways, women come to experience themselves as both shy *and* erotic beings.

In line with Mahmood (2005), I suggest alternative thinking about agency, including embodied capacities and means of subject formation. As with Mahmood's example of veiling, shy behaviour expresses feminine identity correctly. The practice of veiling itself teaches a woman how to conduct herself appropriately. One of Mahmood's interlocutors explained: 'But you must wear the veil, first because it is God's command [ḥukm allah], and then, with time, because your inside learns to feel shy without the veil, and if you take it off, your entire being feels uncomfortable about it'. However, Egyptian women must thus behave modestly even as they must cultivate sexual skills for use during intercourse. The women used other creative forms of body language instead of words to express their sexual desire to their husbands. As one woman clarified: 'A woman shows what she wants by her behaviour. She wears sexy clothes or she cooks special food such as fish, prawns or arugula'. Another older woman told me that she was taught by her aunt how to treat a man: 'I observed her and I learned everything from her'. She recalled that her aunt had used a very soft voice when speaking with her husband and that she had looked into her husband's eyes with a special gaze. She was soft, smooth and coquettish. Her husband melted, she remembered, since he could not resist her and he gave her everything she wanted. She explained to me that a woman who wants her husband sexually should take care of her household perfectly, she should cook food and receive her husband in sexy underwear, a nice dress, high heels, make up and flowing hair, since these are 'the signs'. After some silence, the woman, who I had met countless times, looked at me, my loose shirt and topknot, very carefully and then she asked me:

> You do not look as you do here in your own home, do you? You can catch your husband with your femininity. In your home you can wear whatever you want, you know, but not outside, because then you are extremely impolite. You should look like a man outside.[3]

She then said that she knew some women of her own age who used their femininity to wrap their husbands round their little fingers. They were '*titmara*', which means very sexy. Furthermore, women utilise seductive artefacts in creative ways to fulfil other desires than sexual ones. In all these cases, the body is the locus of moral cultivation by the self and others. However, the FGM discourse undermines various modes of agency among the Egyptian women – in particular, embodied agency among the young generation. The international interventions provoke sexual fear often disproportionate to the young women's lived sexual experience.

The production of sexual mutilation

This was apparent in discussions with Heba, a university student, who asked 'Do you think I am permanently sexually destroyed?', apparently seeking reassurance. This was not the first time she had asked me this. Indeed, many of the young, unmarried women I spoke to would repeatedly raise this issue. Heba had also discussed the matter with her older sister, who had responded despondently that maybe they had both been destroyed for life, but what could they do about it?

The interventionist discourse on FGM engenders this kind of uncertainty in many young women. The mothers in my study did not associate circumcision with sexual dysfunction; they told me that they had not been worried about having been sexually mutilated before marriage.

Furthermore, as Hernlund (2003) found in the Gambia, in contemporary Cairo too the anti-FGM campaigns seem to rephrase the pain of circumcision for younger women, making it intolerable and meaningless (cf. Malmström et al. 2011; UNFPA 2011). These discourses have transformed many young Egyptian women's experiences of ordeals into a new kind of hardship that carries little value since the endurance of pain no longer yields moral merits or generate proper womanhood. To suffer in life has not previously been a question of being unfortunate. Instead, ordeals have been perceived as a crucial part of a woman's life. Still, suffering and pain are, especially among the older women, understood as 'natural' and as expected parts of life. Being able to endure pain and suffering provides highly qualifying merits. This reflects a moral discourse that is closely connected to the gender ideology situated within the context of local understandings. Conversely, many of the young women I met during fieldwork do not any longer consider it to be an essential part of becoming a proper woman. In this way, modernisation has contributed to the reformulation of the significance of pain.

Although young women often see suffering as meaningless, this does not mean that they consider female circumcision meaningless. They reflect upon and criticise the practice but with considerable ambivalence. Women take different stances, and one and the same person may hold contradictory views. The ambivalence and uncertainty evoked by political change and modernisation means that young women in particular shift positions in their pursuit of viable strategies for coping with the conflicting demands they face. In doing so, they become agents in the ongoing reformulation of gender ideology as they both challenge and embrace existing norms.

Conclusion

The need to understand agency as the capacity to act according to the exigencies of the specific socio-cultural has been the main premise of this article; the Egyptian context comprises the complex interaction between the local and a variety of wider global forces (cf. McNay 2004). In this article, I have suggested that the FGM discourse must be understood against this backdrop of post-colonial politics and modernisation, which transform ideals of gender and affect agency and experiences of the body. For today's young Cairene women, these changes have brought greater access to education, later marriages and the birth of fewer children. This means that, even though young women face new challenges in aspiring to be 'modern', many are spared the hardships that coloured their mothers' lives. These factors nurture new ways of thinking about idioms of suffering. The 'new' way of perceiving suffering seems to be to view it as devoid of meaning and as being associated with ideas of sexual mutilation and sickness. The body is always acted upon by others and by a conscious self through various techniques and practices of learning to be a gendered subject, but the interventionist approaches do something else with these women. In fact, the globalisation of intimacy and its political actions are expressed and acted out through the bodies of the women with the effect of reducing or even destroying these young women's agency. The embodied experiences of interventionist discourses actually transform the women's bodies, where the subjects may be incapable of resisting normative inscriptions and inculcations (cf. Bryan and Schofield 2007). It is, therefore, pertinent to ask whether it may be possible for young women to move beyond this new self-definition as a 'destroyed woman' (Malmström 2009a, 2009b).

My concluding argument is that the conception of female circumcision as a form of sexual mutilation is constructed in the same way as sexuality: culturally by different norms shaped by history and context. The idea of the circumcised female body as a mutilated and frigid body is produced by interventionist approaches inculcated by global hegemonic structures of power. The idea of sexual mutilation is derived from post-Freudian Western conceptions of sexuality, in which the clitoris, as the site for experiencing pleasure, lies at the heart of women's emancipation. As Ahmadu (2007) argues, this notion 'is as much a symbolic construction as the idea that its removal suppresses women's sexuality' (Ahmadu 2007, 306). In the Egyptian context, the clitoris is also important, but must be removed in order for a woman to develop respectable female maturity. Thus, it would seem that Egyptian women have the same motivations for performing circumcision as Western women have for not doing so; in both cases, the goal is to gain control over female sexuality and emotions. These ambitions are clearly as important for Egyptian women as they are for the daughters of the modern feminist movement in the West (cf. Malmström 2009a).

Notes

1. Intense pain may be the body's indirect way of protesting against cultural hegemony through physical agency and intentionality (Johansen 2002; Talle 2007).
2. Obviously, there are always multiple discourses of gender in society (Moore 1994) and sometimes also conflicting or ambivalent views, especially in times of rapid political changes. Being a proper woman meant different things to women of different ages.
3. By saying one should look like a man outside, she meant that a woman should not have any feminine decoration or make-up in contrast to how a married woman is supposed to look in her home.

References

Abu-Lughod, L. 1990. "The Romance of Resistance: Tracing Transformations of Power through Bedouin Women." *American Ethnologist* 17 (1): 41–55.

Abu-Lughod, L. 2010. "The Active Social Life of 'Muslim Women's Rights': A Plea for Ethnography, Not Polemic, with Cases from Egypt and Palestine." *Journal of Middle East Women's Studies* 6 (1): 1–45.

Ahmadu, F. 2007. "Ain't I a Woman too? Challenging Myths of Sexual Dysfunction in Circumcised Women." In *Transcultural Bodies: Female Genital Cutting in Global Context*, edited by Y. Hernlund and B. Shell-Duncan. New Brunswick, NJ: Rutgers University Press.

An-Na'im, A. A. 1992. *Human Rights in Cross-Cultural Perspectives: A Quest for Consensus*. Philadelphia, PA: University of Pennsylvania.

Barker-Benfield, G. J. 1976. *The Horrors of the Half-Known Life: Male Attitudes Toward Women and Sexuality in Nineteenth-Century America*. New York: Harper and Row.

Basson, R. 2000. "The Female Sexual Response: A Different Model." *Journal of Sex and Marital Therapy* 26 (1): 51–65.

Berg, R., and E. Denison. 2010. *Psychological, Social and Sexual Consequences of Female Genital Mutilation/Cutting (FGM/C): A Systematic Review of Quantitative Studies*. Oslo: Norwegian Knowledge Centre for the Health Services.

Boddy, J. P. 2007. "Gender Crusades: The Female Circumcision Controversy in Cultural Perspective." In *Transcultural Bodies: Female Genital Cutting in Global Context,* edited by Y. Hernlund and B. Shell-Duncan, 46–66. New Brunswick, NJ: Rutgers University Press.

Bourdieu, P. 1990. *The Logic of Practice*. Cambridge, MA: Polity.

Boyle, H. E. 2002. *Female Genital Cutting: Cultural Conflict in the Global Community*. Baltimore, MD: The John Hopkins University Press.

Bryant, J., and T. Schofield. 2007. "Feminine Sexual Subjectivities: Bodies, Agency and Life History." *Sexualities* 10 (3): 321–340.

Butler, J. 1990. *Gender Trouble: Feminism and the Subversion of Identity*. New York: Routledge.

Cameron, D., and D. Kulick. 2003. *Language and Sexuality*. Cambridge: Cambridge University Press.

Catania, L., O. Abdulcadir, V. Puppo, J. B. Verde, J. Abdulcadir, and D. Abdulcadir. 2007. "Pleasure and Orgasm in Women with Female Genital Mutilation/Cutting (FGM/C)." *Journal of Sexual Medicine* 4 (6): 1666–1678.

Crooks, R., and K. Baur. 2005. *Our Sexuality*. Belmont, CA: Thomson Wadsworth.

De Beauvoir, S. 1953. *The Second Sex*. New York: Vintage Books.

Dellenborg, L. 2004. "The Cultural Meanings of Female Circumcision: Experiences from Fieldwork in Casamance, Southern Senegal." In *Rethinking African Sexualities,* edited by S. Arnfred. Uppsala: Nordic Africa Institute.

Dellenborg, L. 2009. "Moulding Girls into Moral Women – Clitoridectomy and Other Ordeals in Jola Society, Senegal." In *Body Politics and Women Citizens – African Experiences*, edited by A. Schlyter. Sida Studies No. 24. Stockholm: SIDA.

Dopico, M. 2007. "Infibulation and the Orgasm Puzzle: Sexual Experiences of Eritrean Women in Rural Eritrea and Melbourne Australia." In *Transcultural Bodies: Female Genital Cutting in Global Context*, edited by Y. Hernlund and B. Shell-Duncan. New Brunswick, NJ: Rutgers University Press.

El-Defrawy, M. H., G. Lotfy, K. F. Dandash, A. H. Refaat, and M. Eyada. 2001. "Female Genital Mutilation and Its Psychosexual Impact." *Journal of Sex and Marital Therapy* 27: 465–474.

El-Kholy, H. A. 2002. *Defiance and Compliance: Negotiating Gender in Low-Income Cairo*. New York: Berghahn Books.

Elnashar, A. M., K. E. Ibrahim, M. M. El-Desoky, O. M. Ali, and M. E. M. Hassan. 2007. "Female Sexual Dysfunction in Lower Egypt." *British Journal of Obstetrics and Gynaecology* 14 (2): 201–206.

Foucault, M. 2002 [1976]. *Sexualitetens Historia. Band 1: Viljan att Veta*. [Histoire de la Sexualité. La volonté de Savoir]. Göteborg: Daidalos.

Fredriksen, B. D. 2008. "Jomo Kenyatta, Marie Bonaparte and Bronislaw Malinowski on Clitoridectomy and Female Sexuality." *History Workshop Journal* 65: 23–48.

Ghannam, F. 2002. *Remaking the Modern: Space, Relocation, and the Politics of Identity in a Global Cairo*. Berkeley, CA: University of California Press.

Gruenbaum, E. 2001. *The Female Circumcision Controversy: An Anthropological Perspective*. Philadelphia, PA: University of Pennsylvania Press.

Heiman, J. R. 2007. "Orgasmic Disorders in Women." In *Principles and Practice of Sex Therapy,* edited by S. R. Leiblum, 193–214. New York: The Guilford Press.

Hernlund, Y. 2000. "Cutting Without Ritual and Ritual Without Cutting: Female 'Circumcision' and the Re-Ritualization of Initiation in the Gambia." In *Female 'Circumcision' in Africa: Culture, Controversy, and Change*, edited by Y. Hernlund and B. Shell-Duncan, 235–252. London: Lynne Rienner Publishers.

Hernlund, Y. 2003. "Winnowing Culture: Negotiating Female 'Circumcision' in the Gambia." PhD diss., Anthropology, University of Washington, Washington, DC.

Johansen, E. 2007. "Experiencing Sex in Exile: Can Genitals Change Their Gender? On Conceptions and Experiences Related to Female Genital Cutting (FGC) among Somalis in Norway." In *Transcultural Bodies: Female Genital Cutting in Global Context*, edited by Y. Hernlund and B. Shell-Duncan, 248–277. New Brunswick, NJ: Rutgers University Press.

Johnsdotter, S. 2012a. "Kultur och Sexualitet." In *Sexualitetsstudier [Sexuality Studies]*, edited by L. Plantin and S.-A. Månsson. Malmö: Liber Läromedel.

Johnsdotter, S. 2012b. "Diskurs och claims making i sexuallagstiftningsprocesser." In *Sexualitetsstudier [Sexuality Studies],* edited by L. Plantin and S.-A. Månsson. Malmö: Liber Läromedel.

Koso-Thomas, O. 1987. *The Circumcision of Women: A Strategy for Eradication*. London: Zed Press.

Mahmood, S. 2005. *Politics of Piety: The Islamic Revival and the Feminist Subject*. Princeton, NJ: Princeton University Press.

Malmström, M. 2004. "Omskärelse är Sött'. Mat, Kropp och Kvinnlig Omskärelse i Kairo." *Socialmedicinsk Tidskrift* 6: 512–519.

Malmström, M. 2009a. *Just Like Couscous: Gender, Agency and the Politics of Female Circumcision in Cairo*. PhD Diss., Department of Social Anthropology, Göteborg University.

Malmström, M. 2009b. "Bearing the Pain: Changing Views of the Meaning and Morality of Suffering." In *Body Politics and Women Citizens – African Experiences*, edited by A. Schlyter. Stockholm: SIDA.

Malmström, M. 2011. "Gender, Agency, and Embodiment Theories in Relation To Space in Gender, Cities and Local Governance." In *Gouvernance locale dans le monde arabe et en Méditerranée: Quels rôles pour les femmes? Égypt/Monde Arabe 9/3e*, edited by S. Denéfle and S. Monqid. Cairo: Centre d'Études et de Documentation Économiques, Juridiques et Sociales, CEDEJ, 2011.

Malmström, M., N. J. Diop, F. Moneti, C. Donahue, A. Toure, and W. Haug. 2011. "UNFPA-UNICEF Joint Programme on Female Genital Mutilation-Cutting: Accelerating Change.". *Annual Report 2010. Nurturing Change from Within*. New York: UNFPA-UNICEF.

Masters, W. H., and V. E. Johnson. 1966. *Human Sexual Response*. Toronto, ON: Bantam Books.

McNay, L. 2000. *Gender and Agency: Reconfiguring the Subject in Feminist and Social Theory*. Cambridge, MA: Polity Press.

McNay, L. 2004. "Agency and Experience: Gender as a Lived Relation." *Sociological Review* 52 (2): 173–190.

Moore, H. L. 2007. "The Failure of Pluralism." In *Transcultural Bodies: Female Genital Cutting in Global Context*, edited by Y. Hernlund, and B. Shell-Duncan. New Brunswick, NJ: Rutgers University Press.

Obiora, L. A. 1997. "Bridges and Barricades: Rethinking Polemics and Intransigence in the Campaign Against Female Circumcision." *Case Western Reserve Law Review* 47 (2): 275.

Okonofua, F. E., U. Larsen, F. Oronsaye, R. C. Snow, and T. E. Slanger. 2002. "The Association between Female Genital Cutting and Correlates of Sexual and Gynaecological Morbidity in Edo State, Nigeria." *British Journal of Obstetrics and Gynaecology* 109 (10): 1089–1096.

Omoigui, N. 2000. "For the National Assembly to Legislate on Female Circumcision is to Criminalize our Custom." *Vanguard Daily*, February 20.

Peteet, J. M. 1994. "Male Gender and Rituals of Resistance in the Palestinian Intifada: A Cultural Politics of Violence." *American Ethnologist* 21 (1): 31–49.

Schildkrout, E. 2004. "Inscribing the Body." *Annual Review of Anthropology* 33 (1): 319–344.

Sen, A. K. 2004. "Elements of a Theory of Human Rights." *Philosophy and Public Affairs* 32 (4): 315–356.

Spencer, J. 1996. "Modernism, Modernity and Modernization." In *Encyclopaedia of Social and Cultural Anthropology*, edited by J. Spencer and A. Barnard, 376–379. London: Routledge.

Switankowsky, I. 2000. "Dualism and its Importance for Medicine." *Theoretical Medicine* 21: 567–580.

Tiefer, L. 1995. *Sex is not a Natural Act and Other Essays*. Boulder, CO: Westview Press.

UNFPA/UNICEF. 2011. *Women's Rights and Children's Rights: Making the Connection*. New York: UNFPA/UNICEF.

United Nations. 1993. "Declaration on the Elimination of Violence against Women." *General Assembly Resolution 48/104,* December 20.

United Nations Background Note. 1995. *The Challenge of Human Rights and Cultural Diversity*. United Nations Department of Public Information DPI/1627/HR. Accessed July 21, 2011. http://www.un.org/rights/dpi1627e.htm

United Nations Children's Fund. 2005. *Changing a Harmful Social Convention: Female Genital Mutilation/Cutting*. Innocenti Digest 12. Florence: UNICEF Innocenti Research Centre.

United Nations Economic and Social Council. 2004. *Economic, Social and Cultural Rights: The Right of Everyone to the Enjoyment of the Highest Attainable Standard of Physical and Mental Health*, (E/CN.4/2004/49). New York: United Nations ECOSOC.

A reply to 'The production of sexual mutilation among Muslim women in Cairo', by Maria Frederika Malmström

Debra L. DeLaet

Department of Politics and International Relations, Drake University, Des Moines, IA, USA

This is a reply to:

Malmström, Maria Frederika. 2013. "The production of sexual mutilation among Muslim women in Cairo." *Global Discourse.* 3 (2): 306–321. http://dx.doi.org/10.1080/23269995.2013.804752

This article develops the argument that interventionist human rights approaches that condemn 'female genital mutilation' may undermine rather than advance fundamental human rights norms and women's agency by producing a sense of sexual mutilation among women in communities where the practice is prevalent. Specifically, Professor Malmström argues that human rights discourse itself may produce outcomes that undermine rather than advance the fundamental human rights of targeted populations.

The idea that external intervention may produce unintended consequences antithetical to human rights is not new. Many scholars have written about the ways in which human rights interventions by outside actors may produce a backlash that leads targeted communities to embrace cultural practices that are being challenged. In particular, some feminist scholars of human rights have criticized strong forms of universalism as mechanisms for advancing women's rights as human rights. According to these critics, formal laws grounded in a universalist perspective on human rights may be ineffective or, worse, counter-productive (DeLaet 2013). Such efforts can be perceived as arrogant and culturally insensitive, especially when they are pushed by 'outsiders' who are not part of a community. In such cases, members of local communities may embrace cultural practices that are being condemned by outsiders as a form of cultural resistance. In this way, well-intentioned universalism may produce unintended consequences. Such arguments have been made in regards to transnational campaigns to eradicate female genital cutting as a harmful traditional practice. Critics charge that eradication campaigns that have been perceived by local communities as culturally arrogant have sometimes resulted in unintended backlash that encourages local actors to embrace female genital cutting, and other cultural practices depicted as by outsiders as harmful, as a form of resistance against perceived Western imperialism (Hernlund and Shell-Duncan 2007; Thomas 2000).

The argument in this article is different. Instead of simply problematizing the way in which human rights interventions may generate increased support for contested practices, this article suggests that interventionist approaches themselves may directly undermine human rights by producing a sense of 'wrong' about practices that otherwise would be perceived as normal among populations who engage in them. Specifically, the article focuses on the way in which a sense of sexual mutilation among Muslim women in Cairo is constructed in response to outside condemnations of female genital cutting. That women come to perceive themselves as mutilated and damaged – as having potentially had their rights violated – results, in Professor Malmström's view, directly from interventionist human rights discourse rather than from the contested practice of female genital cutting itself. In developing this argument, the author demonstrates the ways in which contested cultural practices are inevitably interpreted through particular social, political and ideological lenses.

Professor Malmström's commitment to giving voice to women represents one of the article's many strengths. Recognizing that the voices of women most directly affected by female genital cutting are too often ignored in debates regarding the practice, she seeks to bring women's perspectives to the centre of the analysis and is motivated by a commitment to protecting and enhancing women's agency. In developing her argument, Professor Malmström conducted ethnographic field work in several low-income neighbourhoods in Cairo, Egypt. This methodological approach allowed her to engage deeply and sympathetically with a particular population of women in a particular place and time. Unlike abstract legal approaches that focus on formal law and debates within international institutions far removed from societies that are often the target of interventionist human rights discourse and policies, the author's participant-observer approach prioritized voices in a community where a contested cultural practice is prevalent. In doing so, this methodological approach has the advantage of providing a local perspective that is resistant to hegemonic global human rights discourses. The insights generated by this sort of methodological approach are undoubtedly valuable, and certainly preferable to a wholly abstract, legalist approach that does not at all consider the importance of the social, political and ideological contexts in which contested cultural practices take place. Further, I found the perspectives of the women interviewed by the author compelling and persuasive.

Yet, despite my sympathies for Professor Malmström's fundamental goals and methodology, critical issues are still open to debate. I found myself asking about the voices of dissident women in societies where some variant of female genital cutting is the norm. Is it truly the case that no women who oppose female genital cutting live within the neighbourhoods that served as the site of the author's fieldwork? If women with dissident perspectives do live within these neighbourhoods, what social and political pressures might make them hesitant to come forward to share their perspectives, either with other women in their community or with an author 'from the outside'? If, in fact, dissident perspectives within these areas do not exist, then is it the case that the perspectives of the women living in these particular neighbourhoods in Cairo represent the viewpoint of women who might be subjected to female genital cutting throughout Egypt or everywhere in the world where the practice is prevalent?

I do not doubt that the perspectives of the women interviewed represent the dominant cultural viewpoint in the area where the author conducted her fieldwork. Nevertheless, human rights are not ultimately about dominant cultural perspectives. Rather, a human rights paradigm asserts fundamental human rights that belong to all individuals *especially* in the face of majority of the viewpoints within a particular culture that suggest otherwise. Indeed, a primary rationale for human rights is the protection of individuals and vulnerable minority groups from repression by majorities, and a human rights framework arguably becomes most critical precisely in cases when persons deviate from the dominant norms that govern the cultural contexts in which they live. In this regard, it is important to point out that hegemonic discourses can come in many forms. The author clearly is resistant to hegemonic human rights discourses at the global level. However, it is worth considering that there are also hegemonic discourses and practices *within* particular societies that silence dissident voices from within and that prevent women – and men – who do not conform to prevailing cultural norms from exercising agency within these contexts.

In this regard, alternative conceptions of power become relevant. For example, Lukes' radical conception of power suggests that a power relationship is at stake, even when a person is acting voluntarily, if that person is acting contrary to her genuine, objective interests. (Lukes 1974). In this conception, a person's perceptions of her interests, values and identities may be manipulated by external forces and actors. Michel Foucault takes this conception of power further yet by asserting that power dynamics themselves produce subjects as well as the interests, values and identities held by these subjects. This subject-producing process occurs in the absence of any intentionality on the part of actors and is relevant to understanding the production of power-holding agents as well as relatively powerless subjects. In this way, Foucault's conception of power 'may be useful in excavating the authoritative realm that forges who we are, what we believe, and how we should behave' (Digeser 1992, 982).

The point here is not to engage in a lengthy digression on the many faces of power. Instead, the point is to draw attention to the reality that research methodologies emphasizing the importance of bringing in the voices of those populations most affected by contested cultural practices – an emphasis with which I agree – do not necessarily settle underlying questions about interpretations of fundamental human rights. On the one hand, Foucault's conception of power, which draws attention to the ways in which language can (re)produce fundamental power dynamics, is consistent with Professor Malmström's critique of the ways in which a universalist human rights discourse might be seen to undermine the rights of particular women who come to see themselves as mutilated via this interventionist human rights discourse. At the same time, this conceptualization of power is in play within as well as across particular societies. Thus, it can be equally used to critique the ways in which fundamental identities and conceptions of rights are (re) produced in particular places, including the low-income neighbourhoods in Cairo which were the focus of Professor Malmström's research.

The work of feminist human rights scholar Arati Rao is relevant here. Rao stresses the ways in which culture is politically and socially constructed and asserts that such constructions have tended to be dominated by the perspectives of male elites. Rao argues that 'the notion of culture favored by international actors must be unmasked for what it is: a falsely rigid, ahistorical, selectively chosen set of self-justificatory texts and practices whose patent partiality raises the question of exactly whose interests are being served and who comes out on top.' (Rao 1995, 174). Ultimately, we still have to wrestle with thorny questions regarding who gets to decide the content of rights. As the author convincingly demonstrates, interventionist human rights approaches may cause harm when they produce a sense of 'wrong' – in this case sexual mutilation – among people who would not otherwise feel that human rights are at stake. At the same time, another danger, not fully explored by the author, is that too ready an acceptance of prevailing cultural norms in a particular social and political context will undermine the agency and human rights of actors in these settings who reject dominant cultural frameworks. Does the risk that interventionist human rights discourse might produce a sense of sexual mutilation among women necessarily outweigh concerns that unquestioning acceptance of contested cultural practices might lead to harm and a sense of violation among people who reject these practices? This question is worth exploring in greater depth.

A consideration of male genital cutting as a contested practice provides an instructive comparison. In societies where male circumcision is prevalent, assertions that male genital cutting violates fundamental rights are generally received with scepticism. It is not hard to imagine that interventionist discourse might produce a sense of sexual mutilation that did not previously exist among some men in these settings. At the same time, the growing 'intactivist' movement among men in countries where male genital cutting is prevalent includes many men who oppose male genital cutting on human rights grounds and who genuinely believe that their rights have been violated due to circumcision procedures performed on them without their consent. Is it necessarily self-evident that concerns about producing a sense of sexual mutilation among men who perceive circumcision as normal should trump the views of men who oppose male genital cutting on human rights grounds and who desire to advocate on behalf of this perspective?

This article makes an important contribution by bringing the voices of particular women to the centre of the analysis, and human rights scholars should welcome and encourage the inclusion of these voices. At the same time, we still need to ask questions about the voices that have been left out. Ultimately, the piece highlights the reality that there is no simple way to achieve consensus on contested cultural practices in pursuit of global human rights. Human rights scholars and activists are faced with a difficult dilemma. Many of us would like to minimize the potential harms produced by non-consensual genital cutting and to enhance the agency of women and men (as well as girls and boys) – even if these men, women and children represent a decided minority in a particular context – who would resist the practice if given authentic opportunities to make their own choices. At the same time, human rights scholars and practitioners attentive to the counter-productive dynamics produced by hegemonic global human rights discourses and concerned about enhancing the agency of all people also want to respect cultural differences and to avoid producing a sense of victimization among women (or men) who have undergone some variant of genital cutting. This balance is very difficult to achieve indeed.

References

DeLaet, D. L. 2013. "The Limitations of Law as a Tool for Responding to Violence against Women." *Politics & Gender* 9 (1): 115–119.

Digeser, P. 1992. "The Fourth Face of Power." *The Journal of Politics* 54 (4): 977–1007.

Hernlund, Y. and B. Shell-Duncan. 2007. "Contingency, Context, and Change: Negotiating Female Genital Cutting in The Gambia and Senegal." *Africa Today* 53 (4): 43–57.

Lukes, S. 1974. *Power: A Radical View*. Houndmills: Macmillan Education.

Rao, A. 1995. "The Politics of Gender and Culture in Human Rights Discourse." In *Women's Rights, Human Rights: International Feminist Perspectives*, edited by J. Peters and A. Wolper, 167–175. New York: Routledge.

Thomas, L. 2000. " '*Ngaitana* (I Will Circumcise Myself)': Lessons from Colonial Campaigns to Ban Excision in Meru, Kenya." In *Female "Circumcision" in Africa: Culture, Controversy, and Change*, edited by B. Shell-Duncan and Y. Hernlund, 129–150. Boulder, CO: Lynne Rienner Publishers.

Symposium on German Court ruling on Circumcision

Thinking about infant male circumcision after the Cologne court decision

Geoffrey Brahm Levey

School of Social Sciences, The University of New South Wales, Sydney, Australia

The Cologne regional court's decision of 26 June 2012 criminalizing circumcisions performed on boys for non-therapeutic reasons sparked extraordinary public controversy in Germany and around the world. Though the German parliament recently responded to that decision by passing a law allowing infant male circumcision for religious reasons when performed by a trained practitioner, the Cologne court decision is instructive for thinking about the issue. First, the Cologne court correctly identified the core liberal concern about the practice: it irrevocably alters an individual's body without his consent. Second, in unilaterally criminalizing a long-standing practice commonly accepted by liberal democracies and endorsed by the World Health Organisation, the Cologne court nevertheless showed how liberal institutions should *not* respond to such practices. Finally, the Cologne court decision raises broader questions about how we think – and should think – about the scope of liberal autonomy in liberal democracies.

On 26 June 2012, a Cologne regional court handed down a decision that shook Germany and reverberated around the world (Landesgericht Köln 2012). The case concerned the circumcision of a 4-year-old Muslim boy by a Muslim doctor at the request of the boy's parents. The court ruled that circumcisions performed on boys for religious reasons at their parents' request breached Germany's protection of bodily integrity and autonomy. The court nevertheless upheld a lower court's acquittal of the doctor, albeit on the grounds that the legal status of the practice was unclear. The court presumably sought to clarify that status with its ruling.

The public reaction to the decision was unfortunate though unsurprising. The Orthodox Conference of European Rabbis in Berlin called it the 'worst attack on Jewish life since the Holocaust' (*Spiegel Online International* 2012). Alan Dershowitz (2012), the prominent Harvard law professor, was more blunt, characterizing the decision as 'old-fashioned anti-Semitism, a term coined by Germans for Germans and against Jews'. Jonathan Sacks (2012), the Chief Rabbi of the United Hebrew Congregations of the Commonwealth, noticed that the case involved a Muslim family and that Muslims outnumber Jews in almost every European country. Rabbi Sacks suggested that the Jews were invidiously caught up in the backlash against the 'misguided' policy of multiculturalism, which accentuated difference and segregation. He seemed to overlook that ritual infant male circumcision in Jewish tradition is all about accentuating difference, being a mark of Abraham's covenant with God and, thus, of Jewish identity. Although the Cologne court decision does not bind other German courts, Germany's Medical

Association advised doctors not to perform circumcisions until the legal situation was resolved, while the German Chancellor, Angela Merkel, promised that her government would legislate to allow circumcision to be continued in Germany (*BBC News* 2012). On 12 December 2012, the German parliament overwhelmingly approved a bill, introduced by Merkel that explicitly affirms the right of parents to have their infant sons circumcised by a trained practitioner, with 434 votes in favor, 100 against, and 46 abstentions (Sidman 2012; Snyder 2012).

The practice of routine infant male circumcision has come under increasing scrutiny in recent times in liberal jurisdictions outside Europe. In 1993, for example, the Law Reform Commission of the Australian state of Queensland sparked debate by including circumcision in its review of juvenile consent to surgery, although the final report did not recommend against the practice (QLRC 1993). More recently, a proposal to outlaw non-medically indicated male circumcisions prior to age 18 was struck from a 2011 San Francisco ballot after a California Superior Court judge ruled that it was contrary to a state law that does not permit municipalities to regulate legitimate medical procedures (*New York Times* 2011). In August 2012, following a 3-year inquiry into non-therapeutic male circumcision, the Tasmania Law Reform Institute recommended in its final report that the state government enact a general prohibition on the circumcision of 'incapable minors' with an exception for 'some well-established religious or ethnicity motivated circumcision' (TLRI 2012, vi). The Tasmanian government is yet to respond to the recommendation.

Such attention in places where infant male circumcision has been commonplace indicates genuine concerns about its continued practice in liberal societies, and not simply, or only, animus toward Jews, Muslims, or minorities and multiculturalism in general. The Cologne court decision has the virtue of identifying the core liberal concern about routine or ritual infant male circumcision: it irrevocably alters an individual's body without his consent.

Other arguments against the practice, such as the infliction of pain on children or the desensitization of the glans and thus diminished sexual experience in later life, or arguments in its support, such as personal hygiene or looking like one's father, may be strongly held by individuals but do not go to the heart of the matter. The reputed health benefits of the practice include diminished risk of urinary tract infection, of penile cancer in later life, and of sexually transmitted diseases, and a lower incidence of cervical cancer among women whose partners are circumcised. Such benefits, coupled with a very low incidence of clinically significant complications in neonatal and infant circumcision (Weiss et al. 2010), are significant in distinguishing the practice from the genital cutting of girls, which has no documented benefits and carries serious health risks in the case of clitoridectomy and infibulation (the two most common forms). The legal prohibition of female genital cutting usually applies to women as well as girls; in contrast, it is rarely argued that male circumcision should be outlawed even for consenting adults. Benatar and Benatar (2004, 36) argue that '[e]xcision of the clitoral prepuce is anatomically neither more nor less radical a procedure than removal of the penile foreskin', and certainly a cut to the clitoris to draw some blood in a symbolic fashion is less severe than removal of the penile foreskin. However, neither of these less invasive forms of female circumcision has any documented health benefit. As I have suggested elsewhere, the health risk/benefit profile of infant male circumcision doubtless contributes to its continued acceptability around the world compared to the genital cutting of girls (Levey 2012).

The primary liberal concerns regarding individual autonomy, bodily integrity and consent are not, however, displaced by the putative health benefits of infant male circumcision. The scientific literature and medical opinion remain divided on the question and the reputed benefits are, in many cases, modest and realized only later in life. In the case of increased protection against HIV, for example, adolescent circumcision could achieve the benefit. In other cases, such as reduced risk of cervical cancer in the partners of circumcised men, the benefit does not accrue directly to those who undergo the procedure. Few argue that the public health benefits are so pressing and of such magnitude that they justify the mandatory circumcision of all males. Nor are the liberal concerns over infant male circumcision simply trumped by the right to religious freedom, as many Jewish commentators after the Cologne decision seemed to believe. All liberal rights and freedoms are subject to whether their exercise involves harming others or violating their freedoms, which is precisely what is in dispute in this case.

The fundamental liberal concern is interference with bodily integrity without the consent of the individual involved. The question is whether this concern is sustainable in the case of infant male circumcision. And if so, how should liberal societies act on the matter?

The first question warrants the kind of careful analysis that was missing in the Cologne court's decision. Such analysis would take into account that consent is obviously unavailable in the case of infants and small children. Parents and guardians are legally entrusted to make decisions in the best interests of their children or charges, on matters ranging from vaccinations and orthodontics to the choice of schooling. A careful analysis would consider whether circumcision is a body alteration that should nevertheless be postponed until the individual is able to make his own decision, as the Cologne court seemed to imply (Heneghan 2012). However, that consideration should also take into account that the pain, discomfort, and anxiety of the operation increase while some of the health benefits diminish when performed later in life (Benatar and Benatar 2004, 26). It would also consider and compare various other practices involving the bodies of youngsters – such as elongating ear lobes, lips, and head shapes, and ear lobe piercing, insertion of studs, and tattooing – that have no associated health benefits and yet are commonly permitted in liberal democracies with little controversy.

Finally, the analysis would consider the weight of religious-cum-cultural identity as a relevant consideration in determining the best interests of a child, even if not overriding. This last factor figured prominently in the conclusion of the American Academy of Pediatrics (AAP) (2012) that although the health benefits of neonatal male circumcision outweigh the risks, the procedure should not be recommended for all boys. The AAP recommended rather that circumcision be available 'for families who choose it' on the grounds that parents are best placed to determine the best interests of their children in this case.

The liberal concern with consent regarding bodily matters may, in the case of male circumcision, ultimately turn on democratic fiat. Public concern over infant male circumcision has gathered force in recent years largely as a result of some men conscientiously resenting what was done to them while in the care of their parents. Various local and international campaign groups maintain that infant male circumcision is a form of child abuse. As Dr George Williams, a Sydney pediatrician and founder of NOCIRC Australia, notes, 'many men feel emotionally and physically scarred by the procedure. They feel betrayed by their parents.... We don't believe parents have a right to alter children's normal genitalia' (Williams quoted in Sweet 1996). Although vocal, these groups still have small memberships compared to the number of men who have been circumcised when young and either do not apparently object to that fact or positively endorse it. Should the number of disaffected men grow significantly, the issue is likely to become even more controversial.

This leads to the second question: even if the preservation of bodily integrity in the absence of the individual's consent is deemed to be ethically paramount in, and seriously compromised by, the practice, how should liberal societies respond to it?

I would argue that the Cologne court here offers instruction in how liberal institutions should *not* respond. Abruptly assigning criminality to an ancient, continuously practiced cultural rite that has hitherto enjoyed domestic legal sanction and also retains the support of most liberal governments, the World Health Organisation, and many medical associations elsewhere, is quixotic and rather illiberal. An appropriate response would instead be cognizant of the divided public and professional opinion on the practice. Moreover, depending on the context, governments have a range of levers or 'nudges' (Thaler and Sunstein 2009) at their disposal for discouraging contested practices. In the United States, for example, where routine male circumcision was until recently the national norm, the incidence of the practice has declined dramatically in states that discontinued Medicaid coverage of it (Berger 2012). Or, as in most Australian states, the practice may be disallowed in public hospitals and clinics while leaving it an option in private settings. In other words, state support for the practice might be withdrawn without criminalizing it. (In the Australian case, banning routine male circumcision would also have ramifications for indigenous rights as many Aboriginal youths continue to be circumcised at young ages in remote areas.)

Governments may also remonstrate with their citizens through advertising campaigns, as they do in discouraging smoking, for example, although what images to use in the case of circumcision may be a tad more challenging. And, of course, governments can more tightly regulate the practice. The New York City Board of Health, for example, recently passed a regulation that requires parents to formally consent to an aspect of Jewish ritual circumcision, still observed by some Orthodox communities, in which the circumciser uses his mouth to draw blood from the wound (Otterman 2012). Insistence on pain mitigation measures is another area that might be better pursued.

Even if all these measures were still judged as inadequate ethical responses, there should at least be an opportunity for public debate about a proposed criminalization of the practice and, pending the outcome of such debate, an advance notice of when the law will change in response to it. In contrast, the Cologne court's unilateral decision amounts to an outburst of a piece with Jewish commentators crying anti-Semitism.

The Cologne court decision raises broader questions of how we think about liberal societies. Many people believe that core liberal values like individual autonomy and informed consent should apply evenly and comprehensively throughout the society. They thus have an expectation that the internal life of private associations will reflect the same liberal democratic ethos of public institutions – what Nancy Rosenblum (1998, 36–41) calls 'congruence' – and a sense of travesty when confronted with incongruence. The trouble with this picture of uniform and congruent values is that liberal democracies deliberately do not conform to it. For example, they typically entertain exemptions from general law, such as those commonly enjoyed by religious associations from some aspects of anti-discrimination legislation in their hiring practices.

In fact, value *incongruence* is normally found not only between public institutions and private associations, but also within public institutions themselves. Although a vital public institution, the military, for example, is scarcely a bastion of autonomous living. Where conscription does not apply, one typically enters the military freely, but exits it prior to one's term of service rarely and only with great difficulty. Liberal revisability doesn't rank highly here. In military life, one takes orders from one's superiors, the flow of information is often deliberately restricted, and *not* questioning the authority is generally considered virtuous. Or consider the presumptive consent at the very heart of the liberal project. Although the authority of liberal institutions is claimed to derive only from the consent of those subject to them, most of us cannot recall when we granted that consent. In recent times, it has become common to ask migrants formally to assent to the governing institutions of their new societies through citizenship tests and pledges, but 'born citizens' typically have no such opportunity.

Such examples highlight how there is considerable variegation in the way that core liberal values apply throughout liberal societies. 'Gaps' abound in the compass of these values and are part of the deep structure of liberal orders (Levey 2013). To recognize this much is an argument neither for relativism nor for complacency regarding particular cases. The history of modern liberalism, after all, can be read as the history of extending rights to liberty and equality, of plugging the gaps, as it were. So there remains a legitimate question of whether the practice of infant male circumcision constitutes the kind of gap in the protection of individual autonomy that warrants fixing. But even framing the question in this way helps put the matter into perspective. Understanding that variegation in the scope of liberal values is integral to liberal orders provides for a more mature and possibly moderating approach to the public controversy.

Brian Barry (2001), the arch-liberal critic of liberal multiculturalism, powerfully argued that legal exemptions for cultural minorities are unjust: either the case for exemption from general law is so compelling that the general law should be scratched for everyone, or the end served by the law is so important that it should apply to everyone. General access to routine infant male circumcision, such as in the United States, effectively satisfies the first part of Barry's contention, while the Cologne court decision effectively interpreted the law in the spirit of the second part. Yet, significantly, Barry allowed that exemptions might be entertained on the basis of prudence or generosity. Such pragmatism is exhibited in the Tasmania Law Reform Institute's recommendation, noted earlier, providing an exemption from a general prohibition on non-therapeutic male circumcision for some well-established religious or cultural circumcision.

Historically, liberal politics arose in an effort to secure peace among warring religious sects. Liberal states ever since have brought a pragmatic temper to their relations with their constituent groups. However, it is not a shambling pragmatism or a boundless generosity but rather a kind of 'principled pragmatism' that has come to define their modus operandi: 'pragmatic' in being responsive to contingency and circumstances, and 'principled' in seeking to show how policy respects or at least is compatible with foundational liberal values (Levey 2008). The current settlement regarding infant male circumcision is a good example of such principled pragmatism in action. The case against the practice as a form of assault or child abuse has not yet convinced most people in light of other allowable non-therapeutic interventions on the bodies of 'incapable minors', and in the light of its health risk/benefit profile. Meanwhile, groups are at liberty to build and agitate a case against the practice. In culturally diverse democracies, where the scope of liberal values is, in any case, deeply variegated, there is rough justice in principled pragmatism.

Acknowledgments

I am grateful to Vicki Dixon, Dirk Moses, Helen Pringle, and David Trigger for helpful comments on an earlier version of this article.

References

American Academy of Pediatrics. 2012. "Circumcision Policy Statement." *Pediatrics* 130: 585–586. Accessed October 4, 2012. http://pediatrics.aappublications.org/content/130/3/585.abstract?rss=1.

Barry, B. 2001. *Culture and Equality*. Cambridge: Polity Press.

BBC News. 2012. "Angela Merkel Backs Circumcision Right After German Ruling." Accessed July 15, 2012. http://www.bbc.co.uk/news/world-europe-18833145.

Benatar, M., and D. Benatar. 2004. "Between Prophylaxis and Child Abuse: The Ethics of Neonatal Male Circumcision." In *Cutting to the Core: Exploring the Ethics of Contested Surgeries*, edited by D. Benatar. Lanham, MD: Rowman & Littlefield.

Berger, P. 2012. "Circumcision Rates Vary Widely in U.S." *The Forward*, August 31. Accessed September 3, 2012. http://forward.com/articles/161642/circumcision-rates-vary-widely-in-us/?p=all.

Dershowitz, A. 2012. "J'Acuse: Shame on Germany for Circumcision Ban." *The Huffington Post*, September 6. Accessed September 10, 2012. http://www.huffingtonpost.com/alan-dershowitz/jacuse-shame-on-germany-f_b_1861252.html.

Heneghan, T. 2012. "German Verdict to Delay Circumcision, Not Ban it, Jurist Says." *Reuters*, June 29. Accessed July 4, 2012. http://www.reuters.com/article/2012/06/29/us-germany-circumcision-jurist-idUSBRE85S0XE20120629.

Landesgericht Köln. 2012. *Urteile des Amtsgerichts und des Landgerichts Köln zur Strafbarkeit von Beschneidungen nicht einwilligungsfähiger Jungen aus rein religiösen Gründe.* [Judgments of the Local District Court and of the Cologne Regional Court on the Criminalization of Circumcision of Non-Consensual Boys for Purely Religious Reasons]. Press Release, June 26, *Justiz-Online*, Decision of May 7, 2012 [in German], Docket No. Az. 151 Ns 169/11.

Levey, G. B. 2008. "Secularism and Religion in a Multicultural Age." In *Secularism, Religion and Multicultural Citizenship*, edited by G. B. Levey and T. Modood. Cambridge: Cambridge University Press.

Levey, G. B. 2012. "Liberal Autonomy as a Pluralistic Value." *The Monist* 95: 103–126.

Levey, G. B. 2013. "The Web of Autonomy." Paper presented at the Midwest Political Science Association Conference, Chicago, IL, April 11–14.

New York Times. 2011. "Judge May Strike Circumcision Ban." July 27. Accessed September 26, 2012. http://www.nytimes.com/2011/07/28/us/28circumcise.html?_r=1.

Otterman, S. 2012. "Board Votes to Regulate Circumcision, Citing Risks" *New York Times*, September 13. Accessed September 15, 2012. http://www.nytimes.com/2012/09/14/nyregion/health-board-votes-to-regulate-jewish-circumcision-ritual.html?_r=0.

QLRC (Queensland Law Reform Commission). 1993. *Circumcision of Male Infants*. Research Report. Brisbane: QLRC.

Rosenblum, N. L. 1998. *Members and Morals: The Personal Uses of Pluralism in America*. Princeton, NJ: Princeton University Press.

Sacks, J. 2012. "'The Europeans' skewed view of circumcision." *The Jerusalem Post*, July 5. Accessed July 8, 2012. http://www.jpost.com/Opinion/Columnists/Article.aspx?id=276439.

Sidman, F. 2012. "Germany Passes Law Legalizing Ritual Circumcision." *The Jewish Voice*, December 19. Accessed April 26, 2013. http://jewishvoiceny.com/index.php?option=com_content&view=article&id=2653:germany-passes-law-legalizing-ritual-circumcision&catid=106:international&Itemid=289.

Snyder, D. 2012. "Circumcision to Remain Legal in Germany." *NBC News*, December 12. Accessed April 26, 2013. http://worldnews.nbcnews.com/_news/2012/12/12/15869347-circumcision-to-remain-legal-in-germany?lite

Spiegel Online International. 2012. "European Jewish Leaders on Circumcision Ruling." Accessed October 2, 2012. http://www.spiegel.de/international/germany/european-jewish-leaders-lambast-german-circumcision-ruling-a-844128.html

Sweet, M. 1996. "The Unkindest Cut." *The Sydney Morning Herald*, February 16.

Tasmania Law Reform Institute. 2012. *Non-Therapeutic Male Circumcision*. Final Report No. 17. Hobart: Tasmania Law Reform Institute.

Thaler, R. H., and C. R. Sunstein. 2009. *Nudge: Improving Decisions About Health, Wealth, and Happiness*. Updated ed. New York: Penguin.

Weiss, H. A., N. Larke, D. Halperin, I. and Schenker. 2010. "Complications of Circumcision in Male Neonates, Infants and Children: A Systematic Review." *BMC Urology* 10 (2): 1471–2490.

Circumcision: what should parents and states do? An essay

Ayelet Banai

Centre for Advanced Study 'Justitia Amplificata', Goethe University, Frankfurt am Main, Germany

In May 2012, the district court in Cologne found that male circumcision was unlawful in Germany. The law has since changed, but the ethical question remains: should parents circumcise their sons? Should states try to stop them? In this essay, I examine seven arguments for circumcision applicable to Jewish parents.

'"For example" is not an argument.'[1]

1. The debate

In May last year, the district court in Cologne found that male circumcision in infants was unlawful in Germany. Congratulatory reactions from proponents of child rights applauded the court for taking a stance against 'violence' against children. These were followed by statements of shock and indignation from the organization of the Jewish communities in Germany and from Rabbinical authorities in various countries. Government and parliament responded with remarkable speed and began working towards legal change.

Meanwhile public debate rambled on in the media, and was quick to become polarized. On the one hand speakers for Jewish and Muslim associations, backed by voices from the Churches, parliamentarians from different parties and commentators of various political leanings argued adamantly against the court, emphasizing: the importance of Jewish life in Germany for the political identity of the Federal Republic; the constitutional right of religious freedom; the constitutional right of parents to raise and educate their children; the supposed medical benefits of the practice; the anti-Jewish and anti-Muslim resentment (and anti-Semitic tenor) of circumcision opponents; the need to respect an old tradition, and a general denial that there could be any ethical or other problem with circumcision at all. Voices from the Churches, Catholic and Protestant criticised the court's hostility to religion and tradition, which according to some is potentially directed against Christianity too. Commentators described the court's ruling as a case of enlightenment fundamentalism, tyranny of justice and values and an expression of an anti-religious Zeitgeist (for some of the arguments, see e.g. Bahners 2012; Bommarius 2012).

On the other hand, supporters of the court's judgement too amassed arguments for a legal ban on male circumcision of infants. Here legal experts and child-rights activists took centre stage, and over the summer received growing support from parliamentarians from different parties. Judging from vox pops public opinion polls,[2] they reflected public sentiment. Defenders of the court emphasized their opposition to the 'unacceptable violence' (Putzke 2012a, 2012b)[3] of the practice, its 'traumatic effects'[4] on the children, not to mention the 'barbarism' of it all. Other arguments for a ban included the rights and well-being of children, their bodily integrity, and the freedom, consent and self-determination of minors (Merkel 2012).[5] By the end of the year, new legislation was adopted by the Bundestag that clearly established the legality of parents' decision to circumcise their newborn sons (under specified conditions).[6]

With the new legislation, the media and press moved on to other topics. But we might stop and ask, what should we actually think about circumcision and its legal status? We might wish to answer this question because it is likely to make a public comeback if and when the legislation is challenged in German courts, or when other European countries move to legislate on the matter. But more importantly, we ought to seek an answer because for some of us – those expected to circumcise their newborn sons, as well as those that care about the legal equality and well-being of their fellow citizens – the question is particularly relevant and the heated media debate is of little help and guidance.

2. The ethical question

What, then, ought we to think about male circumcision and its legal status? It is useful to begin by separating the ethical and legal questions. The ethical question: is it good or bad, right or wrong for parents to have their sons circumcised? The legal question: if circumcision is ethically wrong, is it the kind of wrong that the state ought to prevent by means of a legal ban? I will seek to answer this question only from a Jewish perspective on circumcision; I do not assume that the same considerations apply to other social contexts in which circumcision is practiced (for example, among non-Hispanic white Americans, Muslims and South Koreans).[7] A good place to start our ethical investigation is with the parents. I begin with the following assumptions:

- Most parents who have had and will have their sons circumcised believe that, as a rule, removing pieces of skin, tissue or other organs from their young children for non-medical, non-therapeutic purpose is not a good idea, possibly even a remarkably bad one.
- *Other things being equal* the said parents would strongly object to any such procedures being performed on their children and would probably like to see such actions criminalised and punishable by law.

If these assumptions are correct, the interesting ethical puzzle arises. Circumcision *is* a procedure that involves the removal of body tissues from the newborn for no therapeutic reason. How is it that so many parents do – and are often happy about doing – what they otherwise think is bad and wrong? Is circumcision different? Motivated by personal curiosity, I have gathered anecdotal information on this question in recent years through conversations with friends, relatives and acquaintances who performed the practice due to their Jewish faith or cultural and social affiliations.[8] The following answers emerge.

(1) *The working of a social convention.* Where circumcision is widely practised individual parents often follow the habit and convention without asking themselves whether and why they wish to perform it. Parents do not think of themselves as engaging in action that they would have otherwise disproved of (i.e. removing tissues for non-therapeutic reasons), but as simply doing things the way they are done.

(2) *Social pressure*. Jewish parents both in Israel and in large communities in North America report that they worry about the social exclusion that their sons may suffer, stigmatised as different or outsiders in a social milieu in which male circumcision is the norm.

(3) *Belief in health benefits*. Parents who have had their children circumcised tend to believe that it is beneficial for the baby's health. Specifically the foreskin is perceived as non-hygienic, and its removal is seen as a means of protecting the baby from infections and disease.

(4) *Community expectations*. Jewish parents report that their parents, relatives, friends, colleagues and others in their social environment clearly expect them to have the circumcision performed and celebrated. Since the practice is very widely considered to be a rite of passage allowing entry to the community, it is expected that anyone who wishes to raise their children Jewish would have them circumcised and, as a corollary, contemplating the alternative is seen as strong and radical negation of the values of one's family and society.

(5) *Positive identification; pride in membership and identity*. As circumcision remains one of the most widely practised Jewish rituals and traditions, it is an evident way for parents to express their affiliation to and the pride they take in their Jewish identity; a way to affirm their own sense of belonging to the community, its history, values and cultures.

(6) *Faith and consciousness*. For a religious and believing Jew, circumcision of sons is a clear and unequivocal religious duty. For a person who believes that (parts of) the Torah document are a revelation and that the established orthodox Rabbinical traditions are the authoritative interpretation of that revelation and subsequent religious duties, circumcision of newborn sons is undoubtedly required by faith and consciousness.

(7) *The working of a taboo*. Where circumcision is the norm (in a society or within a group of it), voicing doubts about the practice even in private and certainly in public is often met with strong disapproval. Circumcised men likely feel that if something is wrong with circumcision, then something is wrong with them – and not just with anything, but with their sexuality. Parents strongly wish to avoid the thought that they may have done something wrong to their own children. As a result there are strong social incentives not to raise doubts or questions about the practice, and to deflect them when they are being raised nevertheless. Moreover, the fact that the practice does not seem to prevent so many individuals, groups and societies from doing well in their life, negates concern: if something were really wrong about circumcisions we would have known about it by now.

The next step in the ethical investigation is to ask whether any of the seven considerations by parents listed above overrides the initial '*other things being equal*' judgement that points against circumcision. Before we turn to answer, it is important to clarify what exactly is at stake in the *question*. As mentioned above, I assume that the parents in question do not as a rule consider it unproblematic to perform on their children a procedure to remove skin, tissues or other organs for non-medical non-therapeutic reasons. As a rule, they would judge intervention of this kind as ethically undesirable and object to it. Therefore, the ethical question at hand is whether and why any of the seven considerations above indicates that circumcision is different in a relevant way, which can overturn our initial judgement that, as a rule, procedures of this kind are objectionable. At the same time I assume – based on the available medical information – that to the extent that risks and harms are involved, the practice is not *in and of itself* sufficiently harmful categorically to reject it – irrespective of the reasons the individuals involved might have to perform it.

Do the seven considerations listed above overturn the initial judgement against procedures of this kind? Let us examine them in turn. Recall that answers to the ethical question do not immediately entail any particular answer to the legal question. Some things may be ethically wrong, but not in a way that requires a legislation to prohibit them.

(1) *Social convention*. Broadly liberal ethics expect individuals to reflect upon their actions. From this perspective the fact that any particular action is the convention is not as such a valid reason to perform it. The proverb 'for example is not an argument' captures this idea, as it applies to situations of the following kind.

> Girl: 'Mom, can I please have two dollars to buy ice cream?'
>
> Mother: 'Not today, you already had ice cream this week.'
>
> Girl: 'But why mom? The parents of my friend Ruth, for example, give her money to buy ice cream every day.'
>
> Mother: '"For example" is not an argument.'

From a broadly liberal perspective, the fact of social convention alone is not reason to perform an action. But what about parents who do not generally endorse a liberal or individualist view on ethics? What about the communitarian, conventionalist or moral relativist for whom accepted social conventions are valuable in virtue of being accepted? Communitarians do not generally expect us to avoid reflection. Rather they expect that (1) more often than not, upon reflection, we would find ourselves reconciled with the norms and conventions of our community; (2) we would appreciate the transmission and maintenance of communal value and consider the continuity as such valuable. These, however, are the kind of considerations that belong in reason 5 – identification and affirmation of group identity. For the communitarian too acting upon convention while suspending reflection is not as such valuable.

For the ethical relativist and conventionalist, however, conventions as such matter for ethical judgement. If it is widely believed in a society that circumcision is good and ethical then the acceptance of the ethical convention is as such a ground for its validity. From this perspective, circumcision is seen as ethical in some societies, where it is the accepted convention, and at the same time un-ethical in other societies, where it is not the accepted convention. A parent that adopts moral relativism and lives in a society in which circumcision is the accepted norm has a reason to endorse the practice on ground of its ethical goodness.

Note however, that this ethical judgement in favour of circumcision would be a Pyrrhic victory if endorsed by proponents of practice in the current debates in Germany and elsewhere in Europe. First, the voices in favour of circumcision are not inclined to endorse moral relativism. Indeed some of the participants are, as a rule, supporters of humanism and universal values. Second, in Germany and other European societies circumcision is not the norm. In fact the norm and conventional ethical judgement by the majority supports a legal ban on the practice. Third, the problem at hand is one in which a convention or tradition is being *contested;* one in which societies are conflicted about which norm and ethical position is the right one. Therefore a theory that appeals to what is accepted is ill-equipped to help us form a judgement on ethical conflicts of this kind within one society.

(2) *Social pressure.* Parents who respond to social pressure act upon the fear of future harm to their child in the forms of social exclusion, rejection and disadvantage. Social pressure of this kind is a form of blackmail: the parents are requested to pay a price now in order to prevent greater future harm to their child and to themselves. The question of how real and severe is the perceived threat of future exclusion and harm to the child is relevant for our ethical judgement. Let us suppose that the threat is real and serious – that the social rejection experienced by a non-circumcised child results in greater harm than the circumcision itself. If this condition obtains, parents can justify their decision in favour of circumcision, as choosing a lesser evil for their child. However, they are still required to act to change the situation; they as adults are required then to mobilize other adult members of their society to change the norms, so that future children and their parents will no longer face the threat. Note, that in the case of the debate in Germany and elsewhere in Europe, social pressure of this kind is very unlikely to occur. On the contrary, if there is a social norm and pressure to conform, it points against circumcision. Moreover, if and where social pressure of this kind indeed exists, the pressured parent ought to be in favour of a legal ban – an intervention by the state – that would relieve them from being blackmailed by other members of their society.

(3) *Belief in medical benefits.* In a scene from his film *Sleeper* (a science fiction comedy), Woody Allen experiences life in a future society, where science will have discovered that steak, cream pies and hot fudge are healthy and life prolonging. In the case of circumcision, reliable and accessible information about the risks, complications and benefits of the procedure are clearly missing. There are some medical facts that seem safe enough to cite, but they do not amount to a full picture. Circumcision reduces the risk of urinary tract infections in infants and the risk of contracting certain sexually transmitted viruses (including HIV) in adults.[9] This information alone does not tell us what the risk of contracting any of these infections is without circumcision, and how the risk reduction compares to the risk of circumcision itself and its complications, nor does it mention other available ways to prevent the said diseases. Therefore, when Rabbinical authorities simply affirm that circumcision is good because it is medically beneficial, they do not disclose all the relevant parts of the story. Indeed, no medical body or association *recommends* neonatal circumcision as a routine procedure in the way that certain vaccinations, for example, are generally and routinely recommended.

For parents to make an informed decision, the relevant information needs to be available to them in an accessible form. A pile of medical studies with diverse results and conclusions that very few parents are capable of deciphering and evaluating is unhelpful. Interestingly, it seems that the full picture is not even available to the medical profession. A recent report by the American Academy of Pediatrics recommends, based on evaluation of *current* evidence, that 'the health benefits of newborn circumcision outweigh the risks, and the benefits of newborn male circumcision justify access to this procedure for those families who choose it'.[10] But we also learn from the report that adequate and systematic knowledge of the risks and complications of circumcision is *not* available. We learn that '[t]he true incidence of complications after newborn circumcision is unknown.'[11] 'Based on the data reviewed, it is difficult, if not impossible, to adequately assess the total impact of complications, because the data are scant and inconsistent regarding the severity of complications.'[12] In short, while proponents of circumcision rush to celebrate the medical benefits, they neglect to mention that they do not really know much about the risks and complications. The available medical information gives no reason to overturn our initial 'other things being equal' judgement against circumcision.

(4) *Community expectations.* The ethical weight of community expectations depends in part on parents' own inclinations. For parents who are inclined against circumcision, the question of community expectations is whether, how and why it is right to please some people we care about at the cost of acting against our better judgement and possibly risking disappointing or upsetting someone else we care about (and have a legal obligation to care for) – the child. If the social expectations come with actual or potential serious sanctions then we find ourselves back to point (2) – social pressure. For example, if the grandparents not only express their wish to see their grandchild circumcised, but also threaten to sever contact if the parents do not comply. If the expectation is not accompanied by a threat of sanction, then parents ought to act according to their judgement against removing body tissues from their newborn for non-medical reasons. If on the other hand the parents in and of themselves are inclined to perform circumcision because of their own wish to express their communal affiliation and identification, then communal expectations merely reinforce a decision already taken for other reasons.

(5) *Positive identification and pride in membership.* So far we have focused on situations in which the main motivation or incentive to perform circumcision lies in the parents' environment or society and not in the parents themselves. But there are many Jewish parents who for many very good reasons affirm their cultural and communal affiliation and take pride in it. Given that neonatal circumcision is seen as an important indication of this membership and affiliation, by continuing a tradition that has been kept over many centuries, parents see themselves as affirming and endorsing their identities and histories. 'This is what it means to be Jewish', they say, and 'this is part of who I am and who I wish to be'. Are these parents committing an ethical wrong of bad judgement? It depends. Parents who feel this way and are motived to circumcise their newborn sons by considerations of affirmation of and pride in membership ought to find themselves in a dilemma. The dilemma is between, on the one hand, the wish to keep a tradition, transmit it to their own children and future generations and affirm an affiliation and, on the other hand, their initial judgement that the removal of skin, tissue or other organs for non-therapeutic reasons is very undesirable. Indeed this very judgement makes many parents worried about the procedure – worried about what might go wrong, worried about the possibility of pain inflicted on their child, worried that they might indeed be doing something bad to the child they love.

It is important to understand, however, what exactly the ethical problem is. It is important because of a misconception of the issue both by commentators and the Cologne district court ruling. The court argued that circumcision undermines the self-determination of the child. This was one of the reasons why the parents had no right, according to the court, to have their child circumcised. The child's right to self-determination limits the parents' right to care for and educate their children.[13] Prominent legal scholar Reinhard Merkel argued too, that while parents, in their roles as educators and care givers, are entitled to interfere with their children in many different ways – including through religious education – circumcision is 'not an act of education [...] It is an irreversible physical mark of integration into a religious community. To secure such integration permanently lies beyond the rights of parents.' (Merkel 2012)

The error in this argument is that the fact that circumcision is irreversible does not as such undermine the ability of the grown up individual to defy his parents' wishes and intentions and join another religion or culture. If we were to limit parental education in general only to those actions and decisions that do not leave long term and irreversible marks, traces and impacts, we would be left with an untenable notion of child rearing. Many of our physical traits are predetermined for us by our parents' decision to reproduce and by each parent's choice of a mate. Parents and other care givers also pick for us the language(s) of which we will be native speakers for our entire life. We might choose to learn another language as adults, but the marks and traces of one's native tongue are, for most people, impossible to undo. Our psychological dispositions, for better and worse are determined by early age experiences, and the decisions of our parents. Some indeed argue that because so much is predetermined for us the idea of individual autonomy and self-determination is an illusion. I do not take this view. Rather as argued by philosophers of personal autonomy and freedom, meaningful relationship and affiliations, even if they sometimes leave long term and permanent traces on us, are elements of and important conditions for our ability to be self-determining. Even if, as John Locke thought, we come to world as a blank slate – *tabula rasa* – it is not by remaining this way that we maintain our freedom and self-determination. In sum, whatever is wrong about circumcision, it is not that *because* it is irreversible it undermines personal autonomy and conflicts with it.

My argument in this section so far may have pleased proponents of circumcision. The bad news for this camp, on my view, is that leaving aside the erroneous argument does not make circumcision right or unproblematic. Even if the self-determination of the adult is not hindered merely by the fact of being circumcised, parents who decide to perform it take action that involves the removal of skin and body tissue for non-therapeutic purpose. So parents who agree that removal or skin, body tissues or organs for no therapeutic purpose from their children is objectionable, but still want to affirm their identity and affiliation by circumcision of their sons, ought to find themselves in a dilemma, and to take this dilemma seriously.

The way out of this dilemma is to work to change the practice – to keep the meaning, the cultural transmission and the affirmation of identity, but transform the content of the ritual. Some groups, currently marginal and very small, have begun to do just that. I do not believe that they will have quick and overwhelming success. However, the attempt itself is meaningful. Now, the parents with the dilemma would argue that until a general change in their society and community is achieved, choosing the alternative ritual just would not do: neither they nor their community consider the alternative ceremony as the appropriate way to affirm their membership and identity and take pride in their traditions. At this point, my argument leaves each parent with the voice of his or her consciousness to decide. However, even if they decide for circumcision, it would be ethically wrong to ignore the dilemma. Therefore, they will still have an obligation to work to change the accepted practice, to enquire more about the effects of circumcision, to take action to inform others, to draw their attention to the dilemma and to persuade them to help bring about change.

(6) *Faith and consciousness*. The only argument for circumcision that changes the balance of the 'other things being equal' judgement against the practice is freedom of consciousness. This freedom applies to a much narrower range of activities than the general freedom of religion. For freedom of consciousness to kick in, a person has to be asked to actively violate a strong and important duty or conviction dictated by her consciousness. For those religious Jews that *sincerely believe* in the divine origin of the Torah and of subsequent religious duty,

circumcision of their newborn sons is a serious requirement. They will be violating a clear and unequivocal religious duty, akin to the situation of a pacifist drafted to a military service. This does not apply to any obligation that a believer might take upon herself on religious grounds, but circumcision of sons in Jewish religious law is an important matter. For this subset of parents, who form a minority among Jewish parents, circumcision, until otherwise proven, is an ethically permissible decision.[14]

(7) *The working of a taboo*. Having read and talked about circumcision over the past couple of years, I suspect that there is taboo in the working. Seeking easily accessible and clear information about the procedure and its effects reinforces the suspicion. A parent that raises doubts is immediately confronted with different means of deflections. Soothing reactions: 'there is nothing to worry about, everyone does it, it is fine!' or references to all the beautiful and imaginative Rabbinical and literary interpretations of the symbolic meanings of the rituals. The parent is also soon confronted with discontent that doubts and questions are being raised. If the doubting parent then proceeds to seek information about the medical and physiological aspects of the ritual, s/he has to delve extensively into scientific medical literature. There is no way of predicting where an open conversation might lead us, but it is clearly wrong not to have it.

In sum, the seven considerations above yield the following guidelines on the ethical question of what Jewish parents should do about circumcisions of sons. We began with an 'other things being equal' judgement: with the assumption that, as a rule, parents are strongly inclined to oppose the removal of skin, tissues or organs from their children for non-therapeutic purposes. With the exception of faith and consciousness, no ethical consideration examined above shifts the balance of the 'other things being equal' judgement in favour of circumcision. As far as the ethical question is concerned, unless they truly believe that God has commanded them to perform the ritual, parents ought to rule against circumcision with three caveats: (1) if the parents are sincere moral relativists, they have a reason to favour circumcision where it is the norm. This does not apply to Germany or elsewhere in Europe. (2) If the threat of social exclusion and future sanctions for their child, when not circumcised, is real and serious, a decision to circumcise is ethically permissible (though not desirable). However, parents who circumcise because of blackmail of this kind ought to campaign for a change of the social norm or for a legal ban that would protect them and other parents in the future from this unpleasant situation. This consideration, too, is inapplicable to parents in European societies. (3) For parents who find themselves in a sincere dilemma between their wish to affirm their identity/communal affiliation and the objection to the ritual of circumcision, the ethical judgement is ultimately theirs to make. But even if they rule in favour of circumcision, it remains their obligation to work towards a change of the norm, so that in the future they and other parents will not face the same dilemma. They ought not to choose instead to suppress their doubts and objections and to reconcile themselves with their decision by down-playing the dilemma. Finally, everyone involved ought to seek and provide reliable, accessible and factually unbiased information; it is a good time to let go of a taboo.

3. The legal question

What about states? How ought states to act or forbear regarding male circumcision? An exhaustive discussion of this question will take more than the available space. Two considerations can, nevertheless, move us forward in this discussion. First, it bears to reason that legal systems will vary on this point. Namely, that on grounds of reasonable pluralism and justifiable differences, legal positions and conclusions will vary across states – even across states that are generally committed to individual rights and protection of child interests and well-being. Whereas in Germany, the court found that circumcision contradicted the constitutional provision of bodily integrity, in Israel an appeal to the Supreme Court to ban circumcision on similar grounds was rejected outright. Whereas in Germany, it has been argued that it is inconceivable that a constitutional right to religious freedom would permit a physical interference with another individual, in the United States an initiative to ban circumcision in San Francisco was prohibited by the court because of its implications for religious freedom. We need not assume that either the American or the German lawyers and judges are necessarily wrong when they reach different conclusions on the limits of religious freedom. They operate in two different legal environments that understand religious freedom and its limits in different ways.

Second, we started with the debate about the legal status of circumcision in Germany. While the Cologne court ruling of 2012 included some dubious and even erroneous arguments, it did get one point right. Physical interference for non-medical reasons, of the kind that circumcision is, is incompatible with the requirements of bodily integrity as understood in German law. Therefore, we ought to ask then whether there are reasons to exempt a minuscule Jewish minority in the country from this legal provision, for the specific purpose of neonatal male circumcision. Exemptions on grounds of faith and consciousness are not unheard of under German law. In the time of mandatory military service, individuals were exempt on grounds of pacifism. In another case, a husband who let his wife die instead of taking her to a hospital for treatment was exonerated by the Constitutional Court because of the religious motives of the couple in avoiding medical treatment.[15] Given the commitment of the Federal Republic to encourage the Jewish community to take root in the country, and the fact the number of children involved is tiny, there are good reasons to be in favour of an exemption of this kind.[16]

I suggested elsewhere (Banai 2012) that the change in legislation to make circumcision generally permissible was not the best way to establish the exemption. The law, however, is now changed and I doubt that a campaign to undo the change would be either effective or desirable. Given the new legal situation in Germany and in light of the ethical considerations above, the state ought to see that parents are provided with the pertinent factually impartial information on the procedure, including the risks and alternatives. In the law regulating abortions in Germany a consultation is a required precondition. This regulation should be adopted for circumcision too. Given that the state has now officially delegated the choice to parents, it incurred the responsibility of providing the required information. This responsibility is reinforced by the taboos protecting the issue of circumcision in the communities that practice it.

Notes

1. A Yiddish proverb.
2. On public opinion polls with majorities against the practice, see, for example, 'Deutsche lehnen religiöse Beschneidung ab'; 'Mehrheit der Deutschen gegen Beschneidungsgesetz'.
3. Holm Putzke, a prominent voice in favour of the court from the legal community, referred to male circumcision as an act of violence against children (from which they need to be defended by the society) on different occasions; for example: 'Schutz von Gewalt ist wichtiger als religiöse Riten', and 'Die Politik reagiert reflexhaft, nicht reflektiert'.
4. See, for example, in the report by Birgitta vom Lehm (2012)

5. An open letter to Chancellor Angela Merkel (Franz 2012) signed by some 400 health, lawyers and mental health professionals, referred to the circumcision as a form of sexual violence against children.
6. For the new legislation see paragraph 1631d BGB, 'Beschneidung des männlichen Kindes'.
7. An estimated third of men worldwide is circumcised. Seventy per cent of circumcised men are Muslim. Among white non-Hispanic Americans 80% are circumcised, though there seems to be a trend of decline.
8. Since I employed no scientific sample or interviewing methods, I can claim no scientific validity to my results. However, the information is pertinent as hypotheses for future investigation.
9. I rely here on a recent report of the American Pediatric Association. As a layperson it is impossible for me to judge the quality and full meaning of medical evidence. American Academy of Pediatrics, Technical Report: Male Circumcision, August 2012.
10. *Technical Report: Male Circumcision,* e761.
11. *Technical Report: Male Circumcision,* e772.
12. *Technical Report: Male Circumcision,* e775.
13. Landesgericht Köln Urteil 151 Ns 169/11, 07.05.2012, pp. 5 and 7. This was not the only reason: the court also mentions the right of the child to bodily integrity. I have argued elsewhere (Banai 2012) that in the way bodily integrity is understood in German law, it is hard to see how the court could have concluded otherwise.
14. It does not follow that the practice ought simply to be ignored. It is certainly possible for a state, to provide parents with the relevant information and even require parents to attend a consultation before they decide on the matter. I will return to this point below. It is also possible to leave the parents liable for harms under civil law. I will not discuss this option here.
15. Information about the legal case is available in Gerhard Robbers (2010).
16. In principle, an exemption of this kind should only apply to Orthodox parents. However, I want to assume that the German legal system strongly wishes to avoid testing members of its Jewish community for their Judaism, and so it would make sense pragmatically to opt for the less strict option.

References

Bahners, Patrick. 2012. "Ein Rechenfehler". *Frankfurter Allgemeine Zeitung*. July 22.

Banai, Ayelet. 2012. "Das Dilemma" *Jungle World*, Nr. 31. August 2.

Bommarius, Christian. 2012. "Rechtsschutz für die Beschneidung". *Berliner Zeitung*. September 25.

"Deutsche lehnen religiöse Beschneidung ab". 2012. *Stern*. July 1.

Franz, Matthias. 2012. "Religionsfreiheit kann kein Freibrief für Gewalt Sein". *Frankfurter Allgemeine Zeitung*. July 21.

"Mehrheit der Deutschen Gegen Beschneidungsgesetz." 2012. *Spiegel*. December 22.

Merkel, Reinhard. 2012. "Die Haut eines Anderen". *Süddeutsche Zeitung*. August 30.

Putzke, Holm. 2012a. "Schutz von Gewalt ist wichtiger als religiöse Riten". Interview with Holm Putzke by Veronika Beer and Annette Walter, Bayerischer Rundfunk. June 29.

Putzke, Holm. 2012b. "Die Politik Reagiert Reflexhaft, Nicht Reflektiert". Interview with Holm Putzke in *Focus*. July 24.

Robbers, Gerhard. 2010. *Religion and Law in Germany*, 102. Alphen aan den Rijn: Kluwer Law International.

von Lehm, Birgitta. 2012. "Unterschätztes Trauma-Risiko". *Frankfurter Rundschau*. July 18.

Legislation on male infant circumcision in Europe: a call to avoid paternalism and to promote evidence-based, patient-centred care

Maria Kristiansen[a] and Aziz Sheikh[b]

[a]*Danish Research Centre for Migration, Ethnicity and Health, Department of Public Health, Faculty of Health and Medical Sciences, University of Copenhagen, Copenhagen, Denmark;* [b]*Primary Care Research & Development, Edinburgh Ethnicity and Health Research Group, Centre for Population Health Sciences, The University of Edinburgh, Edinburgh, UK*

Male infant circumcision is a controversial and debated topic in both scientific and public discourses in parts of Western Europe. Debates are heated and it is not always entirely clear what is in the best interest of the male infant. In this article, we discuss the importance of returning to core principles of evidence-based, patient-centred care that may help move the discussion away from the current, increasingly polarised positions. According to principles of evidence-based medicine, systematic retrieval and critical appraisal of the best evidence available should be a core consideration in all decisions regarding healthcare policy and practice. Applying this principle to male infant circumcision, we need a careful, dispassionate critique of the evidence in relation to the benefits and risks associated with the procedure and an assessment of the potential health gains and adverse effects of any interventions (such as legislation) that may be introduced. Currently, the more robust evidence-base has tended to focus on biomedical aspects of male infant circumcision and this shows consistent evidence of important benefits of this practice, but also some risks. However, health is multi-dimensional and when considering male infant circumcision, there is therefore a need to broaden the perspective to also include psycho-social considerations. It is also imperative that those striving to deliver patient-centred care keep the best interests of the patient/family at the heart of their decision-making, promote autonomy and do not inadvertently exceed the fine line between beneficence and medical paternalism.In summary, we argue that a more comprehensive and robust evidence-base is needed to enable evidence-based policy-making and that these uncertainties are communicated to patients/families so they can in the light of this evidence make an informed choice.

Male infant circumcision continues to invoke considerable controversy and debate in parts of Western Europe, not least since the German court ruling deemed male circumcision equivalent to grievous bodily harm in June 2012 (Landesgericht Köln 2012). There are many reasons why it provokes such strong emotions: circumcision is a practice that relates to children who are typically unable to, or in some cases not invited to, provide their informed consent; it involves surgical operations performed for non-therapeutic reasons; and it is a practice that in many cases stems from deeply held religious beliefs, which are for many difficult to grapple with in a now predominantly secular Western Europe (Gatrad and Sheikh 2001). This is however anything but a simple debate between secular and religious perspectives. The complexity of this issue is exemplified by the fact that although a number of medical bodies have criticised the practice on the above grounds and because of concerns related to health risks associated with the procedure, other powerful advocacy and professional bodies such as the World Health Organization (WHO) and the American Academy of Pediatrics (AAP) have strongly argued for the preventive and public health benefits associated with male circumcision (e.g. in reducing heterosexually transmitted HIV infections). This has in the US led to calls for reimbursement of the procedure and promotion of the practice among groups who have no tradition for this specific practice (Baker 2012; Siegfried et al. 2009; Singh-Grewal, Macdessi, and Craig 2005; Task Force on Circumcision 2012). Within this overall highly charged professional and public discourse, it is not always clear what is in the best interests of the child and his family and whether these interests are centre-stage in the minds of the various protagonists.

In this article, we draw on some core principles that should underpin decision-making when seeking to protect and promote public health (Institute of Medicine 2002; International Conference on Primary Health Care 1978; Public Health Leadership Society 2002). In particular, we point to the inherent dangers of medical paternalism, the need for a sufficient evidence-base encompassing not only the biomedical dimensions of male infant circumcision but also the psycho-social considerations, and in libertarian societies the need to ensure that this is then combined with respect for patient perspectives, preferences and autonomy (Illich 1976; Locke 2009; Mill 1859; Skrabanek 1994). Adherence to these core principles is we argue all the more important when considering deeply contested issues in order to ensure sound public policy-making.

Evidence-based medicine is one of the central pillars underpinning modern medicine. It has been defined as 'a systematic approach to clinical problem solving which allows the integration of the best available research evidence with clinical expertise and patient values' (Sackett, Strauss, and Richardson 2000). Systematic retrieval of the best evidence available and a critical appraisal of this evidence should be the basis of all decisions regarding health care policy and practice, although this scenario undeniably remains an ideal rather than a reality (Heneghan and Godlee 2013). At least in principle, promoting or discouraging certain practices should build on both scientific evidence and a principle of proportionality (Lee 2012; Rose 1994). When considering intervening against male infant religious circumcision, we therefore need strong evidence for the health risks associated with the procedure; these risks should then be balanced carefully against the benefits of this practice and the risks of interventions inadvertently resulting in harm. In relation to the health risks and benefits of male circumcision, the more robust evidence-base suggests important benefits, but also some risks. Studies have tended to focus on biomedical considerations including the physiological, prophylactic and to a lesser extent sexual effects of male infant and adult circumcision (Hayashi and Kohri 2013; Pinto 2012; Weiss et al. 2006; Wheeler and Malone 2013). Recently published reviews and the review performed by the AAP Task Force on Circumcision show preventive effects of male circumcision in relation to urinary tract infections, transmission of some sexually transmitted infections (HIV, human papillomavirus and herpes simplex virus type 2) and penile cancer (Hayashi and Kohri 2013; Larke et al. 2011; Task Force on Circumcision 2012). Randomised controlled trials conducted in developing countries have documented benefits of male circumcision on rates of sexually transmitted infections and sexual satisfaction (Kigozi et al. 2008; Krieger et al. 2008; Siegfried et al. 2009; Wawer et al. 2011). The risks associated with the procedure are mainly surgical complications and concerns about psychosexual function, but the key question here is the trade-off between potential benefits and risks (Perera et al. 2010; Siegfried et al. 2009; Task Force on Circumcision 2012; Wheeler and Malone 2013).

According to Sackett's definition of evidence-based medicine, scientific evidence and clinical expertise need to be integrated with patient values if we wish to achieve the goal of providing high-quality health care services that reflect the interests, values and choices of patients (Sackett, Strauss, and Richardson 2000). Patient-centred care is therefore central to evidence-based medicine and so is a multidimensional concept of health as 'a state of complete physical, mental and social well-being and not merely the absence of disease or infirmity' (World Health Organization 1948). This multidimensional concept of health emphasises that health is about more than just physical functioning. When considering male infant circumcision, we therefore need to broaden our gaze beyond just biomedical issues and also include the psycho-social dimensions of it. Parallel with the biomedical research, there is a need to understand the psychological and social effects of male infant religious circumcision including the possible meanings attributed to being circumcised in relation to masculinity, identity and belonging to religious communities, but this remains a very under-developed field of enquiry (Yavuz, Demir, and Dogangün 2012). A narrow focus on possible health risks based on relatively few cases of short or long-term physical complications following male circumcision fail to encompass the diversity of religious, cultural and social factors that influence decision-making surrounding male infant circumcision. In keeping with the WHO concept of health, we therefore need a much broader evidence-base that also investigates the impact of male circumcision on psychological and social well-being among larger populations than is most often the case in current studies. An unbiased summary of this broader evidence base will help families contemplating having their son circumcised for religious or health reasons in deciding what is in the best interest of their child.

Male infant circumcision is a contentious issue and there is a real danger of exceeding the fine line between beneficence and unwarranted medical paternalism. Acting in the best interest of the male infant must be the key concern for both opponents and proponents of male infant circumcision. In the absence of a broad evidence-base, we risk acting on behalf of these children without fully considering whether our understanding of the best interest of the child is adequate or whether our actions build on too narrow understandings of health which have been fashioned on possibly normative grounds. Holding on to standard principles underpinning evidence-based medicine and patient-centred care is therefore important, not least in the current situation with charged 'ugly, messy and nasty' debates surrounding male infant religious circumcision (Collier 2012). We need carefully to balance respect for individual values, interests and autonomy with obligations to prevent harm and protect health. This is even more important when male infant religious circumcision is concerned, since this topic is simultaneously sensitive, concerned with minors, and practised by religious minority groups who may be at particular risk of marginalisation and social exclusion in response to actions on part of majority groups (Grove and Zwi 2005; Inhorn and Serour 2011; Johnson et al. 2004; Sheikh 2007). If we fail to acknowledge the multiple dimensions of male circumcision both on a discursive level and in clinical encounters with families from Jewish or Muslim backgrounds, we risk alienating these families which may negatively affect their trust in and use of health care services in relation to circumcision and perhaps also when other health needs arise (Inhorn and Serour 2011).

Legislation against male circumcision should be a last resort, and in view of the emerging evidence of health benefits and the real risk that prohibition would drive the practice underground, we believe prohibiting male infant religious circumcision to be counter-productive as it is likely to result in net harm. It is unlikely – not least given the considerable controversy on the health aspects of the procedure and the deep-held religious beliefs from which it arise – that male infant religious circumcision will be easily abandoned by Muslim and Jewish communities. Practices that are perceived to be important – even constitutive – for identity, that are normalised and reinforced in interactions within immediate and extended relationships and build on deeply personal beliefs about the existential meaning with the human condition are not changed nor eradicated by simple information or even legislation (Gatrad, Sheikh, and Jacks 2002). The heated discourse on religious circumcision with arguments feeding into debates on multiculturalism and religious diversity in the West only makes the debate even less likely to influence the everyday decisions and practices in families (Laird, de Marrais, and Barnes 2007). It is much more likely that legislation ruling the procedure illegal will drive the practice underground resulting in potentially more harm to the children undergoing this ritual. Even if legal action is not taken, the current discourses on religious circumcision may hinder the trust and mutual understanding that is needed in clinical encounters between parents considering having their child circumcised and health care professionals who still for the most part do not share the religious beliefs of their patients. Also, heated debates may lead to over-sensitivity or reluctance to take up any reasonable concern that could be important and relevant to discuss in these encounters, e.g. in relation to the question of pain or prevention of bleeding and infection. Acknowledging both the importance attached to male circumcision for individual families and the risks associated with this practice will enable the engagement of families that is necessary if poorly performed male circumcision and its negative effects on children are to be prevented. A more balanced, person-centred approach based on a broader evidence-base is therefore needed.

In conclusion, debates on male infant religious circumcision are often heated and resting on a narrow evidence-base pertaining to the effects on the overall well-being of the child. From a medical point of view, adhering to the core principles underpinning evidence-based medicine is of paramount importance for the delivery of high-quality, patient-centred care. For this to happen, we need a more substantial, broader evidence-base that encompasses both biomedical and psycho-social dimensions of male circumcision. This insight should be translated into recommendations thereby ensuring that families considering male infant circumcision are offered impartial, informed choice. In the meantime, sensitive, accessible care should be available for those who choose to have their child circumcised.

We do not call for an anything-goes attitude to this practice, but we do suggest that the current discourses on circumcision – with their at times quite charged perspectives on the practice – risk contributing to a climate that is not conducive to tackling the potential adverse health effects of the practice. Given the charged nature of the debate and the wider religious connotations of it, it is important that legislators, policy-makers and health care professionals avoid turning to unwarranted medical paternalism and instead remain true to the principles that have helped secure Europe's position as a bastion of rationality, liberalism and person-centred care.

References

Baker, M. 2012. "Doctors Back Circumcision." *Nature* 488: 568.

Collier, R. 2012. "Ugly, Messy and Nasty Debate Surrounds Circumcision." *CMAJ* 184: E25–E26.

Gatrad, A. R., and A. Sheikh. 2001. "Muslim Birth Customs." *Archives of Disease in Childhood – Fetal and Neonatal Edition* 84: F6–F8.

Gatrad, A. R., A. Sheikh, and H. Jacks. 2002. "Religious Circumcision and the Human Rights Act." *Archives of Disease in Childhood* 86: 76–78.

Grove, N. J., and A. B. Zwi. 2005. "Our Health and Theirs: Forced Migration, Othering, and Public Health." *Social Science & Medicine* 62: 1931–1942.

Hayashi, Y., and K. Kohri. 2013. "Circumcision Related to Urinary Tract Infections, Sexually Transmitted Infections, Human Immunodeficiency Virus Infections, and Penile and Cervical Cancer." *International Journal of Urology*. doi:10.1111/iju.12154.

Heneghan, C., and F. Godlee. 2013. "Where Next for Evidence Based Healthcare?" *BMJ* 346: F766.

Illich, I. 1976. "The Medicalization of Life." In *Medical Nemesis. The Expropriation of Health*, 39–126. New York: Random House.

Inhorn, M., and G. Serour. 2011. "Islam, Medicine and Arab-Muslim Refugee Health in America after 9/11." *The Lancet* 378: 935–943.

Institute of Medicine. 2002. *The Future of the Public's Health in the 21st Century*. Washington, DC: National Academies Press.

International Conference on Primary Health Care. 1978. "Declaration of Alma Ata." Alma Ata: USSR. Accessed May 14, 2013. http://www.who.int/publications/almaata_declaration_en.pdf

Johnson, J. L., J. L. Bottorff, A. J. Browne, S. Grewal, B. A. Hilton, and H. Clarke. 2004. "Othering and Being Othered in the Context of Health Care Services." *Health Communication* 16: 253–271.

Kigozi, G., S. Watya, C. B. Polis, D. Buwembo, V. Kiggundu, M. J. Wawer, D. Serwadda, F. et al. 2008. "The Effect of Male Circumcision on Sexual Satisfaction and Function, Results from a Randomized Trial of Male Circumcision for Human Immunodeficiency Virus Prevention, Rakai, Uganda." *BJU International* 101: 65–70.

Krieger, J. N., S. D. Mehta, R. C. Bailey, K. Agot, J. O. Ndinya-Achola, C. Parker, and S. Moses. 2008. "Adult Male Circumcision: Effects on Sexual Function and Sexual Satisfaction in Kisumu, Kenya." *Journal of Sexual Medicine* 5: 2610–2622.

Laird, L. D., J. de Marrais, and L. L. Barnes. 2007. "Portraying Islam and Muslims in MEDLINE: A Content Analysis." *Social Science & Medicine* 65: 2425–2439.

Landesgericht Köln. 2012. "Urteile des Amtsgerichts und des Landgerichts Köln zur Strafbarkeit von Beschneidungen nicht einwilligungsfähiger Jungen aus rein religiösen Gründe" [Judgments of the Local District Court and of the Cologne Regional Court on the Criminalization of Circumcision of Non-Consensual Boys for Purely Religious Reasons]. Press Release, June 26, *Justiz-Online*, Decision of May 7, [in German.] Docket No. Az. 151 Ns 169/11.

Larke, N. L., S. L. Thomas, I. dos Santos Silva, and H. A. Weiss. 2011. "Male Circumcision and Penile Cancer: A Systematic Review and Meta-analysis." *Cancer Causes Control* 22: 1097–1110.

Lee, L. M. 2012. "Public Health Ethics Theory: Review and Path to Convergence." *The Journal of Law, Medicine & Ethics* 40: 85–98.

Locke, J. 2009. *A Letter Concerning Toleration*. New York: Classic Books America.

Mill, J. S. 1859. *On Liberty*. 2nd ed. London: John W. Parker and Son.

Perera, C. L., F. H. Bridgewater, P. Thavaneswaran, and G. J. Maddern. 2010. "Safety and Efficacy of Nontherapeutic Male Circumcision: A Systematic Review." *Annals of Family Medicine* 8: 64–72.

Pinto, K. 2012. "Circumcision Controversies." *Pediatric Clinics of North America* 59: 977–986.

Public Health Leadership Society. 2002. "Principles of the Ethical Practice of Public Health." Accessed May 14, 2013: http://www.apha.org/NR/rdonlyres/1CED3CEA-287E-4185-9CBD-BD405FC60856/0/ethicsbrochure.pdf

Rose, G. 1994. *The Strategy of Preventive Medicine*. Oxford: Oxford University Press.

Sackett, D. L., S. E. Strauss, and W. S. Richardson. 2000. *Evidence-Based Medicine: How to Practice and Teach EBM*. London: Churchill-Livingstone.

Sheikh, A. 2007. "Should Muslims have Faith Based Health Services?" *BMJ* 334: 74.

Siegfried, N., M. Muller, J. J. Deeks, and J. Volmink. 2009. "Male Circumcision for Prevention of Heterosexual Acquisition of HIV in Men." *Cochrane Database of Systematic Reviews* 2: CD003362.

Singh-Grewal, D., J. Macdessi, and J. Craig. 2005. "Circumcision for the Prevention of Urinary Tract Infection in Boys: A Systematic Review of Randomised Trials and Observational Studies." *Archives of Disease in Childhood* 90: 853–858.

Skrabanek, P. 1994. *The Death of Humane Medicine and the Rise of Coercive Healthism*. Suffolk: Social Affairs Unit.

Task Force on Circumcision. 2012. "Male Circumcision." *Pediatrics* 130: e756–e785.

Wawer, M. J., A. A. Tobian, G. Kigozi, X. Kong, P. E. Gravitt, D. Serwadda, F. Nalugoda, et al. 2011. "Effect of Circumcision of HIV-Negative Men on Transmission of Human Papillomavirus to HIV-Negative Women: A Randomised Trial in Rakai, Uganda." *Lancet* 377: 209–218.

Weiss, H. A., S. L. Thomas, S. K. Munabi, and R. J. Hayes. 2006. "Male Circumcision and Risk of Syphilis, Chancroid, and Genital Herpes: A Systematic Review and Meta-Analysis." *Sexually Transmitted Infections* 82: 101–110.

Wheeler, R., and P. Malone. 2013. "Male Circumcision: Risk Versus Benefit." *Archives of Disease in Childhood*, 98 (5): 321–332.

World Health Organization. 1948. Preamble to the Constitution of the World Health Organization as Adopted by the International Health Conference, New York, June 19–22, 1946; signed on July 22, 1946 by the representatives of 61 States (Official Records of the World Health Organization, no. 2, p. 100) and entered into force on April 7, 1948.

Yavuz, M., T. Demir, and B. Dogangün. 2012. "The Effect of Circumcision on the Mental Health of Children: A Review." *Turkish Journal of Psychiatry* 23: 63–70.

The goose and the gander: the genital wars

Richard A. Shweder

Department of Comparative Human Development, University of Chicago, Chicago, IL, USA

Should there be gender equity in genital cutting? In Germany (and much of Europe), the native inhabitants tend to argue there is moral equivalence between customary male circumcision and customary female circumcision and both should be proscribed. In Sierra Leone (and several other countries in Africa), the native inhabitants tend to argue there is moral equivalence between customary male circumcision and customary female circumcision and both should be permitted. In the United States, the native inhabitants tend to argue against moral equivalence, permitting customary circumcisions for boys while proscribing them for girls. Who has the better of the argument? And what are the implications of the argument for Jews and other circumcising ethnic groups living in Europe, Africa, and North America?

It is rumored that when God issued the command, Abraham looked up at the heavens and said 'You want us to do what?' According to legend Sarah was not party to the conversation and was not included in the deal. Such stories don't surprise me. I hesitated too when my son was born, at least until the absentee ballots came flooding in from generations of ancestors; for the dead had a vote, including Abraham. And when my daughter was born the thought 'why aren't Jewish women circumcised?' never occurred to my wife. Not once did she look up at the heavens and say 'What kind of justice is this? Shouldn't there be gender equity in genital cutting?'

That however is the question fully considered by Shaye Cohen in *Why Aren't Jewish Women Circumcised?*[1] His book is an exegesis of medieval rabbinic understandings of the genital cutting required of Jewish males in Genesis 17. It is also an eye-opening account of Jewish attempts to respond to early anti-Semitic Christian accusations that neonatal male circumcision is not only gender biased, patriarchal, and exclusionary (of the female half of the Jewish population) but also morally inferior to the ecumenical and gender inclusive practice of Christian baptism. The author, who is a Professor of Hebrew Literature and Philosophy at Harvard University, then brings us up to date by observing that contemporary opponents of Jewish male circumcision 'assume [moral] parity between male circumcision, which is tolerated, and female circumcision, which is proscribed,' with the aim of expanding existing legal prohibitions of female genital mutilation (FGM) to include the male circumcision of minors.[2] What's good for the goose is good for the gander. Or so argue today's opponents of childhood male circumcision.

Even when discussing an ideologically overheated topic, Professor Cohen is admirably respectful of the process of critical reasoning. So, he follows the logic of the gender equity principle where it leads. In the concluding footnote of his book he observes that '…western discourse about female circumcision has been shaped exclusively by its opponents' and he raises some doubts about the validity of that discourse, for example with respect to claims about diminished sexual enjoyment for circumcised women. Making reference to one of my own writings on the topic[3] he remarks 'Perhaps, then, an argument could be made for moral parity between female circumcision and male circumcision, not in order to proscribe them both but in order to tolerate them both….'[4] In the remainder of this essay I hope to at least touch on several sides of that question.

'Equal Rights for All Sexes: Say 'No' to Forced Genital Cutting!'

'Equal Rights for All Sexes: Say 'No' to Forced Genital Cutting!' is the gender equity position of contemporary anti-male circumcision groups in North America and Europe. These activist organizations hope to put an end to the circumcision of male minors, which they describe as genital mutilation and child abuse. They believe that the male surgery is physically and psychologically harmful to boys, and a violation of several human rights, including the right to self-determination and the right to the preservation of physical integrity. In their efforts to abolish the practice they are encouraged by the ubiquitous North American and European news reports, opinion pieces, and NGO advocacy literature denouncing customary female genital surgeries in Africa in precisely those terms; and by the ready embrace by legislators (and by several global organizations too) of legal statutes criminalizing female genital surgeries for minors (and in some countries in Europe even banning the procedure for adult women, if those women are motivated by a desire to uphold their own ethnic traditions).

Simply put, the gender equity argument of the anti-male circumcision groups runs as follows: if it is reasonable to have public policies safeguarding the body of female minors from all medically unnecessary genital modifications, then the principle of gender equity (plus logical consistency) suggests there should be similar policies protecting the male body as well. Therefore, whenever global feminist organizations, public policy advocates, politicians or celebrities speak out against customary female genital modifications, denouncing them as mutilations and child abuse, so too they should speak out against customary male genital modifications, morally condemning them in similar terms; even at the risk of offending Jewish and Muslim supporters of anti-FGM campaigns. Put even more simply: there should be equal protection for boys and girls before the law. If you are an outspoken critic of FGM but then remain silent about male genital mutilation (MGM) you are either biased against men, insufficiently conscientious in the application of your principles, or a hypocrite.[5]

The gender equity argument in Europe

That gender equity argument plays relatively well in countries such as Holland, Sweden, Denmark, and Germany, where neither boys nor girls are customarily circumcised. In 2010, the Royal Dutch Medical Association (KNMG), striving for logical consistency with respect to the issue of gender equity, issued an official policy statement decrying the 'non-therapeutic circumcision of male minors' and calling on Muslims and Jews in Holland to abandon the practice. One of their main announced reasons for speaking up at this time was 'the growing sentiment that there is a discrepancy between the KNMG's firm stance with regard to female genital mutilation and the lack of a stance with regard to the non-therapeutic circumcision of male minors, as the two have a number of similarities.'[6]

In anticipation of the common and predictable retort that male circumcision may offer some distinctive protection against HIV infection, the Royal Dutch Medical Association (KNMG) offered this reply, with a strong emphasis on the general autonomy and physical integrity rights of both males and females: 'Insofar as there are medical benefits, such as a possibly reduced risk of HIV infection, it is reasonable to put off circumcision until the age at which such a risk is relevant and the boy himself can decide about the intervention, or can opt for any available alternatives' (By 'available alternatives' one assumes they had in mind, for example, using condoms or exercising care in the selection of sexual partners or abstinence rather than electing to be circumcised).

And the KNMG offered the following assessment of the evidence:

> the studies into HIV prevention were carried out in sub-Saharan Africa, where transmission mainly takes place through heterosexual contact. In the western world, HIV transmission is much more frequently the result of homosexual contact and the use of contaminated needles. That the relationship between circumcision and transmission of HIV is at the very least unclear is illustrated by the fact that the US combines a high prevalence of STDs and HIV infections with a high percentage of routine circumcisions. The Dutch situation is precisely the reverse: a low prevalence of HIV/AIDS combined with a relatively low number of circumcisions. As such behavioral factors appear to play a far more important role than whether or not one has a foreskin.

Two years later, male circumcision was banned in Germany. Constitutional rights of general applicability – gender inclusive rights to self-determination, physical integrity, and freedom from harm – were invoked by an appellate judge in Cologne in a 2012 court decision criminalizing the circumcision of male minors as customarily practiced by Muslims and Jews. From an historical point of view, the zone of European tolerance for Jewish male circumcision has long been narrow and insecure. Currently, that zone is being contested once again, perhaps fueled in part by self-defensive reactions by dominant European ethnic groups against immigrants from Africa and Asia and perceived threats to the cultural homeland. The recent German court decision concerned a Muslim 4-year-old boy and a Muslim doctor, although Jewish communities and organizations around the world were quick to react. They successfully lobbied German political leaders to legislatively overturn the decision, despite German popular opinion strongly opposed to male circumcision, and with at least some of that popular opinion appealing to modern secular liberal principles of the sort invoked by the judge in Cologne and the physicians in Holland.

The Jewish reaction was hardly surprising, given the Jewish experience in Germany and their historical status as a circumcising minority group living in a not necessarily welcoming non-circumcising German nation. In his book, *Making the Body Beautiful: A Cultural History of Aesthetic Surgery* Sander Gilman remarks:

> Recently there has been a resurgence of the debate about male circumcision that had marked the first generation of [German] Reformed Jewish thinkers in the 1840s. The most radical of these, Samuel Holdheim, had unsuccessfully advocated the abolition of infant male circumcision [in Germany] as a sign of the modernity of Jewish belief. The image of circumcision as a form of barbaric bloodletting dominated this discussion in the nineteenth century. It appeared in the rationale for the ritual murder accusations in the 1890s, that Jews ritually slaughter non-Jewish children for their blood. The argument ran: if the Jews will do this to their own

> children, imagine what they will do to ours! At the end of the twentieth century the accusation has resurfaced in the identification of circumcision as a form of child abuse.[7]

A further (and even more dreadful) historical irony of the recent court decision in Cologne was not lost on the collective memory of many Jews around the world: namely, the ghastly incongruity of witnessing post-WWII constitutionally granted rights to self-determination, physical integrity, and freedom from harm, which were inspired by the ethical lessons of the Holocaust and Nazi era medical experiments, invoked by a German judge with the aim of eradicating a ritualized surgical procedure central to Jewish ethnic identity.

Nevertheless, whatever the alarming ironies of the German court decision, dominant ethnic groups in Europe do have their own traditions and distinctive cultural histories with respect to genital norms for males and females. Many Europeans, even those who are not anti-Muslim or anti-Semitic, react both viscerally and upon reflection with disapproval to the very idea of a non-therapeutic circumcision of male minors. They are primed by virtue of their own long-standing customary habits to be relatively open to the gender equity arguments of anti-male circumcision activists and the Royal Dutch Medical Association calling for a general cessation of all non-therapeutic genital surgeries on minors, both male and female (and as noted many Europeans even support legal bans against genital surgeries by adult African women living in Europe who may wish to uphold their ethnic traditions). It is striking however (because disconcerting and reminiscent of the medieval tensions between Christian theologians and Jewish rabbis examined by Shaye Cohen and mentioned earlier) that the Royal Dutch Medical Association concluded its 2010 scientific report with a discussion of religious freedom in which they managed to draw an invidious comparison between the male circumcision rituals of Jews and Muslims and the baptizing of Christian children (which leaves no trace on a child's physical body, as the Dutch physicians didn't hesitate to point out).

'Nurse, come quickly, there is something terribly wrong with this child!'

The peoples of the world are quite divided in their social norms for genital cutting; and the typical European pattern (where neither boys nor girls modify their genitals) is not a cultural universal. There are no ethnic groups anywhere in the world where only girls modify their genitals. But, there are many where both boys and girls do, and even more where genital modification is exclusively a male prerogative, such as the United States, Israel, South Korea, the Philippines, most of the West Asian Muslim world, and many ethnic groups in Sub-Saharan Africa. In those countries, the gender equity argument of anti-male circumcision groups plays much less well.

In the United States, for example, most boys (and only boys) have their genitals surgically modified. Local social and legal norms proscribe female genital modifications for minors (although cosmetic genital surgeries of various sorts are growing in popularity for women and even teenage girls). Contemporary habits and dominant cultural views are highly permissive of the circumcision of male minors. Anti-male circumcision activists in San Francisco (a city which is arguably the geographical center for this type of activism in the United States) failed miserably in 2011 when they tried to sponsor a ballot initiative banning the surgery within city limits. They never even got on the ballot because their initiative was successfully contested in the courts, where it was judged an unwarranted intrusion into a State licensed medical procedure. The very idea of a ballot initiative of that sort precipitated a broad legislative and cultural backlash highly supportive of male circumcision. Various Jewish and Muslim interest groups and their lobbying organizations expressed concerns about interference with the free exercise of religion, parental rights, and family privacy. (It seems noteworthy that male circumcision in Israel is not officially defined as a medical procedure but rather as a religious ritual).

The experience of a female Jewish American friend of mine illustrates this relatively widespread cultural sensibility in the United States. When she was a young woman in her 20s she started working as an assistant in the neonatal ward of a well-known Boston hospital. On her first day on the job she looked down at a naked newborn child, screamed, called for a nurse and exclaimed (while pointing): 'Nurse come quickly, there is something terribly wrong with this child!' The nurse looked down and replied, 'Haven't you ever seen an uncircumcised penis before?' The answer of course was 'no'. She had grown up in a cultural world in which all the naked males she had encountered had been circumcised. What she had just observed she had spontaneously experienced as a defect of nature or a biological mutation of some kind. The uncircumcised penis of that newborn child deviated strangely from her ideal image of physical integrity and normal genital aesthetics. She did not then, and she does not now, associate that ideal body image with 'genital mutilation' or 'child abuse.' It is the anti-male circumcision groups and their slogans – they refer to themselves as 'intactivists' – that strike her as bizarre, and even a bit alien.

Not surprisingly arguments abound in the United States claiming (in one way or another) that the differences between female and male genital surgeries overwhelm any similarities and that justice requires that different cases should be labeled and treated differently. According to the local dominant cultural attitude in the United States the customary modification of female genitalia is savage, ugly, unnatural, misogynist, harmful, disgusting, and basically horrifying. In the popular imagination it is the kind of thing barbarians do in Africa where (as the nightmare scenario about the 'dark continent' envisions) they maim, murder, and torture their own daughters and deprive them of the capacity for sexual pleasure; while the customary modification of male genitalia is thought to be normal and health promoting and is said to improve the human body – the way it looks (smooth and shapely without any fleshy encumbrance), the way it feels (clean), the way it works (reducing premature ejaculations). As far as I know, unlike some professional medical associations in Europe, no medical association in the United States has disparaged male circumcision by comparing it to FGM or called for its cessation on medical or therapeutic grounds. Imagine the reaction of the readers of the New York Times if the lawyers and language use editors of the newspaper should ever adopt a gender equitable naming policy and begin referring to Jewish circumcision as male genital cutting or start describing the circumcision ceremony of observant Jews (the 'Bris' or the 'Brith') held on the eighth day after the birth of a son as an occasion for male genital mutilation.

Gender equity the other way around

A rather different sort of equity argument has currency in countries such as Egypt, Ethiopia, Mali, Sierra Leone, parts of Malaysia, and Northern Sudan; where it is the dominant cultural view that males and females should be treated alike by modifying the genitals of both; and where the vast majority of females (approximately 80–90% in seven African countries) would be deeply troubled by the exclusion of females from the practice. 'What's good for the goose is good for the gander' gender equity thinking has been around for a long time in many African ethnic groups. Indeed, at the time European explorers first encountered the circumcising ethnic groups of West Africa there were probably a higher percentage of circumcised female chiefs exercising political power in that region than there are female senators in the US Congress today. Some African countries (Kenya and the Sudan, for example) have a history of both female and male resistance to global interventions into their family privacy going back to the British colonial era in the 1920s, when infertility was one of the several morbidities (erroneously) attributed to female genital circumcision. In what is probably the most rigorous piece of scientific research ever conducted on female genital cutting and reproductive health – a 2001 study by the British Medical Research Council – comparing 'cut' and 'uncut' women in the Gambia – 10% of circumcised Gambian women in the study were indeed infertile, but the level of infertility was exactly the same for the uncircumcised Gambian women. The same pattern of findings – no significant difference found between 'cut' and 'uncut' women – held true for most of the reproductive health problems investigated in the study, such as menstrual problems or painful sex. One or two diseases occurred more frequently among 'cut' women; one or two occurred more frequently among 'uncut' women. While the women in the study had many troubling health problems, in general, the ill health of a circumcised Gambian woman could not be attributed to her customary genital surgery. The authors caution activists against exaggerating the morbidity and mortality risks of the practice.[8]

Recall Professor Shaye Cohen's caution that '...western discourse about female genital circumcision has been shaped exclusively by its opponents.' Recall too his observation that if the horrifying claims in that discourse about sexuality and health should turn out to be insufficiently evidence based and inaccurate then 'an argument could be made for moral parity between female circumcision and male circumcision, not in order to proscribe them both but in order to tolerate them both....' That is the argument that holds sway for many highly educated African women who find it perfectly natural to frame the question this way: why shouldn't social norms in Mali, Egypt, or Sierra Leone (or other African countries) respect the principle of gender equity and permit females to be circumcised too?

Jomo Kenyatta, the first president of postcolonial Kenya, was also asking that question back in the 1930s when he wrote his PhD thesis in social anthropology at the London School of Economics. In that thesis, which was later published as a book titled *Facing Mount Kenya* and is still taught in college courses in anthropology and African studies, Kenyatta describes many of the customary practices of his own ethnic group, the Gikuyu. Those customs include premarital sexual experimentation for girls and boys (lots of fondling and rather liberal attitudes towards petting and sexual arousal) and both female and male circumcision. Politely avoiding the question of why Jewish women aren't circumcised Kenyatta explicitly compares the Gikuyu custom to the tradition of circumcision among Jews. He argues that circumcision is a bodily symbol of 'the whole teaching of tribal law, religion and morality' and functions for his ethnic group as a gender inclusive step into responsible adulthood. He notes that 'there is a strong community of educated Gikuyu opinion in defense of this custom.'

Kenyatta's text now seems prescient. As if anticipating the mind-set of UNICEF and other global organizations in the early twenty-first century, he draws our attention to the following international event:

> In 1931 a conference on African children was held in Geneva under the auspices of the Save the Children Fund. In this conference several European delegates urged that the time was ripe when this 'barbarous custom' should be abolished, and that, like all other 'heathen' customs, it should be abolished at once by law.[9]

Kenyatta, of course, went on to be one of the leaders of the 1950s Mau Mau uprising against British colonial rule and spent much of that decade in a British prison in Kenya before becoming the Nelson Mandela of his liberated country. His nationalist movement was bolstered by local resentment over aggressive British attempts to abolish female circumcision and to inspect the genitals of Kenyan girls before letting them attend school.

Not all that much has changed with regard to the international campaign since the 1920s and 1930s, although the era of postcolonial African rule has it own distinctive dynamics. The gender equity argument that was and is commonplace in several African countries calling for parity the other way around (tolerating genital modifications for both females and males) is not an argument that is routinely featured (or even visible) in public policy debates in North America or Europe or at global institutions. Instead, given the way power works in the 'First World' and its influence on global institutions and on post-colonial elites almost everywhere (and despite the overwhelming and persisting popularity of both female and male genital modifications in various East and West African countries), female circumcision has been officially proscribed throughout much of Africa (although without much serious enforcement). This is largely due to the reluctance of local political elites in poor supposedly liberated countries to defy the external pressure of global institutions or refuse the largesse of North American and European donors. Under conditions of unequal bargaining power African political elites take the money and duck. They seem to have the political capacity to ignore popular opinion and the general will of the electorate, mollify the righteous passions of their international patrons, and allegedly accept the strings attached to foreign assistance.

There are, of course, some committed indigenous advocates in countries such as Mali, Sierra Leone, and Egypt who actively oppose local genital norms (at least with regard to females). Although they are a small minority of the general population they are often well-placed. At times they hold influential political positions. They are increasingly well-funded and aligned with benefactors from abroad who support local NGO activities; and they and those NGOs get lots of attention in mainstream media outlets in North America and Europe, and at the United Nations. In December 2012, the United Nations General Assembly took a leaf from that 1931 Save the Children Conference in Geneva and unanimously called for a universal ban on customary female (but not male) genital 'mutilation,' which in the postcolonial UN argot is now dubbed a 'harmful traditional practice' rather than a 'heathen custom.'

Meanwhile, within global organizations and in educated elite networks in North America and Europe, the inflammatory rhetoric of 'mutilation', 'child abuse', 'female castration', 'sexual blinding', 'torture', 'war against women' is preemptive, accusatory, and argument-ending, and effectively silences debate.[10] It misleads even typically skeptical public intellectuals and journalists to think there can't be any other side to this story. It closes down the process of critical reasoning and fact checking; thereby making it easy for inaccurate and hyperbolic claims to be uncontested and blatant falsehoods to go uncorrected; or if contested and corrected to not be heard; or if heard to be ignored or forgotten. No Western journalist wants to be accused of being part of a war against women or of aiding and abetting the mutilators of children. The rhetoric alone has proved powerful enough to convince an educated public in North America and Europe that the African custom is barbaric. The desirability of its eradication seems obvious – a no brainer.

Inflammatory language, legal statutes, and UN resolutions notwithstanding the gender equity argument the other way around continues to appeal to many Africans in East and West Africa. There are far more circumcised African women in the world who embrace their own ethnic practice than there are Jewish men who have no regrets (and most Jewish men have no regrets, at least not with respect to their neonatal circumcision). When challenges have arisen to male circumcision Jewish men have been willing and able to exercise their critical reason and their considerable political and moral influence in defense of their ethnic tradition. This has not been true of the policy shaping abilities of educated circumcised African women. On the global scene and in legislative bodies in North America and Europe they lack visibility and political clout. Yet, they too are attached to (and find meaning and value in) their ethnic traditions. When they ask 'why shouldn't women in Egypt, Mali, or Sierra Leone be circumcised?' it is reasonable for them to expect an informed, logically consistent and evidence-based response rather than emotionally charged polemical finger pointing reminiscent of the nineteenth century accusations against Jews in Germany. Many of these educated circumcised women in Africa and abroad are simply turned off by what they view as Western propaganda castigating their ethnic heritage and slamming them with hyperbolic horror-inducing empirical claims about sexuality and health which they know to be false. At the very least their voices deserve to be heard.

Viewpoint diversity is not only something to be valued on college campuses but should be welcomed in public policy conversations as well. The following views were expressed recently by the editors of the Sierra Leone Telegraph, a West African news outlet. They appeared in an editorial preamble to an outside opinion piece recommending gender equity in genital surgeries. The outside opinion piece was given the title 'The Demonisation of female circumcision: African women fight back,' which the Sierra Leone Telegraph published on 23 February 2013.

The editors wrote:

> Somewhere, buried deep within the sometimes fierce debate [within Sierra Leone] about the merits or otherwise of female circumcision, lies the truth, which is being poisoned by many on both sides of the debate, simply to advance their cause. And the victim of this highly charged and emotive war of words, is 'truth and social justice.' Those arguing against this centuries old cultural practice, say that it is barbaric. They have come to demonise it – with the help of global humanitarian institutions, as 'Female Genital Mutilation (FGM)'; a powerful choice of poisonous words, which many believe to have been constructed by western society to undermine and destroy an African way of life. But is female circumcision a barbaric act, conducted on hapless and defenceless women and children in Africa? Organisations such as the Orchid project are being heavily funded, globally, to bring the practice they refer to as FGM to an end.

The next day, in direct response to the very same outside opinion piece another news outlet in Sierra Leone – The Patriot Vanguard – published the following reader comment:

> Years ago when female circumcision – portrayed as female genital mutilation to condemn it – first took center stage, the powers that be also included male circumcision. In a flash the male side of it died completely without any throes. Why? Because the Jewish lobby in the most sensitive places around the world must have sprung into action, and, perhaps, with the backing of such people as the godly Nelson Mandela [Mandela comes from one of the few male circumcising ethnic groups in South Africa] and other African leaders they told some powerful leaders to desist from going any further. We are now left with the female side of things because Africans are considered gullible, weak and easily cowed. My contention is quite simple: The United Nations should play the role for which it was created after the failure of the League of Nations to prevent the Second World War, which was/still is to foster and maintain peace throughout the world. Delving into long held cultural values of individual nations or whole continents would extensively compromise the integrity of the Organization and sow the seeds of conflict because some tribes or ethnic groups are bound to resist, which may cause certain governments to use force. This is not to say that suggestions should not be made by the U.N. but individual governments should make the final decision to allow or disallow female circumcision based on their unique circumstances.

The outside opinion piece which generated this attention was written by Dr. Fuambai Ahmadu, an American cultural anthropologist of African heritage who is an expert on

West African initiation ceremonies and a health advisor to the Vice President's Office in Sierra Leone. She spent her childhood in Sierra Leone, migrated to Washington, D.C. when she was 6 years old and returned to Sierra Leone in her early twenties with several female relatives to participate in an elaborate, festive, and communal coming of age ceremony, which included genital cutting. She went on to complete a London School of Economics doctoral thesis on the meaning of female initiation in West Africa. For 2 years, she was a postdoctoral fellow in my own department at the University of Chicago.

On 19 February 2013 a respected Australian TV program called 'Insight', hosted by an apparently courageous Australian journalist Jenny Brockie, broke the taboo on having a balanced mainstream media discussion of female genital surgeries. Fuambai Ahmadu was a featured guest. (http://www.sbs.com.au/insight/episode/watchonline/514/Clear-Cut). She was also invited to write an opinion piece which appeared all over Australia the day before the TV program and was published in Africa in the days following the broadcast. (http://www.dailylife.com.au/news-and-views/dl-opinion/defending-fgm-20130218-2em65.html) Her TV appearance was previewed in an interview posted on African news sites. (http://www.newstimeafrica.com/archives/30734)

Fuambai Ahmadu's writings on the topic, including a detailed account of her own initiation ceremony, can be found at this website: http://www.fuambaisiaahmadu.com/).[11] I am circumcised, she proudly tells the world; and so is my sister, my mother, my aunts, my grandmother, my great grandmother, and countless generations of women from my ethnic group. Men in my ethnic group do it too. Why shouldn't we? In her opinion piece (cited above) she addresses what she sees as a rather serious problem with the World Health Organization concept of FGM which WHO defines this way: 'Female Genital Mutilation (FGM) comprises all procedures that involve partial or total removal of the external female genitalia or other injury to the female genital organs for non-medical reasons.'

She writes:

> When I look at the before and after pictures on some FGCS [Female Genital Cosmetic Surgery] websites, I can see that the aesthetic effects of surgeries on white vaginas are conspicuously similar to our supposedly mutilated black vaginas. Exactly who is kidding who – the doctors themselves, the female patients or WHO? Whether done with a laser or a razor; at a high-priced Beverly Hills plastic surgeon's office or at a sacred women's initiation grove in the heat of West Africa; whether no one will find out about our private cosmetic surgery or we join other face-painted initiates in a communal celebration of womanhood; whether we are anesthetized under the modern knife of a male plastic surgeon with fancy framed degrees across the walls of his office or our legs are held open as we display our courage before an experienced traditional Digba, these are 'all procedures that involve partial or total removal of the external female genitalia…for non-medical reasons'.

One hesitates to engage in a full blown semantic analysis of the meaning of the word medical in the phrase 'non-medical reasons' but a brief explication does seem necessary. Narrowly speaking, medical means doing things to the physical body aimed at preventing, alleviating or curing a disease or functional disability. Presumably that is what the authors of the WHO definition had in mind when they distinguished between medical and non-medical reasons for genital surgery (and presumably that is what the physicians at the Royal Dutch Medical Association had in mind when they distinguished between therapeutic and non-therapeutic reasons for male circumcision.)

The WHO definition appears to classify any non-medical modification whatsoever of the external genitalia of a woman as an injury. This is done more or less by definitional fiat and with no interest in providing equal semantic cover to the genitals of males.

Dr. Ahmadu also notices a certain irony in the definition and some hypocrisy as well in its application. She herself is a circumcised woman of West African descent who feels at home in her own ethnic tradition, comfortable with her own body, does not view herself as mutilated, and has written about her own pre-initiation and post-initiation sexuality. The irony: given the WHO definition one ought to conclude that FGM is the fastest growing branch of aesthetic surgery for white middle class women in North America and Europe. The hypocrisy: when North American or European women (even feminists) head to a cosmetic surgeon (typically for non-medical reasons in the narrow sense) for a labiaplasty or cliteroplexy (or any of the other surgical procedures used to shorten a clitoris or smooth out the folds of the labia or tighten the vaginal channel) it is called a vaginal rejuvenation or a designer vagina. Celebrity magazines popularize the trend. The New York Times and the Huffington Post write about the fashion without opprobrium.[12] When similar surgeries take place in Africa they are reported as mutilations.

More broadly speaking, however, 'medical' might mean doing things to the body that improve the body and have a positive effect on a person's sense of well-being. This is a perfectly recognizable and respectable sense of the word. In that sense, a nose job, a breast implant, a face lift, or a sex change operation, might be classified as a medical procedure. If one adheres strictly to the first narrow sense of medical, then American parents are motivated by non-medical reasons when they hire a surgeon to normalize the facial appearance of their Down Syndrome 4-year old or correct a child's lip or cleft palate or even when they subject their daughter to years of painful orthodontic work to achieve a smile displaying a socially pleasing set of straight teeth. On the other hand, one might embrace the second meaning associated with the word medical. In all those examples, the parents are seeking to improve the body of their child for the sake of his or her physical, social, psychological, and spiritual well-being. It seems perfectly sensible to say they are doing it for medical reasons, at least in the broad sense of the term. Rarely (with respect to instances of this sort) are moral or legal complaints registered against the parents for violating the child's fundamental rights to self-determination and the preservation of his or her physical integrity. Their actions are understood and (arguably) judged to be legitimate by reference to a moral and legal framework of guardianship, family privacy, and parental rights.

Whichever the semantics involved, Jews, Muslims, aesthetic surgeons, and the circumcising peoples of Africa have long been concerned to improve the human body; and they believe that there are good reasons to modify human genitals aside from preventing, alleviating, or curing a disease. Some aesthetic surgeons suggest there is a right to be beautiful. Some Jews argue they have a moral obligation to uphold a covenant with their God and they view the foreskin as a blemish on the body or a physical defect that God expects them to correct. Or they view the surgical process itself as a symbolic sacrifice and fleeting ceremonial reenactment of the suffering of the Jewish people, and a way to maintain an unbroken bond with many generations of ancestors.

The gender equitable circumcising peoples of Africa have their reasons too. They too feel attached to generations of ancestors. And some of their other reasons are eye-opening for a North American or European observer. In general, their aim is to improve the form, function, and meaning of male and female sexual organs, and to make the genitals of men and women appear more attractive and more gender appropriate. According to local ideals for beauty in regions of East and West Africa, attractive to the senses means less hairy, less fleshy, fewer folds, more refined, and less animal-like. That aesthetic genital ideal is sometimes described as 'smooth and clean.' With the assistance of the internet the aesthetic ideal appears to be going global. The growing popularity on college campuses in the United

States of Brazilian cuts, total pubic hair removal and even labia trimming may be indicative of the trend. To get a partial sense of this smooth and clean look see the entry on 'vulva' in Wikipedia (http://en.wikipedia.org/wiki/Vulva), where of the four photos the one in the upper left quadrant seems to approximate this particular aesthetic ideal.

Gender appropriate means appropriateness within the terms of some socially constructed definition of male and female. It is characteristic of gender equitable circumcising ethnic traditions that the distinction between being male or being female matters for ones sense of social and personal identity and for the functioning of society. At first blush, it may seem odd to Europeans and North Americans but in many ethnic groups in East and West Africa the foreskin is devalued by males precisely because its fleshy folded appearance reminds them of the look of an uncircumcised vagina. And similarly, the unconcealed part of the clitoris is devalued by women precisely because its protruding appearance reminds them of something male-like that has been pulled out of the body. (There is a concealed and substantially hidden part of the clitoris. It's deeply interior nature has not gone unnoticed in African cosmologies and will inform a discussion of female genital cutting and sexuality later in the essay.)

Odd or not to Western eyes, given that perception of human anatomy, customary gender inclusive African circumcision amounts to standardizing a procedure designed to enhance the intimate physical shape of both males and females. Seen from the insider's point of view one of the several reasons for the ethnic tradition is to sculpt the naturally given body into a culturally improved form. In other words, through customary means, males become aesthetically more masculine by getting rid of an unbidden (and unwanted) female element (the foreskin) and females become aesthetically more feminine by trimming back an unbidden (and unwanted) male element (the exterior protrusions of the clitoris). This way of viewing things may automatically feel unpalatable (or even panic inducing) to members of dominant European or North American ethnic groups, just as they may find it automatically unpalatable (or unnerving) to vicariously step into the shoes of an orthodox Jew who approvingly views his own circumcised penis as evidence of his parent's piety and willingness to obey a divine command and as a sign of his own commitment to uphold a 3000- or 4000-year-old covenant between the Jewish people and their God. But, surely it is not incomprehensible. Nor is it impossible to overcome (or at least mitigate) those spontaneous gut reactions and become impressed by the astonishing scope and power of the human imagination. It just takes a willingness to bracket those emotions so as to be able to do some un-petrified viewing of unfamiliar frames of mind and exercise a little imagination of one's own.

Some feminist theorists may rail against this African imaginary with its premises that gender differences really matter and heterosexuality makes the world go 'round. Some proponents of queer theory in the academy may rail against the premise that bisexuality – the mix of male and female genital elements in every human being – is the state of nature for uninitiated children but is best left behind as one enters responsible adulthood. Yet, perhaps it is still worthwhile to remind ourselves that cultural diversity exists in the world in part because members of different ethnic groups disagree about answers to such basic existential questions as what's male and what's female, and about how best to give bodily expression to one's identity, if at all. And perhaps too, in the service of mutual understanding and the virtues of moderation and tolerance, we should be slow to make moral judgments about unfamiliar others, and push back a bit when a committee at the United Nations issues declarations to a not so culturally flattened world, announcing that they've got it right, and then proposes a universal plan for gender development, sexual relations, and family life that looks very much like some version of the Western way.

'Western discourse about female genital circumcision has been shaped exclusively by its opponents'

Given that Western media coverage of female genital circumcision in Africa has been almost totally reliant on sources from within an opposition movement, it is likely that most readers of this essay will be under the impression (and perhaps even think it self-evident) that girls who have undergone genital surgeries in Africa are sexually impaired: that they are unable to experience orgasm; that they react to sexual intercourse with feelings of pain; that they have a reduced interest in sex in general and suffer in their marriages and other sexual encounters because sex is not pleasurable. When a discourse is shaped entirely by partisans it is unlikely that truth will prevail.

When British colonists and evangelical missionaries first sought to eradicate female circumcision in Africa in the 1920s they did not make strong claims about the effects of genital surgeries on orgasms and sexual pleasure. Cultural attitudes towards erotic activities and sexual encounters inside and outside of marriage are not uniform across the ethnic groups of the world, and it is not just anthropologists who know this. In Kenya, in the 1920s, at least the sexually modest British missionaries seemed to be aware that female initiation ceremonies could be sexually charged festivities. While the British colonists and missionaries disapproved of the public ceremonies as licentious events they were more concerned about the consequence of female circumcision for reproductive success. The British wanted the population in their African colonies to grow for the sake of a large labor force. They advertised what turned out to be erroneous claims about the effects of female circumcision on fertility. These claims still circulate today and get used in the literature of NGO eradication campaigns, despite the evidence mentioned earlier demonstrating no difference in levels of fertility for 'cut' and 'uncut' women in Africa.

These days however claims about the effects of genital surgeries on female sexuality are center stage. Cultural attitudes towards family size, sexual pleasure, and the sexuality of women began to shift in the 1960s in North America and Europe. Thus, with the return in the late twentieth century of foreign campaigns to uplift Africans and liberate them from their ethnic traditions, the advocacy literature calling for the eradication of female genital surgeries has shifted its attention in recent decades to the topic of sex. Featured in the advocacy literature (and advertised in the mainstream press in North America and Europe) are the horrifying and wince-inducing images of female genital cutting as 'female castration' and 'the sexual blinding of women.' According to those who oppose the practice African women in circumcising ethnic groups are sexually disabled.

Similar claims about the negative effects on male sexual pleasure of removing the foreskin have been popularized by anti-male circumcision groups. It is true that the famous twelfth century Jewish rabbi Maimonides and some American physicians in the late nineteenth and early twentieth century (along with some highly educated members of the general public in the United States) endorsed and promoted the practice of male circumcision because they thought it might work as an antidote to uncontrolled erotic impulses and make it easier to be moral and resist the temptation to masturbate (which was viewed as a carnal, worrisome, and even health-depleting indulgence). One can find African women and men in some African ethnic groups today who out of a variety of concerns (including fears about uncontrolled erotic impulses and sexually transmitted diseases) commend female genital surgeries in similar terms. But, Maimonides was wrong! Removing the foreskin does not make men less carnal or reduce the frequency of masturbation. And Maimonides is not the only one who has been wrong about genital cutting and sexuality over the centuries. The best contemporary evidence strongly suggests that circumcised African women have rich sexual lives or at the very least are no more sexually impaired than women in Europe or North America.

Fortunately there are a few high-quality scientific studies on the topic of genital cutting and sexuality. If the truth is to prevail and critical reason brought to bear on a visceral, culturally tabooed, and ideologically charged topic such as genital cutting one must rely on high-quality studies. Methodological rigor and data quality control are essential if one is to fairly and dispassionately assess the validity of empirical claims. A recent commentary by two Swedish researchers, Sara Johnsdotter (an anthropologist) and Birgitta Essén (a MD in gynecology and obstetrics) summarizes the results of the most rigorous and unbiased studies available in the literature. They begin with a bit of history.

> The first actual study to challenge widespread assumptions about lost ability to enjoy sex as an inevitable effect of genital cutting was presented by Lightfoot-Klein [an opponent of the practice] in 1989. Her book was built on interviews with some 300 infibulated Sudanese women. Her interviewees gave testimony of their enjoyment of sex. A high percentage of the women (about 90%) produced convincing accounts of the experience of orgasm.[13]

With regard to the experience of painful sex, Johnsdotter and Essén discuss the large Medical Research Council community-based study in West Africa comparing well over a thousand 'cut' and 'uncut' Gambian women.[14] No significant differences were found between the two groups in reports of painful sex – 15% of 'cut' women versus 14% of 'uncut' women experience pain during sex. With regard to the frequency of coitus in marriage they point to a large population survey of thousands of 'cut' and 'uncut' women in the Central African Republic, where 47% of 'cut' women versus 39% of 'uncut' women report having sexual intercourse more than five times in the last month.[15]

They draw our attention as well to a study comparing the sexual lives of 'cut' African women (mostly from Ethiopia and Somalia) and 'uncut' Italian women who use the services of a health clinic in Florence, Italy (Catania et al. 2007).[16] Eighty-six percent (86%) of the 'cut' African women were found to experience orgasms. With respect to the dimensions of sexuality investigated in the study (desire, arousal, satisfaction, and orgasm) those African women living in Florence led sexual lives that were as rich if not richer than 'uncut' Italian women.

Here, I caution the reader. There are well-recognized difficulties and inhibitions associated with reading and writing about private, intimate, and tabooed parts of the human body and their functions. What follows is a somewhat graphic description of the genital regions of the human body.

If your picture and understanding of the anatomy of the clitoris is the one shared by many educated and sexually experienced adults in North America and Europe (it was once my picture) you are likely to resist the implications of even high-quality scientific studies documenting the rich sexual life of circumcised African women. You might even be inclined to dismiss the findings as implausible. You probably equate the clitoris with that smaller part of its total structure that protrudes beyond the vulva and is visible to the eye or most easily touched. Sigmund Freud and other classical psychoanalysts also made the understandable mistake of accepting that equation. That led them to view the clitoris as a diminutive penis and to the invidious speculation that women experience penis envy. If you hold to that picture of the clitoris it will seem self-evident that female genital surgery must dampen the capacity for orgasm and the experience of sexual pleasure. The picture however is flawed and misleading.

Based on contemporary methods of anatomical analysis it would be far more accurate to imagine a male's penis as an externalized clitoris that has been lifted out of the body; or perhaps alternatively to imagine a female's clitoris as a mostly (but not quite fully) internalized and largely (but not quite completely) concealed penis. The clitoris in its entirety is nearly four inches long and should be visualized as a deeply embedded wishbone shaped structure that surrounds the vaginal wall and is mostly hidden from naked view. Consequently, a massive amount of female erectile tissue and abundant nerve endings enabling the experience of sexual pleasure and the capacity for orgasm reside beneath the surface of the vulva and beyond the scope of any customary African circumcision procedure.

That more accurate picture of female genital anatomy (recognizing the embedded depth of the clitoris and dismissing the naïve equation of the clitoris with its visible external parts) is eye-opening for several reasons. The picture suggests that given the deeply embedded anatomical structure of the clitoris and its intimate connections with the vaginal wall, there may be little value in trying to draw a sharp distinction between a clitoral and a vaginal orgasm. The picture also exposes Freud's error: there is no invidious comparison to be drawn once it is understood that a penis is homologous to a clitoris pulled out of the body. It unmasks as well the grotesque fallacy in the polemical, horror-inducing representations which analogize the African trimming or excision of the visible part of the clitoris to the removal of the entire penis from a man (and in some versions of this nightmarish analogy, the imagined removal involves not just the entire penis, but the scrotum too). (I did caution that this was going to be graphic. The anti-mutilation activists specialize in rousing polemical imagery).

Most importantly, that corrected picture makes it apparent that female genital surgeries (whether in Africa or Beverly Hills) are NEVER designed to remove the clitoris in its entirety but rather to trim back, smooth out or reshape only its most visible external parts. The picture lends some plausibility to the research evidence mentioned earlier which suggests that the sexual life of a circumcised African woman is not typically impaired by the surgery.

Seven things to know about female genital surgeries in Africa

Dispassionate fact checking has not been a strong suit of anti-mutilation activists. And when the conversation turns to female genital cutting in Africa, it has not been a strong suit of mainstream news organizations either. Ever since the revival in the early 1980s of an anti-FGM discourse there has been no free market of ideas in the European Union or in North America. There are exceptions, John Tierney at the *New York Times* for example,[17] but for the most part journalists have shown little interest in debates about the accuracy of the now standardized, media ready, horror-inducing picture of African parents and their relatives: routinely portrayed as mutilators, torturers, misogynists, or child abusers who are wittingly (the brutal African men) or unwittingly (the brainwashed African women) part of a war against women and who cause harm to their daughters and try to control them by depriving them of their capacity for sexual pleasure. Strong moral conclusions are compelled by the very language used in the conversation, which really isn't a conversation at all, but rather a self-affirming (and more often than not self-righteous) accusation which functions to demonize others and proclaim the moral superiority of the speaker (as a good person). Anti-abortion activists begin their 'conversations' this way: are you now or have you ever been in favor of the murder of innocent life? Anti-circumcision activists begin them this way: are you now or have you ever been in favor of mutilation and child abuse?

Recently, however, *The Hastings Center Report*, the bioethics journal, broke the taboo on publicizing facts embarrassing to the cause. In November 2012, they published an advisory statement (of which this author was one of the co-signatories) suggesting that media coverage of female genital surgeries in Africa has been hyperbolic, inaccurate and one-sided, and that the time had come for a more balanced public policy discussion.[18] Titled 'Seven Things to Know About Female Genital Surgeries in Africa' the publication was jointly authored by members of the Public Policy Advisory Network on Female Genital Surgeries in Africa, an informal group of fifteen medical researchers, anthropologists, physicians, legal scholars, African area specialists, and feminists. Their joint statement summarized the highest quality evidence available on the topic, contested the discourse that has dominated conversation among cosmopolitan elites for over 30 years, and supplied readers with relevant source materials. No collective position was taken on public policy towards either male or female circumcision.

What did fact checking by the public policy advisory network reveal? Does the custom of genital cutting in Africa dispossess females of their capacity for orgasm and rob them of sexual pleasure? No! Do the widely publicized claims about the negative reproductive health consequences and medical complications attributed to the custom survive critical scientific assessment and peer review? No! Is the custom restricted to females? No! Is the custom primarily supported and controlled by men? No! Is the custom designed to mutilate females? No!

One might have thought such a document would precipitate a robust debate. In fact, it was largely ignored by the mainstream press, despite the prestige of *The Hastings Center Report*, and despite the obvious relevance of the advisory statement to a prospective United Nations General Assembly vote that was receiving a good deal of media attention. As it turned out (quite coincidentally) The Hastings Center had made the advisory available to the press just a few weeks before years of lobbying efforts by activist organizations was about to produce an uncontested unanimous UN declaration calling for a universal interdiction of 'female genital mutilation.' That ban, endorsed by the UN in December 2012, is now being used to leverage local opinion in countries such as Sierra Leone and Mali and to convince local elites to criminalize their own long-standing gender inclusive norms for genital surgeries, despite the persistent local popularity of the tradition. The hegemony of the Western discourse became conspicuously obvious during the weeks leading up to that UN vote. Watching with some dismay as the mainstream press remained silent, Michael Cook, the editor of a free thinking on-line bioethics journal in Australia, wrote about the advisory statement and the seven things to know about genital surgeries but also wondered whether the topic had become a 'third rail' or 'the ultimate hot potato' for journalists. (http://www.mercatornet.com/articles/view/the_third_rail_of_feminism)

Despite the general silence, or perhaps because of it, Lisa Wade, a sociologist who is an expert on media bias, dared to bring *The Hastings Center Report* publication to the attention of readers of her popular feminist blog 'Sociological Images'. She wrote an opinion piece titled 'A Balanced Look at Female Genital 'Mutilation'' summarizing the central points. She encouraged journalists to think twice about the accuracy of their coverage. (http://thesocietypages.org/socimages/2012/12/10/a-balanced-look-at-fgm/)

Lisa Wade's opinion piece did not precipitate a robust debate either, at least not in the Socratic sense. Instead, despite her feminist credentials, she was slammed and put in the cyber-stocks by startled, enraged, and disgusted readers. Some wanted her to recant. Some threatened to defame her. Some were offended by her suggestion that the rhetoric of mutilation was preemptive, counterproductive, and offensive to African women.

Mutilation is mutilation they seemed to be saying. Beauty is not in the eye of the beholder. Mutilation is not a judgment; it is an objective fact. And it remains mutilation, regardless of the aesthetic judgments of indoctrinated African women; although no one commented on how they themselves aesthetically react to the 'natural' appearance of human genitals, which is a topic well worth exploring.

Having all along assumed that the case against the African practice was open and shut (a 'no brainer') some commentators seemed unprepared for Lisa Wade's revelation of evidence countering their assumptions about health and sexuality. They found themselves at a total loss for words, simply unable to comprehend how the custom could have persisted for so long and remained popular in Africa. Many readers passionately repeated the mutilation, child abuse, war on women horror story they had learned from the activist organizations and the press. Their voices were very much like those of the delegates to that 1931 Save the Fund meeting in Geneva described by Jomo Kenyatta, eager to criminalize and eradicate a heathen custom and sure there could not possibly be another side to the story. Predictably, as often happens when readers send in comments on the topic of FGM, the anti-male mutilation advocates write in too, insisting on gender equity and castigating the global feminists for not denouncing childhood male circumcision as practiced by Muslims, Jews, Nelson Mandela's ethnic group (the Xhosa) or anyone else.

It is likely Lisa Wade was not entirely surprised by her readers' reactions. She herself studies the way hegemonic discourses work to limit the scope of any public challenge. And it was not so long ago that the American Academy of Pediatrics (AAP) set off a moral panic and was instantly and very publically vilified when it dared to put a toe in the policy waters policed by the activist organizations. In a 2010 policy document on female genital cutting they made a modest plea for tactical cultural sensitivity in the treatment of African immigrants to the United States. In the single offending paragraph they wrote:

> Some physicians, including pediatricians, who work closely with immigrant populations in which FGC [female genital cutting] is the norm have voiced concern about the adverse effects of criminalization of the practice on educational efforts. These physicians emphasize the significance of a ceremonial ritual in the initiation of the girl or the adolescent as a community member and advocate nicking or incising the clitoral hood.[19]

In other words the AAP floated the idea of taking a tiny step in the direction of African style gender inclusive genital modification by making available to interested African parents a surgical procedure that was less invasive than a neonatal male circumcision as routinely performed by Jews in the United States. The procedure would be performed under hygienic conditions. The nick or small cut carried no health risks. It probably goes without saying at this point that the sexuality of the girl would not be impaired.

One can expand on the AAP thought experiment. Imagine an African mother who believes that when God issued the command the matriarch of her group (the Sarah of Sierra Leone, for example) as well as the patriarch (the Abraham of Sierra Leone) were both party to the conversation, and bound by the deal. Imagine she believes that her daughters as well as her sons should be circumcised. Why? So as to honor that covenant, improve the bodily appearance of her girls and boys by removing a 'natural' defect, help them develop a healthy sense of their gender identity, and enable them to be seen as socially normal members of their ethnic group. Imagine that her proposed surgical procedure for her daughters is no more substantial from a medical point of view than a customary American male circumcision. Why should we not legally extend that option to West Africans? In light of recent changes in cultural and legal attitudes towards (for example) gay marriage it seems pretty inept to simply reply 'I don't like thinking about it and that is not how we do things here.'

Nevertheless, the general public was ill-prepared for the AAP thought experiment. The nineteenth century colonial discourse about Africa as a land of barbarians engaged in a war against women never really went out of fashion in Europe and North America, or if it did, it is back in full force. So, alarm bells went off as soon as the AAP simply acknowledged the interest of culturally sensitive pediatricians in making available a safe, non-medical genital nick procedure for the families of African girls. Jungle drums could be heard in the distance. The media opened their pages, their websites, and their airwaves to all the predictable polemical and hyperbolic expressions of rage. 'Why are American doctors mutilating girls?' Ayaan Hirsi Ali asked in a widely distributed opinion piece. Why are they supporting a practice designed to control female sexuality? Given the character of media coverage since the early 1980s her rhetorical success was guaranteed. She easily managed to inflame the readers of *The Daily Beast*, inciting feelings of hatred and disgust. Readers sent in comments denouncing ignorant doctors, barbaric men, savage Africans, and, of course, Islam and the Muslims.[20] Reading such slander, I find it hard not to recall Sander Gilman's observations about the blood libel accusations in Germany in the late nineteenth century. The alarming thought is that sooner or later Judaism and the Jews may once again be added to the list.

Perhaps the recent judicial decision in Cologne and the report of the Royal Dutch Medical Association are not harbingers of things to come. Perhaps the liberal 'equal rights for all sexes: say 'no' to forced genital cutting' agenda of the anti-male circumcision advocates will never gain traction, just as the nineteenth century liberal agenda of some German Jews to give up male circumcision as a sign of their modernity and as a way to fully assimilate themselves into German society never gained traction. Perhaps the ethnic and religious minority groups in the United States who circumcise their sons will continue to be part of a circumcising mainstream and gain some protection from secular claims (whether valid or not) about the medical benefits of male circumcision. The disquieting alternative is that global feminism's highly polemical, uncontested, and insufficiently evidence-based eradication campaign targeting ethnic groups in Africa, labeling them mutilators of their daughters, and criminalizing their customs will become an increasingly effective moral and legal springboard for opponents of neonatal male circumcision (first in Europe and ultimately in the United States). Ancient and modern Jewish history is caution enough about the hazards of inflammatory rhetoric and the rush to dark judgments about little known others.

Notes

1. Cohen (2005).
2. Ibid, p. 222.
3. Shweder (2002). Reprinted in Shweder (2003). Also see Shweder (2005).
4. Cohen, p. 271, footnote 41.
5. The anti-male circumcision gender equity argument is discussed and developed by Darby and Svoboda (2007). Versions of the argument frequently appear in anti-male circumcision blog essays and reader comments, for example http://edwardv.livejournal.com/310863.html
6. The KNMG statement can be downloaded from this website: http://knmg.artsennet.nl/Publicaties/KNMGpublicatie/Nontherapeutic-circumcision-of-male-minors-2010.htm
7. Gilman (1999).
8. Morison et al. (2001).
9. Kenyatta (1938).

10. See for example Hosken (1993); Rosenthal (1995). For the influence of this type of inflammatory discourse on political asylum cases in the USA also see Kratz (2002); Martin (2005).
11. Also see Boone (1986) for a detailed ethnographic account of female initiation in West Africa. For a detailed ethnographic account of female initiation in East Africa see Kratz (2004).
12. See for example Navarro (2004) and HuffPost Live interview titled 'Woman Says Labiaplasty Changed Her Life', 9 May 2013 http://live.huffingtonpost.com/r/archive/segment/woman-says-labiaplasty-changed-her-life/517607902b8c2a2799000004
13. Sara Johnsdotter and Birgitta Essén, 'Sexuality After Female Genital Cutting: A Response to Nawal Nour,' (2013) available from Sara Johnsdotter at this e-mail address: sara.johnsdotter@mah.se
14. Morison et al. (2001).
15. Stewart, Morison, and White (2002).
16. Catania et al. (2007).
17. The skeptical iconoclastic Socratic tradition which values controversy and critical debate and follows the argument where it leads even when that means going against the current of received wisdom is still championed by some journalists and John Tierney is one of them. On 30 November 2007 he posted 'A New Debate on Female Circumcision' on his TierneyLab blog of the online Science Section of the New York Times. (http://tierneylab.blogs.nytimes.com/2007/11/30/a-new-debate-on-female-circumcision/). It was the first of six TierneyLab postings on the topic in 2007–2008, including opinion pieces by the World Health Organization, Fuambai Ahmadu, Lucrezia Catania, Bettina Shell-Duncan, and myself.
18. Public Policy Advisory Network on Female Genital Surgeries in Africa (2012).
19. This particular approach to cultural sensitivity in American medicine has a history. See the response of Harbor View Medical Center in Seattle, Washington to the arrival of Somali clients. Coleman (1998).
20. In the face of the controversy The American Academy of Pediatrics eventually decided to withdraw the offending paragraph from their 2010 policy statement.

References

Boone, S. A. 1986. *Radiance From the Waters: Ideals of Feminine Beauty in Mende Art*. New Haven, CT: Yale University Press.

Catania, L. L., O. O. Abdulcadir, V. V. Puppo, J. B. Verde, J. J. Abdulcadir, and D. D. Abdulcadir. 2007. "Pleasure and Orgasm in Women with Female Genital Mutilation/Cutting (FGM/C)." *The Journal of Sexual Medicine* 4 (6): 1666–1678.

Cohen, S. 2005. *Why Aren't Jewish Women Circumcised?* Berkeley, CA: University of California Press.

Coleman, D. 1998. "The Seattle Compromise: Multicultural Sensitivity and Americanization." *Duke Law Review* 47: 717–783.

Darby, R., and J. Steven Svoboda. 2007. "A Rose by Any Other Name?: Rethinking the Similarities and Difference Between Male and Female Genital Cutting." *Medical Anthropology Quarterly* 21 (3): 301–323.

Gilman, S. 1999. *Making the Body Beautiful: A Cultural History of Aesthetic Surgery*, 291. Princeton, NJ: Princeton University Press.

Hosken, F. P. 1993. *The Hosken Report: Genital and Sexual Mutilation of Females*. Lexington, MA: Women's International Network.

Kenyatta, J. 1938. *Facing Mount Kenya: The Tribal Life of the Gikuyu*. London: Secker and Warburg.

Kratz, C. A. 2002. "Circumcision Debates and Asylum Cases: Intersecting Arenas, Contested Values and Tangled Webs." In *Engaging Cultural Differences: The Multicultural Challenge in Liberal Democracies*, edited by R. A. Shweder, M. Minow and H. R. Markus, 309–343. New York: Russell Sage Foundation Press.

Kratz, C. A. 2004. *Affecting Performance: Meaning, Movement, and Experience in Okiek Women's Initiation*. Tucson, AZ: Wheatmark.

Martin, D. A. 2005. "Adelaide Abankwah, Fauziya Kasinga, and the Dilemmas of Political Asylum." In *Immigration Stories*, edited by D. A. Martin and P. H. Schuck, 245–278. New York: Foundations Press.

Morison, L., C. Scherf, G. Ekpo, K. Paine, B. West, R. Coleman, and G. Walraven. 2001. "The Long-Term Reproductive Health Consequences of Female Genital Cutting in Rural Gambia: A Community-Based Survey." *Tropical Medicine and International Health* 6 (8): 643–653.

Navarro, M. 2004. "The Most Private of Makeovers." *New York Times*, November 28. http://query.nytimes.com/gst/fullpage.html?res=9D06E0DA123EF93BA15752C1A9629C8B63

Public Policy Advisory Network on Female Genital Surgeries in Africa. 2012. "Seven Things to Know About Female Genital Surgeries in Africa." *The Hasting Center Report* 42: 19–27. http://www.thehastingscenter.org/Publications/HCR/Detail.aspx?id=6059

Rosenthal, A. M. 1995. "On My Mind: The Possible Dream." *New York Times*, June 13.

Shweder, R. A. 2002. "What About 'Female Genital Mutilation"?: And Why Culture Matters in the First Place." In *Engaging Cultural Differences: The Multicultural Challenge in Liberal Democracies*, edited by R. A. Shweder, M. Minow and H. Markus. New York: Russell Sage Foundation Press.

Shweder, R. A. 2003. *Why Do Men Barbecue? Recipes for Cultural Psychology*. Cambridge, MA: Harvard University Press.

Shweder, R. A. 2005. "When Cultures Collide: Which Rights? Whose Tradition of Values?: A Critique of the Global Anti-FGM Campaign." In *Global Justice and the Bulwarks of Localism: Human Rights in Context*, edited by C. Eisgruber and A. Sajo. Boston, MA: Martinus Nijhoff Publishers.

Stewart, H., L. Morison, and R. White. 2002. "Determinants of Coital Frequency Among Married Women in Central African Republic." *Journal of Biosocial Science* 34: 525–539.

Review symposium on *The New Politics of Male Circumcision: HIV/AIDS, Health Law and Social Justice* by Marie Fox and Michael Thomson

REVIEW SYMPOSIUM: "THE NEW POLITICS OF MALE CIRCUMCISION: HIV/AIDS, HEALTH LAW AND SOCIAL JUSTICE" BY MARIE FOX AND MICHAEL THOMSON

Fox, M., and M. Thomson. 2012. "The New Politics of Male Circumcision: HIV/AIDS, Health Law and Social Justice." *Legal Studies* 32: 255–281.

Review

Sydney Calkin

Introduction

Fox and Thomson highlight some of the considerations that scholars and practitioners must take into account when advocating male circumcision as an HIV/AIDS prevention measure. In particular, their social justice approach highlights overlooked stakeholder groups whose voices must be included in any discussion of HIV/AIDS prevention and male circumcision in particular. Their brief discussion of women among these stakeholders raises several issues that I wish to expand on and connect to broader discourses of women in the development discourse. First, I will briefly remark on the structural nature of the crisis and highlight some linkages between HIV/AIDS and gender inequalities in Sub-Saharan Africa. Second, I will discuss the advocacy for male circumcision as a prevention measure in terms of its location in broader development discourse and the position of women in this discourse; I argue that the 'clamour for circumcision' is reflective of a development culture in which cost-efficiency and short-termism obstruct analysis of structural inequalities. Third, I will discuss possibilities for the engagement of men and boys that male circumcision in HIV/AIDS discourses raise. I want to suggest that social justice approaches to prevention and eradication must engage both sexes in a variety of interventions that span the medical, social, and cultural.

Social justice and structural inequalities

The social justice framework adopted by Fox and Thomson requires analysis of the mutually reinforcing nature of inequalities and the way that patterns of disadvantage are structured; it alerts us to the moral significance of these inequalities (14). It is therefore clear that a social justice approach to the HIV/AIDS crisis will foreground the role of gender inequalities in the spread of the virus and the perpetuation of disadvantage for marginalized groups. Proposed solutions to the crisis must accordingly recognize its structural aspects and look beyond medical procedures to issues of poverty and deprivation.

Gender inequality and women's political, economic, and sexual subordination are 'ingrained' in every aspect of the HIV/AIDS crisis (De Waal 2006, 20). Oppressive sexual relationships (conditioned by economic and political subordination) magnify the risk to women, as sexual relations are often imbricated in women's survival strategies.

Although the gendered aspects of the HIV/AIDS crisis are well-researched, the conclusions bear repeating in the context of the 'clamour for circumcision' that Fox and Thomson explore. The current enthusiasm for circumcision and the accompanying public health advocacy of mass-circumcision policies have the potential to shift the terms of the debate away from broader inequalities, towards medical solutions. While any advances in HIV/AIDS prevention are to be welcomed, it is imperative that we recognize that they constitute one aspect of a broad and embedded crisis. The discourses around male circumcision as a public health 'solution' are problematic for this reason: they circumscribe debate and obscure complementary pieces of the prevention program in favour of a 'one-off' medical protection for men. Although circumcision has been shown to reduce the risk of infection for men, it has the potential to exacerbate gender inequalities if it's not located in a wide range of preventative measures. The spread of HIV/AIDS cannot be attributed solely to the failure to circumcise, nor can its solution be limited to public health advocacy of the procedure.

Women in development

This relationship between gender inequality and public health intervention, in which the search for a 'silver bullet' obscures significant dimensions of analysis, represents a continuation of international development's reductionist and short-termist tendencies. Donor's enthusiasm for male circumcision has been amplified, Fox and Thomson report, by the 'cost-effective, routine' nature of the one-off procedure, thus circumventing the need for the 'heavy investment of time and money entailed by a search for vaccines or therapeutics' (3). The desire for relatively quick and inexpensive solutions to complex problems is a hallmark of development and particularly so in the area of gender. This is an oft cited critique of development efforts, particularly by feminist development scholars who highlight the reductive, short-sighted, and input-driven nature of development solutions (see Kabeer 1994). Correcting the structural inequalities that perpetuate women's subordination is a daunting task and one that requires an enormous commitment of time and investment that is unsuited to the current funding climate. The search for a 'silver bullet' is a perpetual feature of development discourses and practices, although it inevitably produces short-sighted outcomes. We should be wary of this approach and the tendency to advocate universal interventions. This is particularly significant in any discussion of male circumcision, a bodily intervention whose moral significance is highly contested (Fox and Thomson 2009; Johnson 2010).

The public health interventions to promote male circumcision first mirror broader development trends in terms of the focus on investment of time and money and subsequent avoidance of questions of power and inequality; second, the discourse of male circumcision draws on embedded tropes about women as instruments for development. The construction of women in these discourses has revolved around their relationships to men, children, and fetuses: the representation of women-as-mothers and wives places undue weight on their potential to transmit the virus to others (23). The image of woman as 'vector' for disease is laden with sexism and racism, as it robs her of humanity and reduces her to a mechanism for the infection of others. In terms of public health measures, however, the women as 'vector' is situated in instrumentalist discourses whereby intervention targeted at women can promote the health of others (read: men and children).

Given development's tendency to imagine women in relation to their reproductivity, it is little wonder that women emerged in the HIV/AIDS discourses as potential transmitters of the virus to male partners or to their unborn children. Discourses of global development, be it in pursuit of economic growth or public health, tend to construct women as instruments of end goals. Early development theories saw little role for women, who were categorized as 'surplus' population not engaged in wage-work; furthermore, when women became targets of development interventions, it was their reproductive capacity that was foregrounded. Worries about overpopulation led to a recognition of women-as-mothers and the potential for their engagement in these efforts. It was not until the mid 1970s that development institutions and theorists recognized links between poverty, overpopulation, and gender inequality. Despite some advances, development interventions today often couch women's equality in terms of its ability to promote economic growth and family health. Women have often been constructed in terms of their reproductivity across numerous development interventions, from rural agricultural programmes, to microcredit, to maternal health, and now to the AIDS crisis. The discourses and practices around circumcision as a solution to the AIDS crisis are reflective of other development interventions that bypass structural gender issues and instead present partial answers to complex problems. Circumcision may indeed present a significant part of the AIDS prevention process, although it is undoubtedly only part of the solution.

Engaging men and boys

While the debates around male circumcision and public health policies advocating the practice have the potential to reproduce patterns of failed development interventions that neglect structural and gender issues, there is a significant and potentially transformative outcome of the discourse: that male circumcision advocacy promotes the engagement of men and boys in HIV prevention efforts is to be commended. We should welcome the opportunity to theorize a robust role for men and boys as agents in the efforts against HIV/AIDS. The most important thread to draw out from the feminist structural critique of the crisis is the need for a focus on relational inequalities between men and women, a move that necessitates the involvement of both sexes. For too long, 'gender' efforts have meant only women and neglected a critical relational analysis.

However, thus far in feminist debates around engagement of men and boys, discussion has been polarized: many scholars and activists advocate the introduction of men and a critical focus on masculinities as a necessary part of gender equality struggle (Messner 2000), while others warn against the migration of donor funds away from women's programmes and the loss of critical feminist focus that result from the integration of men into gender work (White 2000; Win 2001). The issue of male circumcision in the HIV/AIDS crisis provides us with an opportunity to transcend this debate: rather than asking whether or not to engage men, we can instead focus on *how* to engage them.

A robust challenge to dominant and oppressive sexual cultures can only be mounted with the involvement of men and boys. Part of this challenge must include a critical focus on masculinity and provide the possibility for alternative masculinities as part of a transformation of gender roles. Engagement of men and boys should be inclusive of the diversity of experience among men, highlighting the linkages between rigid masculinities, homophobia, and relational gender inequalities (Peacock n.d.; UN Women n.d.). A relational framework that involves both sexes will work to complicate gender dichotomies (women as victims, men as aggressors) and, related again to the social justice framework at hand, highlight the ways that structural inequalities are manifest in race, class, and gender. Public health advocacy of male circumcision can open up new spaces for the involvement of men and boys in gender equality and HIV/AIDS prevention efforts;

accordingly, we cannot allow the focus on male circumcision to obscure the other complementary aspects of prevention that address social inequalities.

Conclusion

Male circumcision shows promise as a measure to reduce the male-to-female transmission rate and, as such, represents an important medical advance. We cannot overstate its significance, however: male circumcision is one part of a multifaceted approach to HIV/AIDS prevention rather than a solution to the crisis. The adoption of a social justice approach rightly highlights the many groups with interests in the matter and foregrounds the non-medical aspects of the disease's spread and eradication. The 'clamour for circumcision' must not entail the marginalization of analyses that critique structural and gender inequalities that perpetuate deprivation and compound the risks of infection.

References

De Waal, A. 2006. *AIDS and Power: Why There Is No Political Crisis – Yet*. London: Zed Books.
Fox, M., and M. A. Thomson. 2009. "Foreskin is a Feminist Issue." *Australian Feminist Studies* 24: 195–210. http://www.tandfonline.com/doi/abs/10.1080/08164640902852415
Fox, M., and M. Thomson. 2012. "The New Politics of Male Circumcision: HIV/AIDS, Health Law and Social Justice." *Legal Studies* 32: 255–281.
Johnson, M. T. 2010. "Male Genital Mutilation: Beyond the Tolerable?" *Ethnicities* 10: 181–207.
Kabeer, N. 1994. *Reversed Realities: Gender Hierarchies in Development Thought*. London: Verso.
Messner, M. A. 2000. *Politics of Masculinities: Men in Movements*. Lanham, MD: AltaMira Press.
Peacock, D. n.d. "Working with Men and Boys to Achieve Gender Equality and Social Justice." Accessed July 16, 2012. http://www.igwg.org/igwg_media/sympworkwithmen/peacock.pdf
UN Women. n.d. "Virtual Knowledge Centre to End Violence Against Women and Girls: Men and Boys." Accessed July 16, 2012. http://www.endvawnow.org/?men-boys
White, S. 2000. "Did the Earth Move?: The Hazards of Bringing Men and Masculinities Into Gender and Development." *IDS Bulletin* 31: 2.
Win, E. 2001. "Men Are Not My Project: A View from Zimbabwe." *Development* 44 (3): 114–116.

Sydney Calkin
Department of Politics, University of York, York, UK

http://dx.doi.org/10.1080/23269995.2013.804750

Exploring normative space with Fox and Thomson

Richard Mullender

In their response to 'the new politics of male circumcision', Fox and Thomson state their central aim in clear terms. By 'framing circumcision as a public health intervention', they seek to render it 'less private and more politicised' (255, 259). In adopting this approach, they seek to contribute to a debate that will cease to be rooted in a medico-legal context (where, among other things, the assumption that parents may opt to have their children circumcised bulks large) (256, 267). Rather, the debate will (if Fox and Thomson are successful) unfold within a 'social justice paradigm': a context where 'respect for human rights' is a 'foundation of governance' (258, 278).[1] According to Fox and Thomson, this is a context in which we can more adequately grasp the practical significance of programmes of 'mass circumcision' in the lives of adult males and adolescents in sub-Saharan Africa (270–271, 274). Likewise, it provides a context in which we can address the interests of women – a group afflicted by the problem of 'invisibility' as the policy of mass circumcision proceeds in sub-Saharan Africa (276). So too, the social justice paradigm enables us to understand why the circumcision of neonates in the West is 'a body modification' that implicates 'a child's fundamental human rights' (rather than a 'trivial' parental choice) (256).

In their argument for adoption of the 'social justice paradigm', Fox and Thomson identify it as 'opening up' a more adequate 'space' for debate on the new politics of male circumcision (269). The employment of the term 'space' by Fox and Thomson merits close attention. It provides a ground for suggesting that the 'social justice paradigm' is a way of talking about the field of interpretative possibility within which debate concerning the new politics of circumcision is most appropriately located. In this response to Fox and Thomson, we will dwell at length on this field of interpretative possibility.[2] As we will see, a variety of legal norms (most obviously human rights) shape the contours of this normative space or field. So too does an egalitarian philosophy of government (that is itself informed by impulses that have their roots in the Western politico-legal tradition).[3]

The legal norms that secure bodily integrity occupy a prominent position in the field we are considering (257). In addition to securing bodily integrity, these norms also express a commitment to a range of principles and ideals. Among the former, we may number the principles of respect and self-determination; the latter include the ideals of personal autonomy, corrective justice and distributive justice. To circumcise anyone in the absence of informed consent (be they neonates, youths or adults) is to demonstrate a lack of respect for self-determining capacities that they possess or are likely acquire later in life.[4] And to act in this way is to show a lack of regard for the notion of substantial authorship of one's life that is central to the ideal of personal autonomy.[5] In light of these points, those in the groups Fox and Thomson consider have reason to regard themselves as the victims of wrongful harm-infliction.[6] Thus, they have a claim for redress that sounds in corrective justice. They can, moreover, make appeal to the ideal of distributive justice (which specifies that societies should seek to accommodate the interests of all their members defensibly).[7] For circumcision in the circumstances we are contemplating is (or threatens to become) a violation of the human right to bodily integrity and this norm (along with human rights law more generally) advances the agenda of distributive justice. Moreover, the ideal of distributive justice and the human rights that give expression to it make apparent the strongly egalitarian impulses at work in the field of interpretative possibility we are considering. These impulses place limitations on the range of positions that participants in debate may stake out in this field. In order for a position to find a place in this field, it must satisfy the (distributive justice-related) requirement that it adequately accommodates the interests of all those to whom it has relevance.

The legal norms in the field we are considering give expression to a variety of (sometimes antagonistic) moral impulses. For example, the right to bodily integrity gives expression to the deontological assumption that certain goods, interests and states of affairs are intrinsically valuable and merit respect.[8] But the right to bodily integrity is not absolute. For example, in the medical context, a court may authorise involuntary treatment where the benefits of doing so yield compelling reasons for action. Hence, we find a strand of consequentialist moral philosophy at work in the law. This body of moral philosophy specifies that we should assess conduct by reference to its (anticipated or actual) effects (Blackburn 1994, 77). Both consequentialist and deontological moral impulses appear to be at work in the position staked out by Fox and Thomson (257, 271) (since they invoke, in the course of their argument, the qualified right to bodily integrity). This right gives sequential priority to deontological considerations (including respect for the individual and his or her interests).[9] But consequentialist counterarguments may, in a limited range of circumstances, provide grounds for overriding these considerations (275 – on 'compelling' benefits as reasons for action).

In light of these points, we have a basis on which to conclude that a species of qualified deontological moral philosophy informs the thinking of Fox and Thomson.[10] If this conclusion is broadly correct, we can draw a contrast between the position they adopt and that taken up by the proponents of the new politics of circumcision in sub-Saharan Africa (who seek to justify 'clinical research … and … mass public health policy' on the ground that they promise 'an effective response to the [HIV/AIDS] pandemic') (271). Those who espouse the new politics of circumcision in this context, give priority not to deontological considerations but, rather, to consequentialist ones. These considerations have to do with the pursuit of an end that serves the public interest: viz. successfully countering the grave threats constituted by HIV/AIDS (261, 267). This approach prioritises the pursuit of a generally beneficial outcome: i.e. a state of affairs that secures (or that promises to secure) the interests of most members of society (261 – on the so-called 'population-level benefit' of 'promoting circumcision in the African AIDS context'). But in South Africa (the society on which Fox and Thomson fasten their attention most closely), this emphasis on the pursuit of a generally beneficial outcome is accompanied by a lack of regard for deontological considerations. Fox and Thomson drive this point home when they note that informed consent and respect for human rights do not occupy a prominent place in the minds of those pursuing the Zuma administration's 'heavily promoted' health strategy of 'mass' male circumcision (255–256, 272, 274).

Alongside this contrast between the strongly consequentialist orientation of the Zuma regime and the qualified deontological critique offered by Fox and Thomson, we must set a point of intersection between the positions we are considering. South Africa has embraced (indeed, is widely regarded as an exemplar of) the egalitarian philosophy of government.[11] Thus, we have grounds for concluding that Fox and Thomson and those they criticise have broad philosophical commitments in common. But while this appears to be the case, Fox and Thomson alert us to a feature of the new politics of circumcision that greatly reduces its normative appeal. In order to explain why this is so, we must look more closely at the history of the egalitarian philosophy of government. As this philosophy has ramified over recent centuries, the ideal of distributive justice has assumed an increasingly prominent place within it. So too has a conception of government as an agent of benign change.[12] Moreover, 'change' in the context we are considering has to do with ever more adequate approximations of the ideal of distributive justice. As this understanding of government has gained currency, so too has the practice of assessing its performance in consequentialist terms.[13] Alongside this emphasis on outcomes, we must set a further development. This is the tendency for individuals to 'seem smaller' when juxtaposed with 'the whole nation and its practical concerns (De Tocqueville 2003, 78). In light of these points, we can better understand the normative force of the argument against the new politics of circumcision we are considering. The South African government invites its citizens, in consequentialist terms, to embrace the new politics of circumcision (as a means to counter the threat of HIV/AIDS effectively). But to advance the agenda it espouses, it acts in ways that look highly questionable when viewed from the standpoint of human rights law and deontological moral philosophy. Fox and Thomson provide us with an example that illustrates this point vividly. They tell us that the Zuma regime regards those who decline to participate in the programme of mass circumcision as engaging in a 'dereliction of citizenship' (256). But to view citizens in this way is to see them as no more than grit on the governmental flywheel. Thus, we find ourselves contemplating a policy agenda that does not appear to have a home in the field of interpretative possibility where debate should, on the view advanced by Fox and Thomson, proceed.[14]

In response to critique along these lines, the proponents of the new politics of circumcision might make two points with the aim of defending their position as supporters of the egalitarian philosophy of government. Fox and Thomson devote close attention to the first of these points. It takes the form of the argument that the policy pursued by the South African government merits adoption on grounds of practical necessity (since the threat of HIV/AIDS poses a threat to the nation's viability (economically and more generally)) (261, 267, 272). The advocates of mass circumcision might also argue that the critique offered by Fox and Thomson lacks force outside social contexts such as the United Kingdom, where society (for all its imperfections) looks something like a realistic utopia as described by John Rawls. This is a context in which there are grounds for thinking that it is possible to secure the interests of all members of a society defensibly (Rawls 2007, 10–11). Fox and Thomson reject the first of these points and the second seems unlikely to cut much ice with them. Among other things, the first point has to do with governmental ruthlessness (in the sense specified by Thomas Nagel): viz. a readiness to prioritise the public interest broadly conceived at the expense of individuals (Nagel 1979, ch. 6). The second point takes no account of the fact that South Africa, on putting the unhappy history of Apartheid behind it, committed itself to norms that give expression to the egalitarian philosophy of government and are (*ipso facto*) realistically utopian in orientation.[15]

If this analysis is broadly correct, we have grounds for concluding that Fox and Thomson have advanced a critique to which the proponents of the new politics of circumcision cannot make an adequate response. When we scrutinise the arguments advanced by those who espouse the new politics of circumcision, we find that they do not fall within the field of interpretative possibility we examined earlier. But it does not follow from this point that the egalitarian philosophy of government that shapes and finds expression within this field is invariably a source of clear guidance on practical problems.[16] In this brief response to Fox and Thomson, we have touched on points that reveal tensions within it. One such source of tension merits examination before we draw this discussion to a close. As it has developed, the egalitarian philosophy of government has encouraged a view of the state as an active agent of social progress. But to view the state in this (active/interventionist) light is to put the interests of individuals at risk in a wide range of circumstances. While pursuing the outcomes it identifies as benign, the state may fail (as Fox and Thomson demonstrate) to pay adequate regard to the interests of individuals. This prompts the thought that when we embrace this understanding of government, our thinking tends in a Utopian (rather than a realistically utopian) direction,[17] for we harbour the hope that those who wield the levers of power will deliver perfect government while those to whom the law applies enjoy perfect freedom.[18]

Acknowledgements

I am grateful to T.T. Arvind, Patrick O'Callaghan and Ole Pedersen for their comments on various of the points I make in this response.

Notes

1. Drawing on Annas (1999, 37).
2. Since our concern is with a field of interpretative possibility within which debate concerning social justice takes place, we will not consider the many other issues addressed by Fox and Thomson: e.g. the diverse range of interests that have shaped the new politics of circumcision (278–279), the '"blowback" effect' that mass circumcision and associated research programmes in Africa are having on professional policy in the USA (279), and the way in which 'the normalisation and medicalisation of male circumcision in the USA' has exerted a (meme-like) influence ('the "circumcision solution"') in various African jurisdictions (278, 280).
3. On the Western politico-legal tradition and the development within it of an egalitarian philosophy of government, see Mullender (2009).
4. On the circumcision of neonates (in line with parental wishes), Fox and Thomson (256) offer a more guarded view than the one set out in the text. They describe circumcision (of a neonate) as 'a body modification implicating a child's fundamental human rights'. (The guardedness exhibited by Fox and Thomson would seem to reflect their sensitivity to the fact that parental decisions to circumcise their offspring are often an expression of religious commitment. In such circumstances, the communitarian argument that '[w]e are (all of us) culture-producing creatures' who 'make and inhabit meaningful worlds' has some [but not overriding] force (see Walzer 1983, 314). See also Fox and Thomson (267n 1) (noting the 'irreversible' character of the procedure). (While we cannot pursue the matter in detail here, the point made in the text applies, *mutatis mutandis*, to the practice of female genital cutting.)
5. See Raz (1986, 154) on (personally) 'autonomous agents' as people who 'adopt personal projects, develop relationships, and accept commitments to causes, through which their personal integrity and sense of dignity and self-respect' find 'concrete' expression.
6. In Germany, a regional court in Cologne recently concluded that the circumcision of a child for religious reasons can constitute a criminal offence. See Evans (2012). The court found support for its decision in, among other things, the child's right to self-determination, the child's right to physical integrity (as protected by Article 2(2) of the Basic Law (*Grundgesetz*)) and the inability of the defendant to run the defence of consent (on account of the child's lack of maturity).
7. On distributive justice, see Rawls (1971, 4 *et seq.*).
8. On deontology, see Blackburn (1994, 100).
9. On the sequential ordering of distinct moral impulses, see Chapman (1998, 1487).
10. See also Fox and Thomson (274), where the authors invoke the Nuffield Council on Bioethics (2007, para 2.24), stating that normal consent measures should not be overridden in the absence of explicit justification.
11. The Constitution of the Republic of South Africa 1996, Preamble, identifies South Africa as 'a society based on democratic values, social justice and fundamental human rights' and as oriented towards 'improv[ing] the quality of life of *all* citizens' so as to 'free the potential of each person' [emphasis added]. See also Fredman (2008, 114–115).
12. For an early account of this view of government, see De Tocqueville (2003, 778–779), in which the author notes that, 'as social conditions become more equal', a view of government as 'enlighten[ed]', 'wis[e]', and 'caring' gains currency. While a deontological concern with individuals and their interests is a feature of the analysis set out by Fox and Thomson, so too is an outcome-focused conception of government. This is, for example, apparent when they argue that efforts to combat HIV/AIDs in sub-Saharan Africa should focus on the pursuit of social justice. See Fox and Thomson (270).
13. See Dicey (1905, 259) on the 'fundamental principle' that 'benefit derived by the mass of the people' provides an appropriate (and perhaps even adequate) basis on which to assess governmental activity.
14. A field of interpretative possibility of the sort we are considering is politico-legal. We can see its legal aspect in the form of a system of lower-order and higher-order norms that derive their

validity from a highest-order norm (a rule of recognition, to use Hart's term). But this system is political insofar as it is a space that can accommodate a range of norms that are the stuff of competing practical agendas. For further discussion of these points, see Hart (1994, ch. 5 – on law as a system), and Mullender (2012, 919 – on law as a field of interpretative possibility and site of political conflict).
15. See The Constitution of the Republic of South Africa 1996, Preamble, and associated text.
16. See Fox and Thomson (2012, 269) on the indeterminacy of human rights and social justice.
17. Cf. Taylor (2007, 785n 15), where he argues that the (Rawlsian) realistic utopia/Utopia distinction may be too sharp since the notion of Utopia gives expression to the belief that 'these things are really possible in the sense that they lie in the bent of human nature'.
18. See Leff (1979, 1229): '[w]hat we want is simultaneously to be perfectly ruled and perfectly free'.

References

Annas, G. J. 1999. "The Impact of Health Policies on Human Rights: AIDS and TB Control." In *Health and Human Rights: A Reader*, edited by M. Mann, S. Gruskin, M. Grodin, and G. Annas, 37–45. New York: Routledge.
Blackburn, S. 1994. *The Oxford Dictionary of Philosophy*. Oxford: Oxford University Press.
Chapman, B. 1998. "Law, Incommensurability, and Conceptually-Sequenced Argument." *University of Pennsylvania Law Review* 146: 1487–1528.
De Tocqueville, A. 2003. *Democracy in America and Two Essays on America*. London: Penguin Books.
Dicey, A. V. 1905. *Lectures on the Relation Between Law & Public Opinion in England During the Nineteenth Century*. London: Macmillan & Co.
Evans, S. 2012. "German Circumcision Ban: Is it a Parent's Right to Choose?" July 13. Accessed September 10, 2012. http://www.bbc.co.uk/news/magazine-18793842
Fredman, S. 2008. *Human Rights Transformed: Positive Rights and Positive Duties*. Oxford: Oxford University Press.
Hart, H. L. A. 1994. *The Concept of Law*. 2nd ed. Oxford: Clarendon Press.
Leff, A. A. 1979. "Unspeakable Ethics, Unnatural Law." *Duke Law Journal* 28: 1229–1250.
Mullender, R. 2009. "Law, Morality and the Egalitarian Philosophy of Government." *Oxford Journal of Legal Studies* 29: 289–411.
Mullender, R. 2012. "Judging and Jurisprudence in the USA." *Modern Law Review* 75: 914–935.
Nagel, T. 1979. *Mortal Reasons*. Cambridge: Cambridge University Press.
Nuffield Council on Bioethics. 2007. *Public Health: Ethical Issues*. Cambridge: Cambridge Publishers.
Rawls, J. 1971. *A Theory of Justice*. Oxford: Oxford University Press.
Rawls, J. 2007. *Lectures on the History of Political Philosophy*. Cambridge, MA: Harvard University Press.
Raz, J. 1986. *The Morality of Freedom*. Oxford: Clarendon Press.
Taylor, C. 2007. *A Secular Age*. Cambridge, MA: Harvard University Press.
Walzer, M. 1983. *Spheres of Justice: A Defence of Pluralism and Equality*. Oxford: Basil Blackwell.

Richard Mullender
Newcastle Law School, Newcastle University, Tyne and Wear, UK

http://dx.doi.org/10.1080/23269995.2013.806420

Review

Sander L. Gilman

I am delighted to respond to the paper by Marie Fox and Michael Thomson on 'The new politics of male circumcision: HIV/AIDS, health law and social justice.' While they stress the question of a version of informed consent for the application of infant male circumcision as a public health intervention, they seem to bracket the politics of the CDC claims to the efficacy of such procedures. I want to address this question and leave the broader claims of individual rights aside. Certainly the debates about this question, so substantially raised in the proposal to it 'unlawful to circumcise, excise, cut, or mutilate the whole or any part of the foreskin, testicles, or penis' of anyone 17 or younger in San Francisco in the spring of 2011, aired a litany of 'human rights' claims from freedom of religion to the question of bodily integration to the problem of informed consent of such practices on infants. As a result, Governor Jerry Brown signed a bill into law that prevents California communities from banning the practice of circumcision on infant males. Assembly Bill 768, which was introduced after a San Francisco initiative on the topic of circumcision gained momentum, passed the state legislature in late August of 2011 that argued that anti-circumcision measures would infringe on the medical, religious and personal freedoms of parents. Sadly the complexity of these interrelated questions was ignored by the legislature. Fox and Thomson have continued this debate in a substantial and more nuanced manner.

Let me turn to the politics of HIV/AIDS and circumcision that triggered their paper. Under George W. Bush, American financial support for HIV/AIDS intervention in sub-Saharan Africa increased over the terms of his office, but the corollary was the expansion of the Republican 'abstinence only' program to counter HIV/AIDS and STIs in the United States spread to the global marketplace. The Bush administration re-structured the Uganda model for the combating of HIV/AIDS (then perceived to be successful) as an 'abstinence only' intervention in the spread of HIV/AIDS. They eliminated the 'C' (Condoms) from the Uganda ABC model: As one of the Uganda daily papers summarized: 'Sexual **Abstinence** until marriage; secondly, advising those who are sexually active to **Be faithful** to a single partner or to reduce their number of partners; and finally, especially if you have more than one sexual partner, always use a **Condom**.'

By eliminating the B and the C, 'abstinence only' clearly was not going to work any better in sub-Saharan Africa than it did among those who had taken the pledge of abstinence in George Bush's America.

The CDC studies of 'abstinent' teenagers in the United States showed that they had equal rates of gonorrhea as sexually active ones (albeit primarily in the form of oral and anal infections, which have caused a major spike in oral cancers over the past decade). At the major annual CDC conference on STDs in 2006, which I keynoted speaking on the perils of such claims in the sexual marketplace, the panel following my talk on 'Are abstinence-only-until-marriage programs a threat to public health?' was censored by the administration. Rep. Mark Edward Souder (R-Ind.), a supporter of such programs, intervened to achieve 'some balance on this panel.' A speaker was canceled and two advocacy speakers were added to the newly renamed panel on 'Public Health Strategies of Abstinence Programs for Youth.' Abstinence only was the only path for sex education for the Republicans… even if the scientific evidence refuted that.

While this approach is now being reversed by the policies of the Obama's administration and a broader and more comprehensive sex education model has been recently advocated, the legacy of the Bush sex wars in Africa remains. And they remain in ways that are rather frightening because they evoke a historical moment that leads to quite devastating results. For as money increased under George Bush but the options decreased public health authorities rediscovered one of the hoariest public health myths concerning STIs: the efficacy of circumcision as a means of reducing infection. If you have lots of money and the most effective of the three major approaches of your model (condoms) is blocked, then you will have to figure out how to spend the money you have on some type of public health invention. When American foreign policy demanded 'abstinence only' in combating HIV/AIDS in sub-Saharan Africa, the nineteenth-century bromide of circumcision as a major prophylactic against STIs (which proved to be universally ineffective) was reinvented to combat HIV/AIDS even though the studies that argued for this were seriously flawed. The CDC studies assumed a causality between adult circumcision and reduced rates of infection in all populations and they looked at populations of circumcising religions, including indigenous ones, without asking whether belonging to a self-policing religious or social group might be a cause for less risky sexual behavior because of a decreased rate of exposure. Equally unnerving was the CDC's refusal to report the 'serious adverse event data' resulting from circumcision itself. And this was true in the United States as well as in Africa.

The debates about circumcision as a prophylaxis against syphilis (and other STIs) had been a staple of the late nineteenth-century hygiene debates. Indeed, it lay at the center of why the United States became a medically circumcising culture (even with a decrease in rates today) while much of the rest of the Western world did not. The debates about circumcision were always countered with the claim that the very act of ritual circumcision actually transmitted syphilis through ritual practice and often caused death or impairment through the surgery itself. When in the 1930s there was a debate in Great Britain to require infant male circumcision, the arguments were repeated ad nauseam. One writer, F.G., held that 'if the removal of the prepuce lessens the incidence of syphilis...then circumcision is surely a duty in all cases.' BUT another, C.E. Gauthier-Smith, stated, 'no convincing evidence yet presented of less incidence of syphilis in the circumcised.' Need less to say, infant male circumcision never became state policy in Great Britain because the science of the time did not support it. The clearest result of the some one hundred and fifty years of debates about the efficacy of circumcision as a prophylaxis against infectious disease is the determination, both anecdotally and epidemiologically, that such a procedure has little or no effect on STI transmission in Western cultures. Indeed, the American practice began during the late nineteenth century and continued with other medical rationales (reduced cases of penile cancer and uterine cancer in sexual partners) after the introduction of antibiotics for the treatment of STIs. Yet the idea of arguing for an expansion of this practice based on a reduction of the rate of HIV/AIDS in the United States has not been advocated by the CDC. Indeed, this debate was suggested but then officially avoided. The rates of STIs among those ritually or medically circumcised in the United States showed no difference in rates of infection that could be attributed to circumcision. Indeed, among certain groups of ultra-Orthodox Jews the ritual accompanying infant male circumcision has again lead to infections and deaths by herpes to the extent that the New York City Health department is now discussing mandating that parents be informed of the health risk to their newborn infants prior to the ritual practice of circumcision.

The Bush administration was at least successful in destroying the one model for HIV/AIDs intervention that seemed to have some promise. The increase in HIV/AIDs in Uganda today is because '... old-fashioned prevention has flopped. Too few people, particularly in Africa, are using the "ABC" approach pioneered here in Uganda: abstain, be faithful, use condoms,' as the *New York Times* reported on 11 May 2010. The article continued: 'Science has produced no magic bullet – no cure, no vaccine, no widely accepted female condom. Every proposal for controlling the epidemic with current tools – like circumcising every man in the third world... is impractical.' And one can add, not proven in terms of any one's science. What is needed in Uganda and elsewhere is what was and is successful in the global West: public education tied to specific groups that has reduced in many cases risky behaviors and the funding of HAART (highly active antiretroviral therapy) therapy, now the standard of care in the United States, that has dramatically changed the experience of being infected with HIV by offering a means to 'live' with a once terminal disease. This works; circumcision simply does not.

Sander L. Gilman
Emory University

http://dx.doi.org/10.1080/23269995.2013.806428

Response to Calkin, Gilman and Mullender

Marie Fox and Michael Thomson

We wish to begin by thanking Sydney Calkin (2013), Sander Gilman (2013) and Richard Mullender (2013) for their close engagement with our paper. We also extend our thanks to Matthew Johnson and *Global Discourse* for facilitating what we hope will be an on-going dialogue about the future orientation of public health law and policies as well as the politics and ethics of male circumcision. The responses of these scholars have offered us new insights, suggested avenues for future research and forced us to think more deeply about some of the concepts we addressed in the original paper. While each of the respondents takes up different aspects of the politics of circumcision that we identified in our paper, in this short response we seek to draw out some of the themes underpinning these responses and suggest ways in which they have influenced our thinking.

The significance of gender

Calkin's intervention highlights how the social justice framework we advocate requires us to analyse the pattern of disadvantage and the mutually reinforcing nature of inequalities. Noting how gender inequalities and women's subordination is implicated in the HIV/AIDs crisis, she emphasises the importance of addressing this aspect of the drive to circumcision and of locating it in the context of feminist critiques of reductive and short-sighted public health policies. She concludes that 'discourses and practices around circumcision as a solution to the AIDS crisis are reflective of other developmental interventions that bypass structural gender issues and instead present partial answers to complex problems' (Calkin 2013, 369). We agree, although we would add that given concerns about the internal and external validity of the trials (Fox and Thomson 2010), and the evidence that circumcision can increase the risk of infection to women (Wawer et al. 2009), it is in our view doubtful whether it can or should 'present a significant part of the AIDS prevention process' (Calkin 2013, 369). In work we have undertaken subsequent to the publication of the *Legal Studies* paper, we have sought to tease out the negative implications of this public health intervention – and other responses to the HIV/AIDS crisis – for women (Fox and Thomson forthcoming, 2013). In this regard, we have argued that an uncritical advocacy of male circumcision can actually compound women's inequality rather than help ameliorate it. Indeed, as Sander Gilman (2013) notes, throughout its history, the very act of circumcision has been a mechanism for transmitting sexually transmitted infections and has always lacked scientific credibility as a means of reducing disease. We agree with Gilman that we need to be attentive to the history of circumcision as a public health intervention to properly understand the (re)turn to circumcision in this context.

Nevertheless, while questioning the promotion of circumcision, we concur with Calkin on the need to address carefully how men and boys can be encouraged to take responsibility for HIV prevention. However, we would question the appropriateness of circumcision as the vehicle for more fully engaging men. As some of our earlier work has argued, circumcision is deeply embedded in the model of masculinity that has been identified as contributing to the epidemiology of the disease. Moreover, we would question the wisdom of advocating such a flawed intervention that might well increase the gender inequalities that Calkin quite rightly foregrounds. At the same time, we agree that engaging men needs to be part of a broader strategy to reframe masculinity and foster more egalitarian relations between sexual partners. Indeed, as we have sought to demonstrate in our later work, public health initiatives like the circumcision programmes frequently target individuals as part of a project to make them responsible, thereby imposing a greater burden on women who are more likely to lack power in making such choices. In this regard, while we certainly agree with Calkin about the necessity of engaging men, we would nevertheless stress the need to empower women and girls so that choices which affect their health can be more effectively negotiated.

The role of the external agents

In his response, Sander Gilman (2013) states that we 'bracket' the politics of the US Centers for Disease Control and Prevention (CDC) claims to the efficacy of circumcision. Certainly, we had no intention of underplaying the key role of the CDC in promoting the procedure in Africa and the US. As we have stressed, it is crucial to interrogate the role of international organisations and to question their stake in advocating circumcision. Our analysis points towards the need to address the role of bodies such as the CDC, but also supra-national and non-governmental organisations, corporations and the increasingly influential philanthropic institutions. Looking to the involvement of US agencies and organisations, including the CDC, we suggest that part of their motivation may have been to bolster the practice of male circumcision at this juncture where its popularity has radically declined in the US. Our thesis would seem to be supported by the fact that when the American Association of Pediatrics' (AAP) revised guidance on male circumcision was issued in 2012, it relied heavily on 'new' evidence derived from the African studies we analysed to justify its conclusion that the benefits of the procedure outweigh any risks that it poses. It recommended that the purported benefits are 'sufficient' to 'justify access to this procedure for families choosing it' (a significant shift from the position taken in its 1999 guidance that the medical data as to risk and benefits was 'not sufficient to recommend routine neonatal circumcision'). The AAP's reasoning has been extensively criticised elsewhere (Earp 2013; Svoboda and Van Howe 2013). Here, we simply want to note how revisions to its guidance lend support to our prediction about the 'blow back' effect of the trials in Africa and to suggest the difficulties inherent in drawing a bright line between scientific data and its interpretation (AAP 2012). As Gilman persuasively shows in examining the pernicious legacy of the Bush administration, the formulation of measures to combat HIV/AIDS, whether as part of public health policy or the drafting of professional guidance, is necessarily a political process.

Bodily integrity

In campaigns such as that in San Francisco in 2011 that Gilman refers to, the language of bodily or genital integrity is frequently invoked by campaigners, and as Richard Mullender (2013) notes, the 'legal norms that secure bodily integrity occupy a prominent position in the field we are considering' (371). However, he also observes that any right to bodily integrity is not absolute – something which becomes abundantly clear when one considers English law's reluctance to engage with the legitimacy of male circumcision. Mullender is right that the discourse of bodily integrity is prominent in circumcision debates, but we suggest that in legal scholarship there is little engagement with the issue of why bodily integrity is a value worth protecting or indeed what it means to do so. In our current project, we are attempting to analyse how bodily integrity is utilised in cases of surgical modification of children's bodies. We suggest that the concept is potentially valuable in highlighting the harms of non-consensual and non-therapeutic bodily interventions, which are often obscured in conventional best interests assessments. However, we are mindful that traditionally bodily integrity discourse has been mobilised in quite problematic ways – for instance, to justify imposing criminal sanctions. We therefore suggest that bodily integrity and the prominent position it has assumed in health and criminal law needs to be critically interrogated and rethought. Our own rethinking of bodily integrity relies on an ethics of embodiment that recognises embodied beings as existing at the intersection of the corporeal, the discursive and the institutional. In this, we remain engaged with the institutional and discursive sites that we critique in the *Legal Studies* piece and our other work.

The role of the state in promoting social justice and human rights

Bodily integrity is one of a number of human rights at stake in the circumcision debates. However, as Mullender notes, such rights risk being imperiled by the sheer scale of the HIV/AIDS crisis in sub-Saharan Africa which seems to mandate action on the part of governments – as Mullender traces in the case of South Africa. Although we did not frame our position in the language of moral philosophy, we would accept his designation of our position as a qualified deontological one, which would constrain consequentialist reasoning and rule out certain policies as falling outside the field of interpretive possibility that Mullender helpfully sketches. Our later work seeks to develop this social justice framework by drawing on Amartya Sen's capabilities approach to argue that the state does have a key role to play in realising the capabilities of its citizens, including the capability to be healthy. As we suggested in our recent *Medical Law Review* paper, one of the attractions of the capabilities approach for us is how it directs policy-makers to attend to the varying needs of individuals if they are to become capable of an equal level of functioning, an emphasis in keeping with a qualified deontological approach and the concern with gender equality that we share with Calkin. In seeking to respond to systemic disadvantages, the capabilities approach recognises the state as instrumental in securing social justice, while also insisting that the individual must be the object of concern in any analysis. We would suggest that this also fits with Mullender's discussion of governments as agents of benign change. To this, we would add that analysis of the global politics of circumcision reveals that in the context of responding to the HIV/AIDS pandemic, the state itself is only one amongst many players, and that promoting social justice requires us to take account of all the actors in this process, including corporations, NGOs and private philanthropic organisations.

We would like to end by thanking the three commentators again for their thoughtful engagement with our work. This process will undoubtedly have a positive impact on our future research as we continue to consider the place of health and the regulation of bodies in the context of social justice.

References

AAP (American Academy of Pediatrics). 2012. "Circumcision Policy Statement 1999." *Pediatrics* 103: 686–692.

American Academy of Pediatrics Task Force on Circumcision. 2012. "Technical Report: Male Circumcision." *Pediatrics* 130: e757–e785.

Calkin, S. 2013. "'The New Politics of Male Circumcision: HIV/AIDS, Health Law and Social Justice'. Review." *Global Discourse* 3 (2): 367–370.

Earp, B. 2013. "The AAP Report on Circumcision: Bad Science + Bad Ethics = Bad Medicine." *Practical Ethics*. Accessed May 16, 2013. http://blog.practicalethics.ox.ac.uk/2012/08/the-aap-report-on-circumcision-bad-science-bad-ethics-bad-medicine/

Fox, M., and M. Thomson. 2010. "HIV/AIDS and Circumcision: Lost in Translation." *Journal of Medical Ethics* 36 (12): 798–801.

Fox, M., and M. Thomson. 2013. "Realising Social Justice in Public Health Law. *Medical Law Review* 21: 278–309.

Fox, M., and M. Thomson. Forthcoming. "HIV/AIDS and Male Circumcision: Discourses of Race and Masculinity." In *Exploring Masculinities: Feminist Legal Theory Reflections*, edited by M. A. Fineman and M. Thomson. Chesterfield: Ashgate.

Gilman, S. L. 2013. "'The New Politics of Male Circumcision: HIV/AIDS, Health Law and Social Justice'. Review." *Global Discourse* 3 (2): 376–378.

Mullender, R. 2013. "Exploring Normative Space with Fox and Thomson." *Global Discourse* 3 (2): 370–375.

Svoboda, J. S., and R. S. Van Howe. 2013. "Out of Step: Fatal Flaws in the Latest AAP Policy Report on Neonatal Circumcision." *Journal of Medical Ethics*. doi:10.1136/medethics-2013-101346.

Wawer, M. J., F. Makumbi, G. Kigozi, D. Servadda, S. Watya, F. Nalugoda, D. Buwembo, et al. 2009. "Circumcision in HIV-Infected Men and its Effect on HIV Transmission to Female Partners in Rakai, Uganda: A Randomised Controlled Trial." *Lancet* 374: 229–37.

Marie Fox
Birmingham Law School, University of Birmingham, UK

Michael Thomson
School of Law, University of Leeds, UK

http://dx.doi.org/10.1080/23269995.2013.811945

Index

Note:
Page numbers followed by 'n' refer to notes

abstinence 172, 173
Abu-Sahlieh, S.A. 35
abuse: child 121, 123, 142, 145, 147, 154
adolescent circumcision 120–1
adults: incompetent 14n
aesthetics: genital 145
Africa 37, 58, 62, 64, 102, 145, 150, 153; anti-HIV intervention 67; barbarity 40; Botswana 75, 77; circumcision 56, 151, 154; customary female genital surgery 142; female circumcision 147, 148, 152; female genital surgery 154–7; gender equity 147; genital modification 60, 68; labioplasty 38; male genital cutting (MGC) 31; medical care 91; Public Policy Advisory Network on Female Genital Surgeries 1, 155; Uganda 172, 173–4; West 149; women 40, *see also* Lesotho; Sierra Leone; South Africa; sub-Saharan Africa; Sudan; Uganda
African Charter on the Rights and Welfare of the Child (1990) 101
Agence Nationale de recherche su la SIDA 75
agency 97, 98, 108, 115; Egypt 107; embodied 98, 107
agents: external 175–6
aggregation rites 81
Ahmadu, F. 61, 67, 108, 148–9, 150
aid: economic 103
AIDS 31, 75, 165; Lesotho 79, 84, *see also* HIV/AIDS
Alsibiani, S.A.: and Rouzi, A. 53n
American Academy of Pediatrics (AAP) 8, 14, 25, 34, 64, 121, 129, 156, 157, 175, 176; Committee on Bioethics 35–6; Task Force 15n, 136
American College of Obstetricians and Gynecologists (ACOG) 38
American male circumcision 63–5
American Medical Association (AMA): ethical principles 38
amputation: clitoral 48, 52n
anaesthesia 8, 90
anatomy 52; female genital 154
Androus, Z.T. 2, 56–70; reply to 71–3
Ansell, J.S.: and Rajfer, J. 48
anthropological cultural relativism 59
anthropology: critical medical 59
anti-retroviral treatments 79
anti-Semitism 1, 119, 122, 125, 141
Apartheid 169; struggle 92
Apesos, J.: *et al* 33
Aristotle 57
Ashwell, S. 31
Australia: male circumcision 122; Queensland Law Reform Commission 120; Tasmania 120, 123
authority: moral 12; parental 7, 20
autonomy: genital 2, 27–45; liberal 119

Bambara 32
Banai, A. 2, 125–34
banning: circumcision 24–5; female genital mutilation (FGM) 155
baptism: Christian 141, 144
Barr, M.: and Ehrenreich, N. 37, 52n
Barry, B. 123
basic liberties 10, 11
basic rights 7, 10, 11, 12; children 7, 11, 13
Basotho culture 79, 84, 85
Bell, K. 38–9, 40, 50
belonging: cultural 27, 28, 32
Benatar, M.: and Benatar, D. 120
benefits: non-medical 8
Berg, R.C.: and Denison, E. 51; *et al* 49, 51
Bill and Melinda Gates Foundation 75
biocommunicability 76
bioethics 4
biomedical knowledge 56, 76
biomedical medical male circumcision (MMC) 83–5
biomedical perspective 57, 58
biomedicine 57, 60, 74, 85, 87, 90
biopower 76
bisexuality 151
blood shed 91

Boddy, J. 29, 68
bodily integrity 6, 14n, 101, 119, 121, 133, 167, 176; children 24; right to 4, 5, 10, 11, 13; violation 22
body mutilation 30
Boldt v Boldt (2004) 39
Botswana 75, 77
Bourdieu, P. 103
Brahm Levey, G. 2, 119–24
Braun, V.: and Tiefer, L. 37, 38
Briggs, C.L. 76
Brit Shalom 26
Britain: infant male circumcision 173
British Medical Association (BMA) 1, 36
British Medical Research Council (MRC) 146
Brown, S.G.A. 36
Bryant, J.: and Schofield, T. 99
Bulled, N.L. 2, 74–89; reply to 90–5
burden of proof fallacy 14n
Burkina Faso: female genital cutting (FGC) 33
Bush, G.W. 172
Butler, J. 97

Cairo 112–15; Muslim women 96–111
Caldwell, P.: Caldwell, J. and Orubuloye, I.O. 67
California: Assembly Bill (768) 31; Tri Valley Plastic Surgery 38
Calkin, S. 2, 163–6; reply to 174–5, 177
Cameroon 64
cancer 59, 64; cervical 120, 121; penile 120, 136
capabilities approach 176–7
care: patient-centred 135, 137, 138
Carpenter, R.C. 40
castration: female 152
Catania, L.: *et al* 99
Central African Republic (CAR) 153
cervical cancer 120, 121
Chase, C. 35
child abuse 142, 145, 147, 154; and infant male circumcision 121, 123
childbirth: medicalization 31
children: basic rights 7, 11, 13; bodily integrity 24; fundamental human rights 167; interests 11–12; intersex 47–8; moral standing 4–5; rights 20, 39, 101, 125; rights violations 39; self-determination 130; sexuality 30
choice: informed 135; parental 24, 25, 64, 121, 126, 167
Christian baptism 141, 144
circumcision 90; critiquing 56–70; definition 58; rates 1; reasonable 6
citizenship tests 123
clinical biomedicine 57
clinical need: circumcision 36
cliteroplexy 150
clitoral amputation 48, 52n
clitoral prick 35–6
clitoral reduction 37, 47
clitoral repositioning 47
clitoridectomy 31, 41, 47, 48, 52n, 60, 61, 120
clitoriplasty 47
clitoris 96, 97, 108, 151, 153, 154; function 31; orgasm 48
Coffman, J. 2, 71–3
Cohen, S. 141, 142, 144, 146
collectivism 82
Collier, R. 137
Cologne Regional Court 1, 2, 5, 119–24, 125, 130, 133, 135, 143
Colombia: Constitutional Court 39
communitarians 128
communities 26; Jewish 138; Muslim 138; religious 1, 130, 137
community expectations 127, 130
complications 6, 9, 75, 91
comprehensive doctrines 12, 13, 23
conditioning: cultural 15n
condoms 75, 84, 172, 173
confidentiality 75
congruence 122
conscience: liberty of 11, 12
consciousness: and faith 127, 131, 132, 133; freedom of 131
consent 25, 119, 121; informed 4, 31, 39, 75, 122, 135; juvenile 120
considered judgment 9
constructivism: social 97, 98–101
control: sexual 27, 28, 32–4, 157; social 27, 28, 32–4
Convention on the Rights of the Child (1989) 4, 11, 101
Cook, M. 155
cosmetic female genital cutting (CFGC) 27–8, 33, 36, 47, 149; complications 37; law 39; social norms 37–8
cosmetic surgery: genital 149; sex assignment 35
courts 13
Crawford, J.D.: Hendren, W.H. and Donahoe, P.K. 34
critical medical anthropology 59
cross-cultural analyses 58
cultural belonging 27, 28, 32
cultural conditioning 15n
cultural hegemony 109n
cultural norms 114; sexuality 97
cultural practices 2, 57, 80–3, 112, 113; contested 114–15; Lesotho 84
cultural relativism 39–40, 60; anthropological 59

cultural resistance 112
cultural rights 101–2
cultural rites 122
cultural sensitivity 75, 158n
cultural value 2
culture 59, 114; preindustrial 29; and sexual pleasure 50–2; traditional 90
customary circumcision: female/male 141
customary genital mutilation: universal ban 147

Daniels, J.: and Veale, D. 47
Darby, R. 31; and Svoboda, J.S. 48
De Tocqueville, A. 168
decision-making: proxy 7; public health 136
DeLaet, D.L. 112–15
democracy 12, 96; deliberative 12, 23; liberal 119, 121, 122
Denison, E.: and Berg, R.C. 51
Denmark 142
deontological moral philosophy 168, 169
Dershowitz, A. 119
desire: sexual 51, 106–7
determinism: genital 46, 47, 50–2
developing countries 1
development: women in 164–5
Dewhurst, C.J.: and Gordon, R.R. 34
Diamond, M. 35
Digeser, P. 114
dimorphism 37
discrimination: freedom from 40
dissident women 113
doctrines: comprehensive 12, 13, 23; fundamentalist religious 23
Dogon 32
Donahoe, P.K.: Crawford, J.D. and Hendren, W.H. 34
Dopico, M. 100
doxa 103–5
Dwyer, J.G. 6–7

economic aid 103
economic inequality 77
education: sex 172–3
Egypt 145, 146, 147, 148; Cairo 96–111, 112–15; democracy 96; embodied agency 107; female circumcision 96–111, 112–15; female genital cutting (FGC) 2; female genital mutilation (FGM) 97; human rights 96; modernization 103–5; privatization 105; Salafi politicians 106; structural adjustment policies 104, 105
Ehrenreich, N. 40; and Barr, M. 37, 52n
Elchalal, U.: *et al* 47
emancipation: women 97
embodied agency 98, 107
embodiment 97, 98
enlightenment fundamentalism 125
epilepsy 59
equal protection 40
equality: gender 177
equity: ethnic 46, *see also* gender equity
Eskridge, B. 31
essentialism 98–101
esthetic values 72
ethical question 126–32
ethics: Kantian 39; medical 28, 38–41
Ethiopia 145, 153
ethnic equity 46
ethnic identity 144
Europe: gender equity 142–4; infant male circumcision legislation 135–40; Jews 24
Evans, M. 48
evidence-based medicine 136, 137, 138
evidence-based patient-centred care 135
external agents: role 175–6

faith: and consciousness 127, 131, 132, 133; religious 20
family: basic rights 7
female castration 152
female circumcision 35, 46, 48, 56, 96, 142, 146; Africa 147, 148, 152; customary 141; Egypt 96–111, 112–15; fertility 152; health benefits 120; Kenya 62, 146–7; libido 99; medicalization 61; painful sex 153; politicization 105–6; politics 96, 97; politics of knowledge 61; Rendille women 61; sexual pleasure 47, 49; sexuality 49, 98–101; Sudan 99; Western discourse 152–4
female genital cosmetic surgery (FGCS) 149
female genital cutting (FGC) 1, 2, 27, 28–30, 32–4, 35–7, 113, 156; Burkina Faso 33; cosmetic (CFGC) 27–8, 33, 36, 37–8, 39, 47; Egypt 2; ethical perspective 38–9; law 39; legal prohibition 120; medicalization 32; morbidity/mortality 146; reproductive health 146
female genital modification 56
female genital mutilation (FGM) 47, 60, 72, 96, 112, 141, 148, 156; anti-FGM campaigns 60, 61, 62, 107, 142; banning 155; children's rights 101; definition 149, 150; Egypt 97; eradication 102, 103; human rights 39, 57, 101; sexual problems 49
female genital surgery: Africa 154–7
female initiation ceremonies: Kenya 152
female orgasm 97
Female Sexual Function Index 53n
feminine identity 106
femininity 94
fertility 152
First Amendment (US): rights 1

forced genital cutting 142
Ford, K-K. 34, 38
foreskin 38, 67, 150, 151; function 31
Foucault, M. 87
Fox, M.: and Thomson, M. 2, 163–78
fraternal interest group theory 80
freedom 131; of consciousness 131; from discrimination 40; from torture 101; individual 4; religious 5, 121, 125, 133, 144, 172; of thought 11, 12
Freud, S. 99, 153, 154
Frisch, M. 53n
fundamentalism: enlightenment 125
fundamentalist religious doctrines 23

Gagnon, J.H.: and Simon, W. 51
Gambia 107, 146, 153
Gauthier-Smith, C.E. 173
Geertz, C. 73
gender 27, 28, 32, 33, 46, 57, 71, 72, 108, 174–5; ambiguity 37; assignment 41; binary ideas 29; dimorphism 37; equality 177; and genital modification 57–8, 60–3, 71, 72; identity 34; inequality 163–4, 165; norms 37
gender equity 141, 145–51, 148, 151; Africa 147; Europe 142–4
genital aesthetics 145
genital anatomy: female 154
genital autonomy 2, 27–45
genital cosmetic surgery: female (FGCS) 149
genital cutting 27–45; forced 142; intersex (IGC) 27, 28, 29, 32–4, 34–5, 39, 40; non-consensual 115; sexuality 153; social norms 144, *see also* female genital cutting (FGC); male genital cutting (MGC)
genital determinism 47; fallacy 46, 50–2
genital integrity: children 46
genital modification 46–55, 56–70; Africa 60, 68; alternative framework 65–7; developmental stage 66; extent 66–7; female 56; gender 57–8, 71, 72; gender exclusivity 60–3; geography 57–8, 71, 72; global scale 58, 59; initiatory 58–9; local meaning 65–6, 68; Maasai 58–9; new paradigm 71–3; preindustrial cultures 29; as rites of passage 60; sexual effects 46–8; sexual pleasure 48–50
genital mutilation 35, 145; child abuse 142; customary 147; and sexual pleasure 28, *see also* female genital mutilation (FGM)
genital sensitivity 37
genital surgery: cosmetic 35, 149; female 154–7; medical 149–50; non-medical 149–50; nonconsensual 27; reconstructive 50
genital wars 141–59
genitals: aesthetic ideal 150–1; ambiguous 27, 48; role 52
Germany 133, 141, 142; circumcision 133; Constitution 24; Constitutional Court 133; courts 24, 39; Jews 25; male circumcision 125–34, 143; Medical Association 119–20
Ghannam, F. 102, 105
Gikuyu 146
Gilman, S.L. 2, 143–4, 157, 172–4; reply to 174, 175–6
Gini index 77
Global Fund 75
Gollaher, D.L. 35
Golombok-Rust Inventory of Sexual Satisfaction 53n
Gordon, R.R.: and Dewhurst, C.J. 34
governmentality 76
Greenberg, J.A. 35
Griffin, M. 2, 24–6
group identity 128
Gruenbaum, E. 61
El Guindi, F. 33, 40
Gunning, I. 29, 34

HAART 174
harm 9–10, 20, 21, 24, 25, 40, 57, 58; freedom from 143, 144; paradigm cases 22
Hastings Center report 155
Hayes, R.O. 36
healers: traditional 79–80, 84, 85–6, 91
health 137, 156; education 76; public 2, 63, 67, 86, 91, 121, 166, 174, 175, 176; public and male circumcision 136, 164, 172; reproductive 146
health benefits 127; female circumcision 120; infant male circumcision 120, 121; newborn circumcision 129
Hegarty, P. 35
hegemony: cultural 109n
Hellsten, S. 39
Hendren, W.H.: Donahoe, P.K. and Crawford, J.D. 34
Hernlund, Y. 101; and Shell-Duncan, B. 36, 61
herpes 136
Herzfeld, S. 24
heterosexism: hidden 32
Hinton, D.E.: *et al* 52
Hippocrates 57
Hitler, A. 25
HIV 59, 77, 129, 136; anti-HIV intervention 56; anti-retroviral treatments 79; Cameroon 64; developing countries 1; directives 77; Lesotho 64, 78, 79, 80, 84–5; Malawi 64; screening 75; sub-Saharan Africa 62–3; transmission 84, 87n, 143; treatment 75, 79

HIV prevention 80, 87, 120–1, 175; Lesotho 74–89, 90–5; and male circumcision 60, 62–5, 74, 78, 86, 143, 163, 165, 166, 169; medical male circumcision (MMC) 83
HIV/AIDS 172; American financial support 172; Botswana 77; crisis 174, 175; Lesotho 77; pandemic 168, 177; prevention 164; social justice approach 163; South Africa 169; sub-Saharan Africa 173, 176; therapeutics 164; Uganda ABC model 172, 173–4; USA 173; vaccines 164
Holdheim, S. 143
Holland 142
Holocaust 144
Horton, J. 22
Hosken, F.P. 61, 101
hospital circumcision 91–2
Human Development Index (HDI) 76
human papillomavirus 136
human rights 5, 28, 38–41, 46, 97, 102, 115, 172; children 167; doctrines 13; Egypt 96; and female genital mutilation (FGM) 39, 57, 101; fundamental 113; international 6, 96, 97; interventions 112–15; law 169; North Africa 102; state role 176–7
human rights violations 10–11, 12, 13, 71, 72, 142; male genital cutting (MGC) 40
hygiene 120
hymen 106
hysteria 98

identity 137, 138; construction 98; feminine 106; gender 34; group 128; Jewish male 25; Jews 119, 144; male national 74; national 76; sexual 34; urban 82
immigrant groups 59
imperialism: Western 112
incapable minors 123
incompetent adults 14n
indigenous rights 122
individual freedom 4
individualism 82; liberal 21
inequality: economic 77; gender 163–4, 165; structural 163–4
infant male circumcision 4–19, 20–3, 39, 46, 119–24, 156; abolition 143; Britain 173; child abuse 121, 123; European legislation 135–40; health benefits 120, 121; religious 119, 136–7, 138
infertility 146
infibulation 38, 99–100, 120
informed choice 135
informed consent 4, 31, 75, 122, 135; lack of 39
initiation 65, 75, 90, 93; blood shed 91; female ceremonies 152; Lesotho 83, 84; West Africa 149
initiation rites 80, 81; Lesotho 79, 82, 84, 85
initiation schools: Lesotho 78, 80, 82, 84, 85
initiation-embedded circumcision 78
initiatory genital modification 58–9
initiatory male circumcision: Songhoi 60
intactivism 1, 24–6, 115
integrity: child genital 46; physical 143, 145, *see also* bodily integrity
international human rights 6, 96, 97
International Inter-governmental Organization (IGO) 103
International Monetary Fund (IMF) 103
intersex children 47–8
intersex genital cutting (IGC) 27, 28, 29, 32–4, 34–5, 39, 40
intersex surgery 34–5, 37, 52n
intersexuality 34
invasive surgery 1, 2
irrationality 12
Islam 20, 22, 25, 103, 157; political 104, 105, 106
Islamization 97
Islamophobia 1
Israel 144; Supreme Court 133

Jews 25; circumcision 141, 145; communities 138; ethnic identity 144; Europe 24; Germany 25; identity 119; parents and circumcision 125–34
Jhpiego 75, 80, 87n
Jirovsky, E. 33
Johansen, E. 100
Johnsdotter, S. 2, 36, 46–55, 99, 153
Judaism 20, 22, 157; male identity 25
judgment: considered 9; substitute 7–8
justice: as fairness 4, 5, 9, 10, 15n; political 13; principles 23, *see also* social justice
justification 8
juvenile consent 120

Kantian ethics 39
Karkazis, K. 41
Kennedy, J.G. 60
Kenya 75, 85, 146; female circumcision 62, 146–7; female initiation ceremonies 152; Gikuyu 146; Kikuyu 51; Mau Mau uprising 146; Meru initiation practices 62; Rendille 61
Kenyatta, J. 146–7, 156
Kikuyu 51
Kinsey, A. 99
Kirby, V. 41
Kistler, S.L. 31
Kleinman, A. 57, 58, 60
knowledge: biomedical 56, 76; politics of 61
Kono 32; women 61, 72
Korea, South 144

Kristiansen, M.: and Sheikh, A. 2, 135–40
Kuhn, T.S. 58

labia majora: remodeling 37
labia minora: hypertrophy 38; reduction (labioplasty) 37, 38, 150
labia reduction 38
labioplasty 37, 38, 150; Africa 38
law 28, 38–41, 169, 174
League of Nations 148
lebollo: Lesotho 75, 76, 78, 82, 84, 85, 86
legal prohibition: female genital cutting (FGC) 120
legal question 132–3
legal rights 9
legislation 5
Lephowa, T. 80
Lesotho 2; AIDS 84; AIDs Program Coordinating Agency 79; Basotho culture 79, 84, 85; College of Education 77; cultural practices 84; Defence Force 80; Demographic and Health Survey (DHS) 78, 82; economic inequality 77; Gini index 77; government responses 76; HIV 64, 78, 79, 80, 84–5; HIV prevention 74–89, 90–5; HIV/AIDS 77; Human Development Index 76; initiation 83, 84; initiation rites 79, 82, 84, 85; initiation schools 78, 80, 82, 84, 85; *lebollo* 75, 76, 78, 82, 84, 85, 86; life expectancy 77; male national identity 74; Ministry of Health and Social Welfare (MoHSW) 78, 79, 90; modernization 83; national identity 76; national male circumcision policy 78, 79, 80; neonatal circumcision 79; Planned Parenthood Association 80; Population Services International (PSI) 80; public health 85; Tlokoa 82; traditional healers 79–80, 84, 85–6; urban youth 82–3; urbanization 83
liberal autonomy 119
liberal democracies 119, 121, 122
liberal individualism 21
liberal multiculturalism 123
liberal societies 122, 123
liberalism 21, 123; political 2, 12, 20, 22, 23
liberty: basic 10, 11; of conscience 11, 12; religious 20, 22
libido 47, 50, 51, 99
Lightfoot-Klein, H. 34, 36–7, 51
liposuction: pubic 37, 47
Lock, M.M.: and Scheper-Hughes, N. 57
Locke, J. 131
Lockhat, R.: and Stevens, G. 82
Lukes, S. 114

Maasai genital modification 58–9
McNay, L. 98
Mahmood, S. 98
Malawi 64
Malaysia 145
male circumcision 35, 48, 56; advocacy 165; American 63–5; Australia 122; customary 141; fundamental rights 115; Germany 125–34, 143; guidance 175–6; HIV prevention 60, 62–5, 74, 78, 86, 143, 163, 165, 166, 169; initiatory 60; medical justifications 59; medicalized 60; methods 79; neonatal 64, 65, 141; orgasm difficulties 50; politics and ethics 174; public health 136, 164, 172; religious infant 136–7, 138; sexual pleasure 49–50; South Africa 168–9; USA 122, 123, 144–5, *see also* infant male circumcision; medical male circumcision (MMC)
male genital cutting (MGC) 27, 28–30, 32–4, 35–7; Africa 31; ethical perspective 38–9; human rights violation 40; loyalty 33; medicalization 27; South Africa 39; submission 33; Sweden 39
male genital mutilation (MGM) 72, 142; human rights 39
males: newborn 29
Mali 145, 146, 147, 148, 155; Bambara 32; Dogon 32
Malmström, M.F. 2, 50, 96–111; reply to 112–15
Man who is Not a Man, A (Mgqolozana) 93–4
Mandela, M. 92–3
Mandela, N. 81, 148
Mandinka women 61
marginal rites 81
marriageability 61
masculinity 93, 94, 137, 165
masturbation 4, 30, 31, 59, 63, 152
maternal mortality 1
Matlock, D. 37
Mau Mau uprising 46
Mbiti, J. 91
meatal stenosis 9
media bias 155
Medicaid 26, 122
medical circumcision 90
medical ethics 28, 38–41
medical institutions 26
medical male circumcision (MMC) 74, 75, 79; biomedical 83–5; cultural acceptability 75; HIV prevention 83; Lesotho 83, 86
medical organizations 8, 14
medical paternalism 136, 137
Medical Research Council 91, 153
medicalization 2, 4, 30–2; childbirth 31; female circumcision 61; female genital

cutting (FGC) 32; male genital cutting (MGC) 27
medicine 87; evidence-based 136, 137, 138
Mendus, S. 2, 20–3
mental illness 98
Merkel, A. 120
Merkel, R. 130
Meyers, D.T. 40
Mgqolozana, T. 93–4
Middle East: human rights 102; women 40
military service 81, 133
Mill, J.S. 22
Miner, H. 60
minors: basic liberties 4; incapable 123
modernity 74, 75, 77, 90, 102
modernization 97, 102, 108; Egypt 103–5; Lesotho 83
Momoti, N. 91
Monaheng, M. 79
Moore, H. 30
moral authority 12
moral philosophy: aim 5; deontological 168, 169
moral relativism 128
moral rights 9, 10
moral standing: children 4–5
morbidity 146
mortality 1, 46
Moteetee, M. 79
Mullender, R. 2, 166–71; reply to 174, 176–7
multiculturalism 119, 120; liberal 123
Muruli, L.A.: Shell-Duncan, B. and Obiero, W.O. 61
Muscarella, F.: and Szuchman, L.T. 28
Muslim Brotherhood 106
Muslim communities 138
Muslim women: Cairo 96–111; rights 102; sexual mutilation 112–15
mutilation 154, 155, 156; body 30; sexual 96–111, 112–15, *see also* female genital mutilation (FGM); genital mutilation

Namibia 75
national identity: Lesotho 76
National Organization of Circumcision Information Resource Centers International Symposium 59
neonatal circumcision 129, 130; definition 170n; Lesotho 79; male 64, 65, 141; USA 63
nervous disorders 63
New York City Board of Health 122
New York Times 174
newborn circumcision 59, 129
newborn males 29
Nigeria: Yoruba people 67
Njambi, W.N. 51
non-governmental organizations (NGOs) 60
non-medical circumcision 13, 24
normative space 166–71
norms: cultural 97, 114; gender 37; social 37–8, 144
North Africa: human rights 102
Northern Sudan 145
Nour, N.M. 49
Nubian practices 60
Nyaka, L. 78
nymphomania 31

Obermeyer, C.M. 49
Obiero, W.O.: Muruli, L.A. and Shell-Duncan, B. 61
Oregon Supreme Court 39
orgasm 48, 50, 53n, 97, 152, 153, 154; infibulated women 99–100
original position 9, 10
Orthodox Conference of European Rabbis (Berlin 2012) 119
Orubuloye, I.O.: Caldwell, P. and Caldwell, J. 67

Paige, K.E.: and Paige, J.M. 32–3, 34, 80
pain 8, 11
painful sex 153
pandemic: HIV/AIDS 168, 177
paralysis 59
parental authority 7, 20
parental choice 24, 64, 121, 126, 167; smoking 25
parental duty 21
parental power 10
parental rights 6–8, 11–12, 20, 21, 145
parents: Jewish 125–34
paternalism 135; medical 136, 137
patient-centred care 135, 137, 138
patriarchy 1
penile cancer 120, 136
penis envy 153
perinatal mortality 1
Philippines 144
philosophy: moral 5, 168, 169
physical integrity 143, 145
physical pain: freedom from 11
physiology 52
pleasure *see* sexual pleasure
pluralism 5
political Islam 104, 105, 106
political justice 13
political liberalism 2, 12, 20, 22, 23
politicians: Salafi 106
politicization: female circumcision 105–6
politics: female circumcision 96, 97; of knowledge 61
Pollack, M. 32, 33

positive identification 127, 130
potential benefits 64
poverty 165
power 10, 27, 28, 32, 33, 114
pragmatism: principled 123
preindustrial cultures 29
preindustrial societies 32–3
presexual state 38
pressure: social 127, 129
principle of equal consideration of interests (Singer) 16n
principled pragmatism 123
privatization 105
protection: equal 40
proxy decision-making 7
pubic liposuction 37, 47
public health 2, 86, 121, 164; campaigns 67; decision-making 136; facilities 91; interventions 175; law 174; policy 176
public policy 4, 5, 20, 155
Public Policy Advisory Network on Female Genital Surgeries in Africa 1, 155
public reason 4–19, 20–3
Putzke, H. 125–6

Queensland: Law Reform Commission 120
queer theory 151

racism 164
Raftery, I. 5
Rajfer, J.: and Ansell, J.S. 48
Rao, A. 114
rationality 10, 12, 21
Rawls, J. 4–19, 20–3, 169
re-inbulation 100
reason: public 4–19, 20–3
reasonable doctrines 12
reasonableness 5, 9–10, 12, 15n
reconstructive genital surgery 50
reiteration 97–8
relativism: anthropological cultural 59; cultural 39–40, 59, 60; moral 128
religion 12–13, 20
religious belief 4, 12, 21, 22–3
religious circumcision: infant male 119, 136–7, 138
religious communities 1, 130, 137
religious doctrines: fundamentalist 23
religious faith 20
religious freedom 5, 125, 144, 172; right to 121, 133
religious groups 26
religious liberty 20, 22
religious obligations 10
religious practices 13
Rendille women 61
repression 113
reproductive health: and female genital cutting (FGC) 146
resistance: cultural 112
Richardson, W.S.: Sackett, D.L. and Strauss, S.E. 136
Richters, J. 52
rights: basic 7, 10, 11, 12, 13; bodily integrity 4, 5, 10, 11, 13; children 7, 11, 13, 20, 39, 101, 125, 167; cultural 101–2; First Amendment 12; human 102; indigenous 122; legal 9; moral 9, 10; Muslim women 102; parental 6–8, 11–12, 20, 21, 145; religious freedom 121, 133, *see also* human rights
Riner, R.D. 29
rites: circumcision 25; cultural 122; marginal 81; separation 81
rites of passage 60, 65, 72
ritual circumcision 27, 90, 173; Jewish 122
rituals 80
Robertson, C.C. 40
Roen, K. 37
Rosenblum, N.L. 122
Rouzi, A.: and Alsibiani, S.A. 53n
Royal Dutch Medical Association (KNMG) 1, 142–3, 144, 157
Russell, A. 91
Rwanda 75

Sackett, D.L.: Strauss, S.E. and Richardson, W.S. 136
Sacks, J. 24, 119
Salafi politicians 106
satisfaction: sexual 51
Save the Children Fund 146
Scheper-Hughes, N.: and Lock, M.M. 57
Schlemmer, L.: and Wilson, J. 91
Schofield, T.: and Bryant, J. 99
scientific evidence 137
scientific paradigm 57
self-determination 12, 131, 143, 144, 167; children 130
Sen, A. 176
Senegambia 33
sensitivity: cultural 75, 158n
sensory meaning 52
separation rites 81
serfdom 11
sex: and gender 27; painful 153
sex assignment surgery: cosmetic 35
sex education 172–3
sexism 164
sexual control 27, 28, 32–4, 157
sexual desire 51; and creative agency 106–7
sexual dysfunction 107
sexual identity 34

sexual mutilation: Muslim women 96–111, 112–15; production 107–8
sexual pleasure 46–55, 152; and culture 50–2; and female circumcision 47, 49; and genital modification 48–50; and genital mutilation 28; and male circumcision 49–50
sexual problems 51; and female genital mutilation (FGM) 49; medicalized view 37–8
sexual satisfaction 51
sexual scripting theory 51
sexuality 108, 156; alternative 27, 28, 32, 37; children 30; construction 50, 52; cultural norms 97; and female circumcision 49, 98–101; and genital cutting 153; normative 32, 37; Sudan 100
sexually transmitted diseases (STDs) 64, 120, 129, 136, 143, 152, 172–3, 175
Shaalan, M. 32
Sheikh, A.: and Kristiansen, M. 2, 135–40
Sheldon, S.: and Wilkinson, S. 38
Shell-Duncan, B. 33; and Hernlund, Y. 36, 61; Obiero, W.O. and Muruli, L.A. 61
Shorter, E. 31
Shweder, R.A. 2, 30, 32, 46, 141–59
Sierra Leone 141, 145, 146, 147, 149, 155; Kono 32; *Patriot Vanguard* 148; *Sierra Leone Telegraph* 148
Silverman, E. 91
Simon, W.: and Gagnon, J.H. 51
Singer, P. 16n
slavery 11, 15n
Smith, J. 40
smoking 25
social actions: symbolic dimensions 73
social constructivism 97, 98–101
social control 27, 28, 32–4
social convention 126, 128
social justice 2, 167, 172; state role 176–7; structural inequalities 163–4
social norms 37–8, 144
social practices 57
social pressure 127, 129
social virginity 106
societies: preindustrial 32–3
Sociological Images 155
Somalia 32, 153; infibulated women 100
Somerville, M. 29
Songhoi 60
South Africa 75, 76, 85, 176; anti-Apartheid struggle 92; Application of Health Standards in Traditional Circumcision Act No 6 (2001) 78, 85; Constitution 171n; doctors 91; HIV/AIDS 169; male circumcision 168–9; male genital cutting (MGC) 39; masculinity 93; traditional healers 91; urban youth 82; Xhosa 82, 156; youth identity 82; Zulus 81
South Korea 144
Spiegel Online International 119
Spratling, E. 30
stakeholder groups 163
state role: human rights 176–7; social justice 176–7
Stevens, G.: and Lockhat, R. 82
Strauss, S.E.: Richardson, W.S. and Sackett, D.L. 136
structural adjustment policies: Egypt 104, 105
structural inequalities: social justice 163–4
sub-Saharan Africa 75, 163, 167; circumcision 168; HIV 62–3, 143; HIV/AIDS 173, 176; male circumcision 80
subjectivity 97
subordination: women 164
substitute judgment approach 7–8
Sudan 51, 145, 146; female circumcision 99; Nubian region 68; sexuality 100; virginity 36, 38
surgery: intersex 34–5, 37, 52n; invasive 1, 2; sex assignment 35, *see also* genital surgery
surgical normalization 31
Svoboda, J.S. 2, 27–45; and Darby, R. 48; reply to 46–55
Swaziland 75, 77
Sweden 39, 142
syphilis 59, 173
Szasz, T. 29
Szuchman, L.T.: and Muscarella, F. 28

taboo 127, 132
Tamir, Y. 2
Tanzania 75
Tasmania: Law Reform Institute 120, 123
Thomas, L. 62
Thomson, M.: and Fox, M. 2, 163–78
thought: freedom of 11, 12
Tiefer, L. 99; and Braun, V. 37, 38
Tierney, J. 158n
Tlokoa 82
Torah 131
torture: freedom from 101
traditional healers 91; Lesotho 79–80, 84, 85–6
Turkey 66

Uganda: ABC model 172, 173–4; HIV/AIDS 173–4
UNAIDS 74, 75
UNICEF 146
United Hebrew Congregations of the Commonwealth 119
United Nations (UN) 40, 102–3, 148, 151; Convention on the Elimination of All

Forms of Discrimination Against Women (CEDAW 1992) 101; Decade for Women 72; Declaration on Violence Against Women (DEVAW 1993) 101; General Assembly 147, 155; High Commission on Refugees Statement Against Gender-Based Violence (1996) 101; International Conference on Population and Development (ICPD) 105
United States of America (USA) 39, 141, 144; African immigrants 156; California 31, 38; Centers for Disease Control and Prevention (CDC) 172, 173, 175; circumcision 56; civilization 40; foreign policy 173; HIV/AIDS 173; male circumcision 63, 122, 123, 144–5; National Health and Nutrition examination Survey 63; National Institutes of Health 75; neonatal circumcision 63; newborn circumcision 59; President's Emergency Plan for AIDS Relief (PEPFAR) 75
Universal Declaration of Human Rights (1948) 12, 101
universalism 112
urban youth 82–3
urbanization: Lesotho 83
urinary tract infections (UTIs) 59, 120, 129, 136
utilitarianism 5, 9, 14n

vaccinations 24, 121
vaccines: HIV/AIDS 164
vagina: reconstruction 48; tightening 47
values: cultural 2; esthetic 72; incongruence 122
Van Howe, R. 2, 4–19; reply to 20–3, 24–6
Veale, D.: and Daniels, J. 47
veiling 106
Viens, A.M. 5–13, 20, 21, 22
Vincent, L. 2, 82, 85–6, 87, 90–5
violation: bodily integrity 22; children's rights 39; human rights 10–11, 12, 13, 40, 71, 72, 142
virginity: social 106; Sudan 36, 38
Vraun, V. 47
vulva 151

Wade, L. 155, 156
Walley, C.J. 61–2
wars: genital 141–59
West Africa: initiation 149
Western discourse: female circumcision 152–4
Western epistemology 57
Western imperialism 112
Wilkinson, S.: and Sheldon, S. 38
Will/Power Theory 11, 15n
Wilson, J.: and Schlemmer, L. 91
Wilson, M.: *et al* 91
women 40; agency 108, 112, 113; in development 164–5; dissident 113; emancipation 97; empowerment 33; infibulated 99–100; Kono 61, 72; Mandinka 61; Middle East 40; Muslim 96–111, 112–15; Rendille 61; rights violations 103; sexuality 28, 33, 46, 61, 96, 97, 157; subordination 164
Woodhouse, C.R.J. 48
World Bank 76, 103
World Conference on Human Rights Declaration and Programme of Action (1993) 101
World Health Organization (WHO) 1, 32, 39, 49, 60, 74, 75, 103, 119, 122, 136, 137, 149, 150

Xhosa 82, 156

Yoruba people 67; men 72
youth: identity 82; urban 82–3

Zambia 75
Zulus 81